OB-GYN Pathology for the Clinician

Debra S. Heller

OB-GYN Pathology for the Clinician

A Practical Review with Clinical Correlations

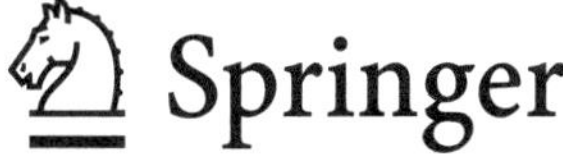 Springer

Debra S. Heller
Department of Pathology
Rutgers-New Jersey Medical School
Newark, NJ, USA

ISBN 978-3-319-36251-9   ISBN 978-3-319-15422-0   (eBook)
DOI 10.1007/978-3-319-15422-0

Springer Cham Heidelberg New York Dordrecht London
© Springer International Publishing Switzerland 2015
Softcover reprint of the hardcover 1st edition 2015

Printed on acid-free paper

Springer International Publishing AG Switzerland is part of Springer Science+Business Media
(www.springer.com)

Foreword

The evolution of training programs in obstetrics and gynecology has led to gains and losses. In former years, the residency in obstetrics and gynecology was usually preceded by a year of internship, either in medicine or in surgery or in a rotating multidisciplinary program. That separate internship has virtually disappeared, and the residency programs now include attention to subjects which were unknown or nascent in former years and are now competing for the time spent in obstetrics and gynecology. In years past, many residency programs in obstetrics and gynecology included a fixed assignment to study gynecologic pathology and the professional organization examinations, the board examinations, included questions on gross pathology and histology. Other subjects have crowded out the pathology study. With the advent and addition of more sophisticated diagnosis and treatment in maternal and fetal medicine as well as reproductive endocrinology, gynecologic neoplastic disease, gynecologic urology, and other subspecialties, formal training in gynecologic pathology has virtually disappeared from obstetrics and gynecology.

Without a grounding in gynecologic pathology for the clinician, pathologists may be dictating clinical care as the clinicians react to pathology reports with algorithms of care, unsupported by a more complete knowledge of the relation between the pathology, the disease, the patient, and treatment. There are occasional sophisticated gynecologic pathology diagnoses, where the subject is unknown to the clinician, e.g., the size of a lesion above which endometrial carcinoma can be diagnosed or the rare germ cell tumors. The progress and dependability of sonographic analysis has frequently eliminated endometrial aspiration biopsies, further divorcing the gynecologic clinician from the pathology from which a decision will be made for treatment. To the best of my knowledge, there is no residency program which now gives formal training in cervical cytology and the clinician is completely dependent on the cytologists/pathologists, although management of the clinical situation where there is abnormal cytology is universally taught. A recurrent theme is the change in names of common and/or unusual diseases, e.g., basal cell hyperplasia, dysplasia, condyloma, carcinoma in situ, class 2 cytology, ASCUS, LGSI, LSIL, carcinosarcoma, and MMMT. The change in focus in the training programs has led to diminished attention to pathology in the American Board examinations. The time available for study of gynecologic pathology has been diminished because of the overall pressures on the training programs to comply with work-hour rules, and participate in newer training programs in endoscopy, simulation laboratories, etc. The impact of these changes weakens what was once one of the greatest strengths of obstetrics and gynecology, the understanding of and familiarity with the nature of the disease processes.

For all these reasons, it is appropriate (for the clinicians, investigators, and teachers) to focus attention again on gynecologic pathology and the powerful and important relation between the obstetrician–gynecologist and the gynecologic pathologist. This book valiantly helps to rebuild the valuable and important bridge between the clinical arena and the pathological laboratory.

New York, NY, USA   Robert C. Wallach, M.D., F.A.C.O.G., F.A.C.S.

Preface

Providers of obstetrical and gynecological care need to understand the pathology of the female genital tract in order to provide optimal patient care. A rotation through the Pathology Department was a prior requirement of an Ob/Gyn residency, but has fallen to the wayside with current time constraints in training. The decreased exposure to pathology may make interpretation of pathology reports more difficult for the clinician at times, as a basic understanding may not have been developed. The pathologist–gynecologist interaction requires good communication, with both understanding the other's point of view.

This is a very personal text. I was originally a practicing obstetrician gynecologist, who retrained as an anatomic pathologist with subspecialty training in obstetrical and gynecological pathology. During my Ob/Gyn residency, my chairman told us that if we didn't review the pathology with the pathologist after we operated, that we were merely functioning as technicians. When I first switched to pathology, I, like many of my clinical colleagues, viewed the pathology process as similar to an ATM. You enter some information, and the "money" comes spitting out. I was surprised to learn that this is not the case. Pathology diagnosis is a physician-to-physician consultation. In addition, the pathologic diagnosis is not always black and white, much to my shock at the time. There are nuances, shades of gray, artifacts and insufficient or poorly oriented tissue, and lesions that don't look like the textbook. This is something a clinician who communicates with his/her pathologist understands, and through conversations, both sides continue their education and the best answer is arrived at. This monograph is thus aimed to meet two needs. One is to establish a fundamental knowledge source of Ob/Gyn pathology for the clinician. The other is to enhance communication between the two specialties, in order to accomplish the goal of us all, to provide the best patient care.

Newark, NJ, USA   Debra S. Heller, M.D.

Contents

Getting the Best Answer: Specimen Handling and a Quick Review of the Workings of the Pathology Laboratory

1.1 The Anatomic Pathology Laboratory

What happens when a surgical specimen reaches the pathology laboratory? A quick tour is in order and will help explain timing of receipt of results by clinicians, as well as what is needed from clinicians to assist with diagnosis. There are a number of steps, all of which have processes in place in the laboratory to avoid error. These include accessioning, gross dissection, processing, embedding, cutting of sections, staining, and labeling [1].

1.1.1 The Requisition Sheet

It is important for the clinician to provide a pertinent clinical history in addition to the usual demographics, which would include patient age and gender. This does not "prejudice" the pathologist, but allows for the best interpretation (Table 1.1). Slides from prior procedures, if within the same institution, are often reviewed, particularly in cases of malignancy, and so prior history of related surgery should be indicated. If the prior surgery occurred at a different institution, slides can be obtained for review, if necessary for diagnosis. This is particularly recommended in oncology cases, where often the biopsy occurs at one hospital, and the definitive surgery at another. Items to put on the requisition sheet include parity, the reason for the procedure, last menstrual period if pertinent, related medications (such as progestational agents, which may alter endometrium), prior therapy such as radiation or chemotherapy, which can induce tissue changes, and orientation of the specimen as applicable. This is particularly important in cases such as a vulvar excision for VIN, where re-excision of a positive margin may rest on where the positive margin was located. In addition, any specific requests the clinician has for the pathologist should be noted, i.e., "please rule out toxoplasmosis" for a patient with a pregnancy loss and a history of cats in the house.

© Springer International Publishing Switzerland 2015
D.S. Heller, *OB-GYN Pathology for the Clinician*,
DOI 10.1007/978-3-319-15422-0_1

Table 1.1 Information needed by pathologist and clinician

Information the pathologist needs from the clinician
• Pertinent clinical history
Age, parity, date of last menstrual period
Why procedure is being performed
Any prior surgery relating to the current disease process?
Orientation of specimen as appropriate
Any pertinent medications?
Any prior therapy?
Any specific questions?
Information the clinician needs from the pathologist
• Short turnaround time
• Understandable report that can be discussed with patient
• Findings in format that can be correlated with clinical findings

1.1.2 Accessioning

The case is given a unique requisition number on arrival, which usually has the year, and then the unique identifier (i.e., S14-12,345, where S stands for surgical). This involves checking both the specimen jar and the requisition, to make sure they match the correct (same) patient, and creation of a computer record of the specimen. Each jar received on a case gets a separate subdesignation (i.e., S14-12345A, S14-12345B) and a separate diagnosis within the report. If two fragments of tissue are in the same jar (i.e., 2 cervical biopsies), it will not be possible to distinguish which came from where. Similarly, if adnexae are submitted detached from the uterus, laterality will not be possible to assign if they arrive in the uterine bucket. Separate jars with designation should be used if separate cervical diagnoses, or adnexal laterality matters in such cases.

1.1.3 Gross Examination

Gross examination involves the initial examination of the specimen, which includes measuring, and possibly weighing, and describing what is seen by the naked eye. A description is created which goes into the report, separate from the final diagnosis. An example from a leiomyomatous uterus can be seen in Table 1.2. The specimen is again checked for identification and labeling at this point. Pertinent areas of the specimen are selected for processing and slide preparation. For small specimens, such as biopsies, the tissue is usually entirely submitted. For larger specimens, representative sections are submitted, after being cut to fit into tissue cassettes, which are small plastic boxes with lids. Whether the tissue is entirely submitted or representative sections are submitted is noted in the gross description, as well as a list of what is in each tissue cassette (Fig. 1.1). For representative sectioning, additional

Table 1.2 Sample gross description

• Cassette A1—anterior cervix
• Cassette A2—posterior cervix
• Cassette A3—anterior lower uterine segment
• Cassette A4—posterior lower uterine segment
• Cassette A5—anterior endomyometrium
• Cassette A6—posterior endomyometrium
• Cassette A7—largest mass, possible portion which was protruding through cervix
• Cassettes A8–A9—largest mass, two (2) sections
• Cassette A10—smaller masses

The specimen is labeled, "Uterine Fibroid and Uterus." Received in formalin is a 3,500 g specimen including an opened, distorted, and dilated uterus and cervix. The uterus measures approximately $11 \times 8 \times 4$ cm. The cervix measures 7.5×5 cm with a dilated os, measuring 7 cm. The uterine cavity measures approximately 7.5×7 cm. Separate from the uterus is large fibroid, measuring $22.5 \times 17 \times 14.5$ cm. There are also multiple intramural and subserosal well-circumscribed white, whorled masses ranging in size from 4.3 to 0.4 cm in greatest dimension. Representative sections are submitted in ten (10) cassettes

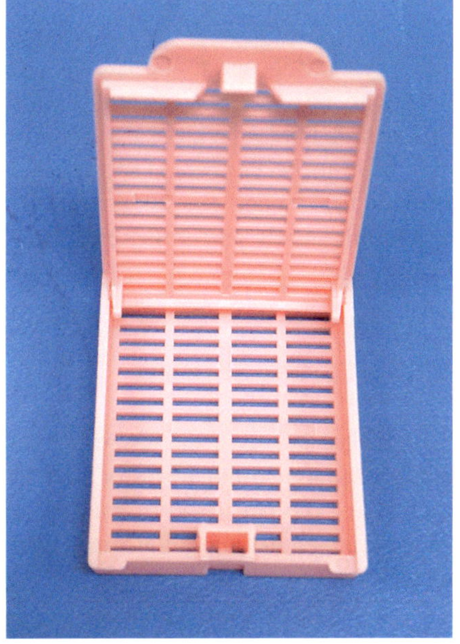

Fig. 1.1 Tissue cassette. The selected tissue is placed in a tissue cassette and then goes into a processor for dehydration prior to embedding the tissue in paraffin

sections can be submitted after initial slide review for the period of time the laboratory keeps specimens. An example would be additional tissue submitted to identify endometrium in a morcellated uterus. Specimens are usually kept for a period of time after a case is signed out. Inking of the specimen may occur if margins are important, as the ink used survives processing, and can be seen on the slides. If there is tumor at the ink, the margin is considered positive. Some specimens may need to be fixed in formalin prior to selecting areas for submission, which may introduce additional time into receipt of diagnosis by the clinician. An example is a cone biopsy, which is difficult to cut into well-oriented sections fresh.

1.1.4   Processing

The tissue cassettes are placed in formalin for primary or additional fixation. After this, they are loaded onto a tissue processor, which is usually automated. The processor goes through a number of steps to dehydrate the tissue. This process takes several hours and may be run overnight in some laboratories. In our laboratory, one of our processors is held for "rush" specimens received by a certain cutoff time. This is why it is better to call the laboratory rather than just submit a specimen that is labeled "rush," so that the nature of the rush, and how it can be integrated into the processing schedule can be best achieved.

1.1.5   Embedding

After processing, the tissue is embedded in paraffin and becomes a block which resides on the outside of the tissue cassette (Fig. 1.2). There are regulations that vary by location, but tissue blocks are kept for many years, so can be gone back to. This may need to be performed at the time of initial diagnosis; however, sometimes sections are needed for studies many years later. An example of this would be a molecular study performed on a tumor many years later, to guide therapy for a recurrence.

1.1.6   Cutting Sections

Sections are cut from the tissue block on an instrument called a microtome. The block goes up and down across a blade, and a thin section (around 4.5 μm) is cut each time. The cut tissue in paraffin comes off as a ribbon of multiple sections, which are then floated in a warm water bath. Slides are swiped underneath to pick up the sections and allowed to dry prior to staining (Figs. 1.3, 1.4, and 1.5).

1.1.7   Staining

Routine staining is with hematoxylin and eosin; however, a large variety of special stains are available that can be performed on the same tissue, by cutting additional sections from the same block.

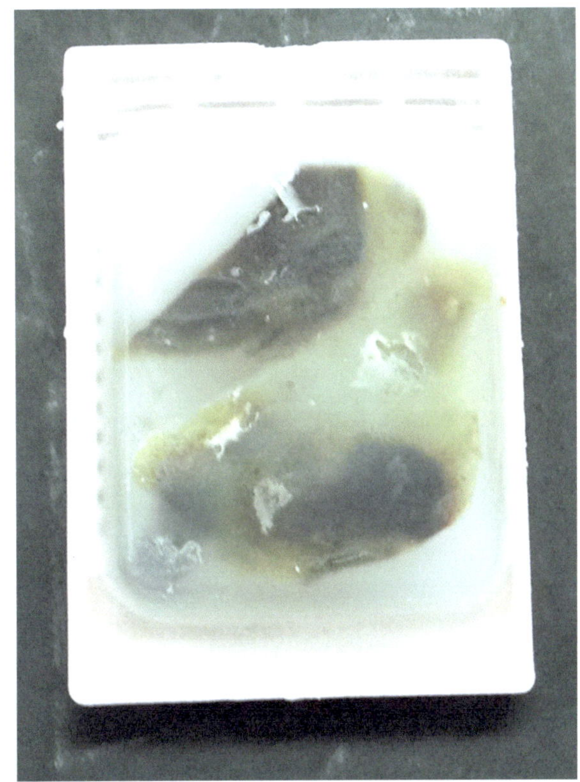

Fig. 1.2 Tissue block. After the tissue has been dehydrated, it is taken out of the cassette and embedded in paraffin. The tissue is now on the outside of the plastic cassette and is now a tissue block from which sections can be cut

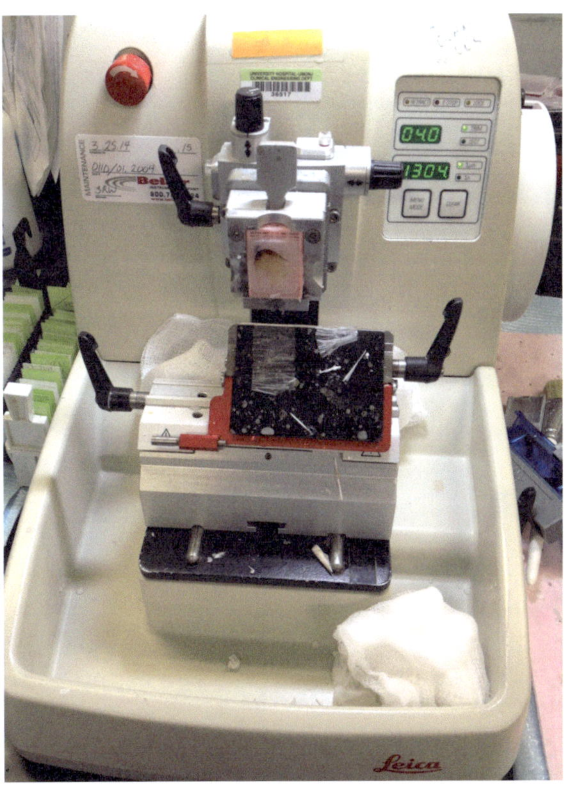

Fig. 1.3 Microtome. This instrument is used to cut extremely thin sections from the paraffin block. Duplicate sections come off attached to each other as a ribbon

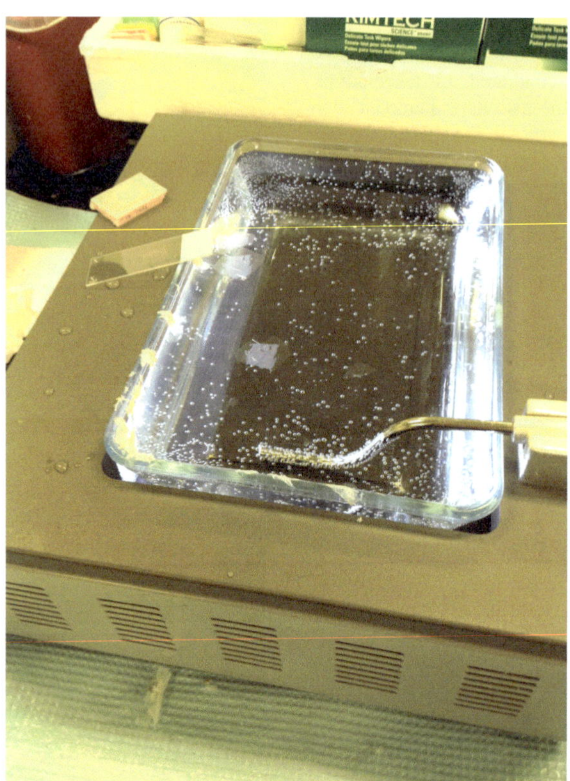

Fig. 1.4 Water bath. The ribbon of sections cut from the block are floated on a warm water bath for pickup onto slides passed underneath the sections

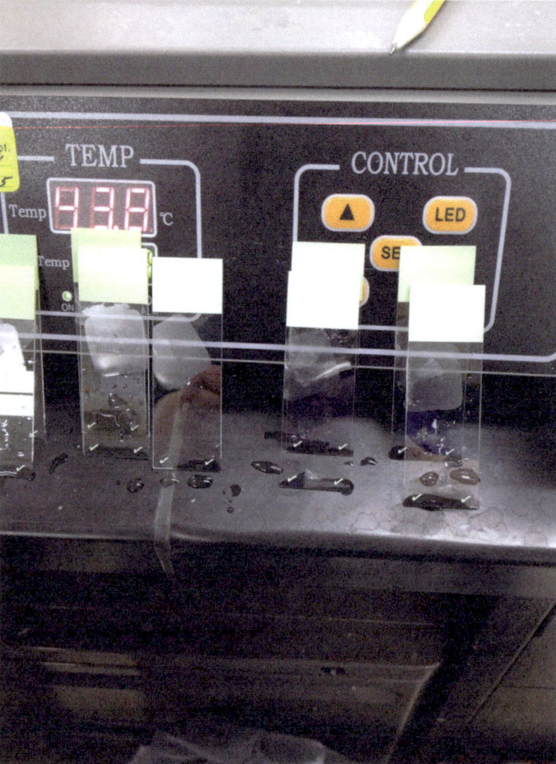

Fig. 1.5 Unstained sections. After the sections are picked up onto slides passed under them in the water bath, and drying of these slides, they are ready for staining

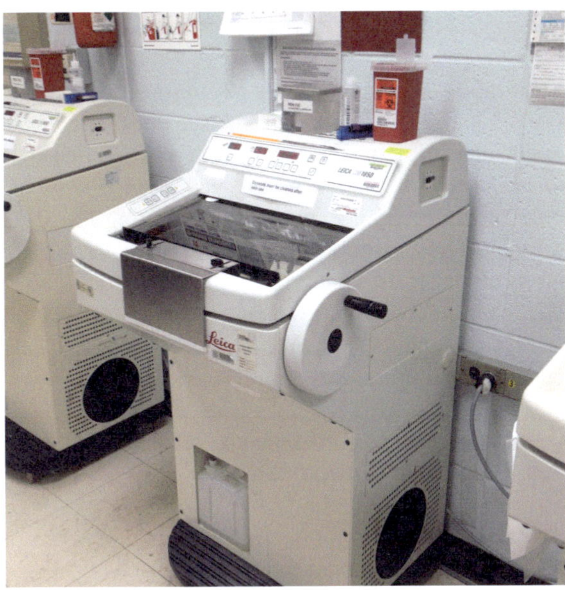

Fig. 1.6 Frozen section machine. This machine makes a rapid tissue block using a special nonpermanent embedding medium that freezes, and then sections are cut and stained

1.1.8 Labeling

The slides have a handwritten label on top of the glass slide during preparation, but now receive a paper label covering it, are matched with the requisition sheet, and are ready for reading.

1.2 Recuts and Levels

A tissue block can be cut multiple times, and each time a section of about 4–5 μm is produced. For large specimens, such as placenta, each "recut," which is usually the next section, is not likely to be significantly different from section to section. However, for smaller specimens, such as a cervical biopsy, each cut may vary in terms of what is seen on the slide. This is used to advantage when a possible site of superficial invasion is seen, as cutting deeper into the block may delineate the finding. Levels are similar to recuts, but instead of sequential sections, these are skip sections, to get deeper into the block, in an attempt to delineate a finding. Occasionally levels and recuts reveal an unexpected finding. This may occasionally occur after the case has been signed out, if recuts are performed, for example, for adjunct studies or outside consultation.

1.3   "Floaters" and Contaminants

Laboratories have procedures to minimize the occurrence of floaters and contaminants. Floaters are fragments of tissue in either the water bath or one of the solutions either not belonging to the patient whose slide it is, or occurring secondary to displacement of fragile tissue, such as fragments of ovarian carcinoma relocated onto the surface of a specimen. Recutting the slide will eliminate these. More difficult at times are contaminants within the paraffin block, which will not disappear on recutting. If the contaminant or floater could in no way be part of the specimen (i.e., chorionic villi in a 90-year-old woman), this is not a real problem, but it can be an issue. Meticulous attention to cleanliness and laboratory procedure minimizes but cannot eliminate this circumstance.

1.4   "Rush" Specimens

As mentioned, usually there is a schedule of when processors are run. As such, a rush specimen may derail the schedule, delaying other patients' slides and diagnoses. Therefore, a rush request should be used judiciously. A phone call to the pathologist to explain the reason for the rush may provide the clinician with a reasonable solution. As an example, if a same day rush cannot be reasonably provided, a result provided first thing the next morning, instead of in the afternoon, may meet the clinical need and avoid difficulty.

1.5   Special Studies and Fixation

Although this comes up less frequently in ob/gyn pathology than in some other subspecialties, sometimes special studies that need tissue submitted a specific way come up. Examples are cytogenetics or flow cytometry, where the tissue needs to be submitted fresh, rather than in formalin, for placement in specific media. Immunofluorescence is performed on frozen sections, so the tissue needs to be received fresh and cut into frozen section slides. For small biopsies, placing the tissue immediately in fixative is preservative and prevents an artifact known as autolysis where the tissue breaks down and is difficult to interpret. For large specimens, appropriate handling by the clinician may depend on the time of the day the specimen becomes available. During the day, most pathology departments receive several shipments from their operating rooms, and fresh tissue can be handled immediately. Pathologists may prefer not to have the surgeon cut into a specimen, which may interfere with analysis. However, if the specimen is coming out late, alternatives include refrigeration or fixation. For a uterus, endometrium autolyzes very rapidly, even with refrigeration, so opening the uterus and fixing it may be a better choice. Fixation should be in a generous amount of formalin, ideally in a 10:1

ratio, fixative to tissue. Discussion between the pathology department and the clinicians in advance will allow for creation of protocols that can handle these specimens.

1.6   Frozen Sections: Uses and Limitations

Frozen sections are prepared on a special machine that freezes the tissue in a non-permanent embedding medium that later can be melted, so tissue can later be embedded in paraffin. The process allows for cutting of the tissue with a microtome housed within the freezer (Fig. 1.6). Frozen sections should be used judiciously, but are very useful in some situations in obstetrics and gynecology (Table 1.3). They are intended to guide the current procedure, not to assuage clinician or patient curiosity. Frozen section diagnosis is not perfect. The frozen section slide is not of as good quality as a slide that has been made from processed tissue, and accuracy may be decreased. In addition, because of the time-consuming nature of frozen section preparation, usually only one or at most two sections are feasible on a large specimen. If extensive sampling is needed, the frozen section may not reveal the salient finding. Mitotic activity in a smooth muscle tumor of the uterus may be difficult to appreciate and count on frozen section. An ovarian tumor suspected of being at least low malignant potential (borderline) requires a section per centimeter to rule out frank invasion, and this cannot be accomplished at frozen section. The freezing of tissue may introduce a tissue artifact that makes later reading of the permanent section limited. Some tissues, such as fat or bone, do not cut well during a frozen section (Table 1.4). Pathologists are trained to give as little information on a frozen

Table 1.3 Frozen sections with potential value

• Results will determine the extent of current procedure
• Margin status
• To establish that diagnostic tissue obtained
• Depth of invasion of endometrial carcinoma
• Unexpected finding
• Fresh or frozen tissue needed for special studies
• Unique and individualized circumstances

Table 1.4 Frozen sections with potential limitations

• Multiloculated mucinous cystic neoplasms requiring extensive sampling
• Worrisome smooth muscle neoplasms requiring extensive sampling
• Other specimens where extensive sampling required
• Tiny biopsies
• Special studies needed to establish diagnosis
• Technical difficulties—tissue that doesn't cut, such as fat or bone

Table 1.5 Pathology terms with different degrees of uncertainty

• Cannot rule out
• Consistent with
• At least
• Suggestive of
• Suspicious for
• Defer to permanent section

section as possible, to avoid error. Deferral of a diagnosis is an option. There are also a variety of terms used by a pathologist when a diagnosis is not certain (see Table 1.5), both for frozen section and permanent section diagnosis. It is considered better to have a patient require a second procedure, than to overdiagnose and be the instrument of too-aggressive surgery.

Occasionally, a situation will arise where a frozen section diagnosis is requested on a specimen not usually frozen. An example would be a cone biopsy. As this requires many sections to embed all the tissue, and cervical tissue is difficult to cut well-oriented slices fresh, it is usually not feasible to perform frozen sections and may introduce tissue artifacts making later permanent section analysis difficult. However, a conversation may change this. An example would be a patient who had a prior biopsy suspicious for invasive cervical carcinoma. The patient cannot tolerate another office biopsy, nor a second anesthesia well. The surgeon wants to perform a radical hysterectomy at the time of the cone biopsy, but needs a firm cancer diagnosis to do so. A conversation between the clinician and pathologist in advance of the procedure will allow for these unique circumstances to best be dealt with.

On a final note, a frozen section represents a separate charge for the patient. It is a physician service. It should be used wisely.

1.7   Special Studies

Special studies may be needed on fresh, frozen, or formalin-fixed tissue. Fresh tissue may be needed for cytogenetics, or flow cytometry, for example. Frozen section slides are used for immunofluorescence and so the tissue must be submitted fresh. In general, it is better to call the pathology laboratory in advance of any unusual non-routine study, if known, to make sure the appropriate fixative is available, or even that the test is available. It is far better to have this arranged in advance than to have the chicken without a head situation of trying to find the right fixative after the procedure has been performed.

With formalin-fixed tissue, time is not usually of the essence to the same degree, although over time, immunohistochemical stains are less effective in fixed tissue, as antigenicity decreases over time for tissue immersed in formalin. A large number of histochemical and immunohistochemical stains are available to pathologists. These may be used for purposes such as to determine the origin of a neoplasm, delineate characteristics of a neoplasm, or identify an infectious organism. The pathologist determines which stains best serve the individual case. For example, in the absence of inflammation, a stain for microorganisms tends to be of no use and generates an additional charge for the patient. Hence, pathologists appreciate clinicians who request "rule out tuberculosis" on a requisition, rather than "Do acid fast bacillus stain." The anatomic pathology analysis is a consultation between professionals, not a laboratory test checked off on a list of blood tests. Certain exceptions are the rule, of course, as clinicians are expected to request HPV testing on pap smears where it is needed but not reflex.

1.8 Slide Review

If a biopsy diagnosis of malignancy was made elsewhere from where the major resection is occurring, it is important to have the biopsy slides reviewed at the institution where the major surgery will occur prior to the procedure. This may prevent significant error [2]. Slide review also occurs within a hospital, among pathology colleagues (pathology is a very collaborative specialty), as well as in interdisciplinary conferences.

1.9 Conclusion

The pathology consultation can be enhanced by good communication between the clinician and the pathologist. The telephone can be as powerful an instrument as a scalpel or microscope.

References

1. Morelli P, Porazzi E, Ruspini M, Restelli U, Banfi G. Analysis of errors in histology by root cause analysis: a pilot study. J Prev Med Hyg. 2013;54:90–6.
2. Santoso JTA, Coleman RL, Voet RL, Bernstein SG, Lifshitz S, Miller D. Pathology review in gynecologic oncology. Obstet Gynecol. 1998;91:730–4.

Normal Histology of the Female Genital Tract

2

2.1 Embryology

An in-depth discussion of embryology and anomalies of the female genital tract is beyond the scope of this text, and interested readers are referred to embryology texts; however, a brief review is in order. In the early first trimester, the external genitalia are not differentiated towards either gender. Both the Müllerian (paramesonephric) and Wolffian (mesonephric) ducts are present in parallel. Genetics determine which duct develops and which regresses. For XX individuals, the Müllerian ducts continue to develop, and the Wolffian ducts regress. Müllerian duct development relies on a number of genes in addition to absence of anti-Müllerian hormone (Müllerian inhibiting substance, MIS) [1], and the differentiation into a female is not merely becoming "not male." Knock-out mice missing a variety of these female-determining genes have a variety of genital anomalies [1]. Differentiation of the embryo begins at about 8 weeks. The external genitalia and lower third of the vagina are formed by the urogenital sinus. The upper two thirds of the vagina, cervix, uterus, and fallopian tubes are formed by the fusion of the two Müllerian (paramesonephric) ducts. After fusion of the Müllerian ducts, the septum between them dissolves. When the urogenital sinus meets the Müllerian ducts, a vaginal plate is formed which subsequently canalizes, forming the patent and lined vagina. In a female, the Wolffian (mesonephric) ducts regress, but remnants may remain and be identified later in life.

The ovaries are indifferent in early embryonic life as well. At about 8 weeks of gestational age, the gonads can be reliably distinguished. This histologic distinction can be extremely important to make when examining an immature fetus from an unsuccessful or terminated pregnancy. Inexperienced clinicians and pathologists tend to mistake the external genitalia of late first/early second trimester female fetuses as male due to the prominence of the clitoris and not looking behind it to see the labia and patent vaginal opening rather than scrotum. Histopathology of the gonads can provide the gonadal gender (Fig. 2.1a, b). Migration of germ cells occurs along the midline along the dorsal mesentery of the hindgut [2], populating the ovaries, which

© Springer International Publishing Switzerland 2015
D.S. Heller, *OB-GYN Pathology for the Clinician*,
DOI 10.1007/978-3-319-15422-0_2

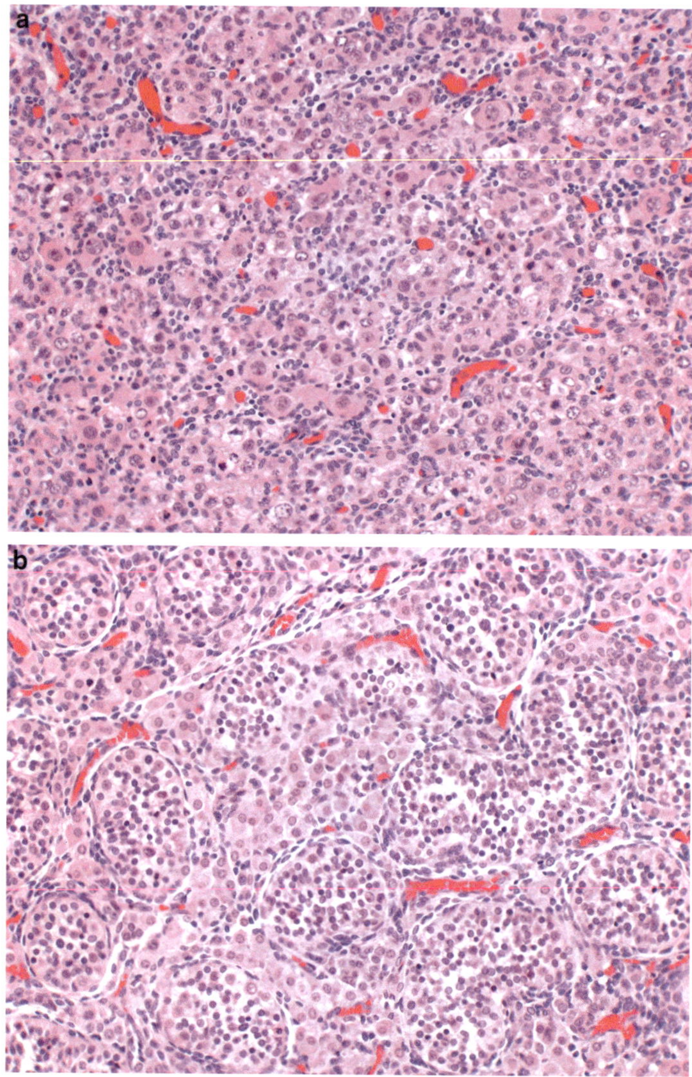

Fig. 2.1 Fetal gonads. The fetal ovary (**a**) shows diffuse distribution of germ cells. The fetal testis (**b**) shows distinct tubules containing Sertoli and germ cells, with intervening Leydig cells

are formed from the gonadal ridges [3]. It is because of this pattern of migration that germ cell neoplasms can occur anywhere in the body along the midline. No additional oogonia develop after birth, and some degenerate prior to birth, the rest enlarging prior to birth into primary oocytes, surrounded by a single flat layer of follicular cells forming the primordial follicle (Fig. 2.2). Therefore, a female is born with all the two to four million oocytes she will ever have. The maternal hormones may persist in the female infant, leading to cystic follicles (Fig. 2.3), which eventually regress in childhood until puberty. The XO fetus may occasionally show a streak gonad devoid of germ cells at birth, but germ cell loss may occur later (Fig. 2.4).

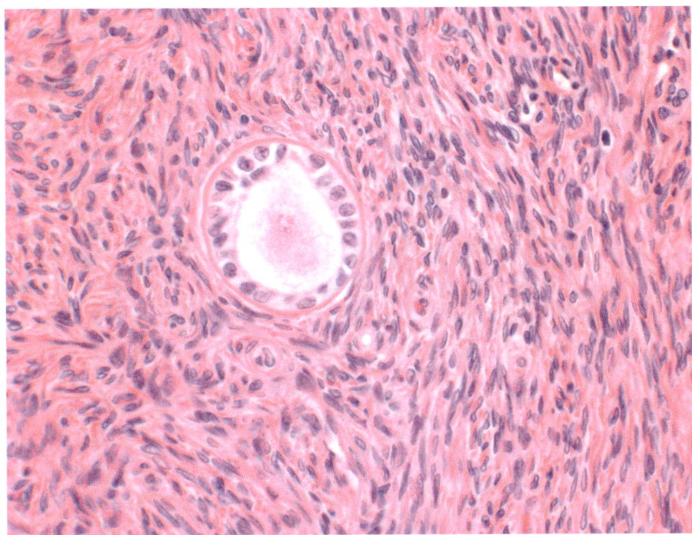

Fig. 2.2 The primordial follicle is composed of the ovum surrounded by a single layer of supporting follicular cells

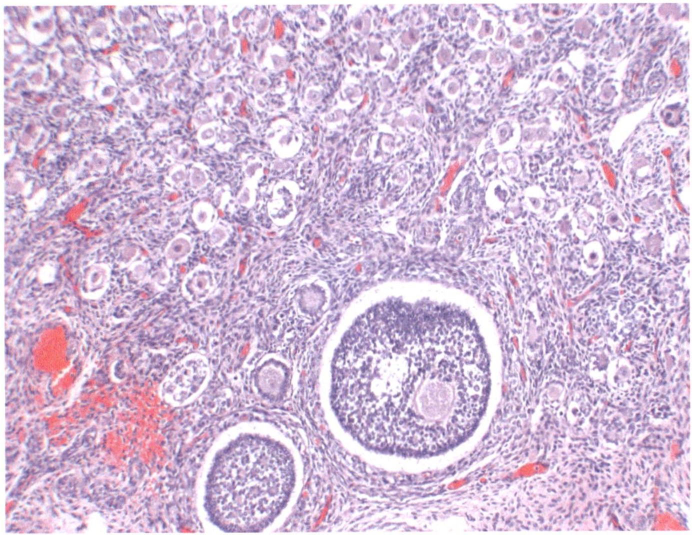

Fig. 2.3 The newborn ovary shows fewer primordial follicles than the fetal ovary, and follicular development as seen at the bottom of the image is a reflection of maternal hormonal effect

Aside from agenesis or hypoplasia, many of the anomalies of the female genital tract can be explained by defects in canalization of the urogenital sinus, or defects in either fusion of the Müllerian ducts or later dissolution of the intervening septum.

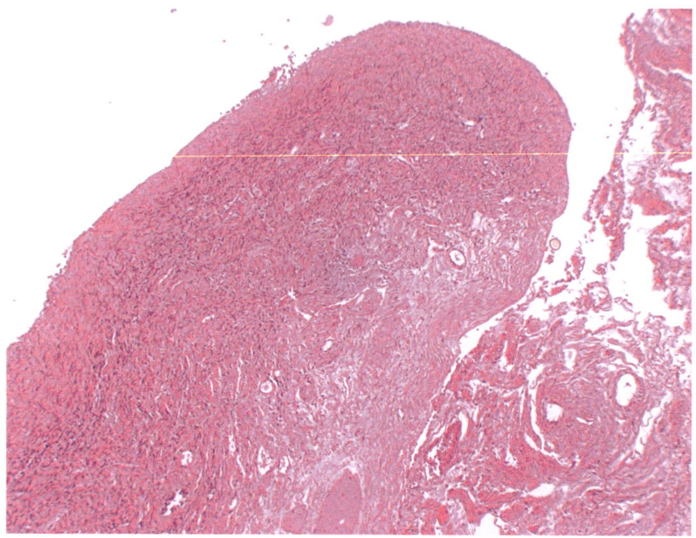

Fig. 2.4 Streak ovary devoid of germ cells

2.2 Histology of the Vulva

2.2.1 Labia Majora

The labia majora are similar to skin elsewhere on the body and are lined by a keratinized stratified squamous epithelium (Fig. 2.5). The dermis is less delineable into papillary and reticular dermis than skin elsewhere on the body, which is the basis of the modification of Clark's levels used for skin to vulvar Chung's levels for evaluating melanoma [4]. The labia majora contain hair follicles, apocrine, and eccrine glands confined to the outer portion of the labia majora only, and sebaceous glands in both outer and inner portions (Figs. 2.6, 2.7, and 2.8).

Labia minora—The labia minor are lined by squamous epithelium with a thin keratin layer outside, none inside, no hair, and fewer glands than the labia majora. These glands are comprised of sebaceous glands, with no apocrine or eccrine glands, hair follicles, or fat in the dermis. The dermis contains collagen and elastic fibers, blood vessels, and nerves.

Vestibule—The vestibule is the area above Hart's line, external to the hymen. Sebaceous glands end external to Hart's line, and there are generally no sweat glands in the vestibule. Minor vestibular glands comprised of acini lined by mucinous columnar epithelium may be present. The vestibule contains the openings of Bartholin's ducts, vagina, and urethra and is lined by a non-keratinized stratified squamous epithelium.

Fig. 2.5 Labia majora lined by keratinized stratified squamous epithelium. The basal pigmentation seen here corresponds to clinically appreciable pigmented skin

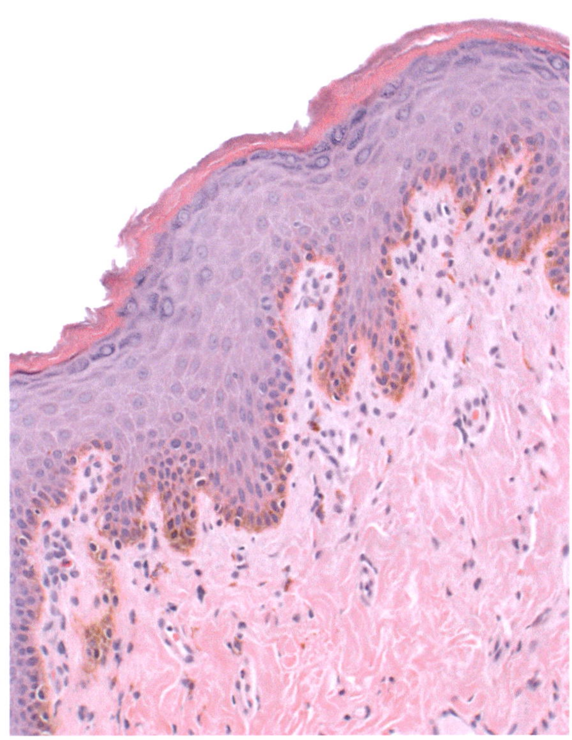

Bartholin's glands—The Bartholin's glands contain three types of epithelium. The glands are composed of acini lined by mucinous columnar epithelium. This merges in the ducts with a transitional epithelium and becomes squamous epithelium at the ostia which open onto the 4 o'clock and 8 o'clock positions of the vestibule (Fig. 2.9).

Clitoris—The clitoris is lined by keratinized stratified squamous epithelium, without dermal appendages. Erectile tissue is abundant beneath the epithelium and is composed of abundant vascular spaces (Fig. 2.10).

Perineum—The perineum is lined by keratinized stratified squamous epithelium. The perineum contains apocrine and mammary-like glands (Fig. 2.11). It used to be thought that there was accessory breast tissue along the milk line. This is now recognized as being anogenital mammary glands, which can also be present at the interlabial sulcus. These glands can give rise to neoplasms similar to those seen in the breast.

Mons pubis—The mons pubis is a fat pad covered by hair-bearing skin.

Hymen—The non-keratinized squamous epithelium of the hymen covers a loose fibroelastic tissue.

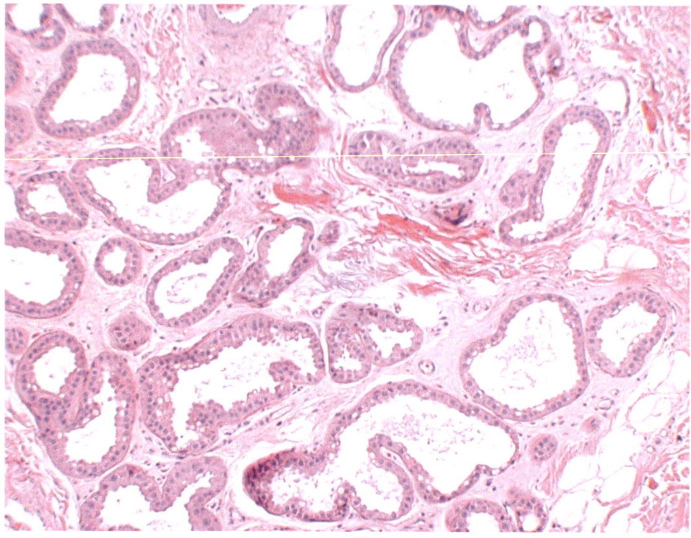

Fig. 2.6 Labia majora. Apocrine glands showing abundant eosinophilic cytoplasm

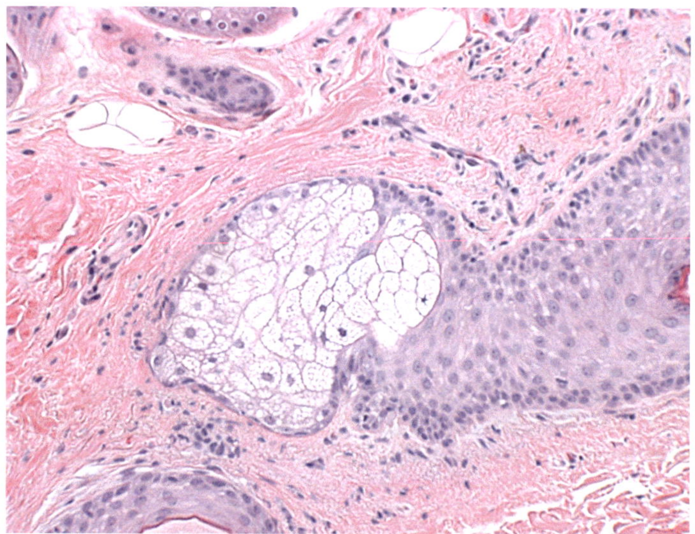

Fig. 2.7 Labia majora. A sebaceous gland is seen

Skene's ducts and glands—The Skene's glands are composed of mucinous columnar epithelium which drains via transitional ducts out on either side of the urethra, where the epithelium blends with the squamous epithelium of the vestibule. It is also thought that branches of the duct drain into the urethra. The Skene's glands are considered analogous to the male prostate.

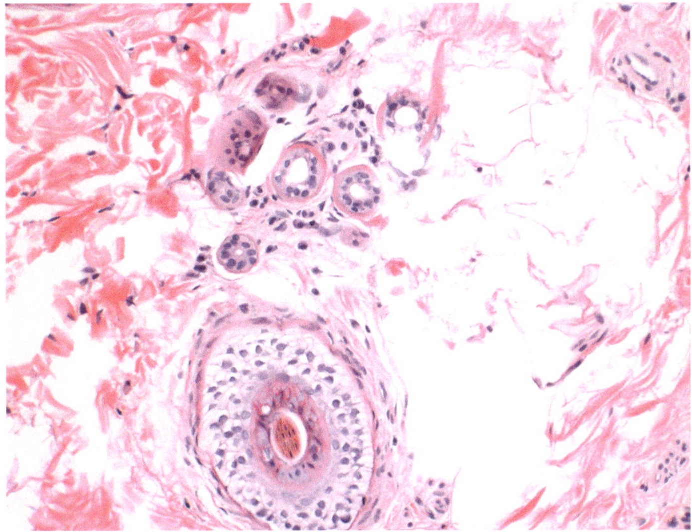

Fig. 2.8 Labia majora. A hair follicle is present at the bottom of the image, with eccrine glands above

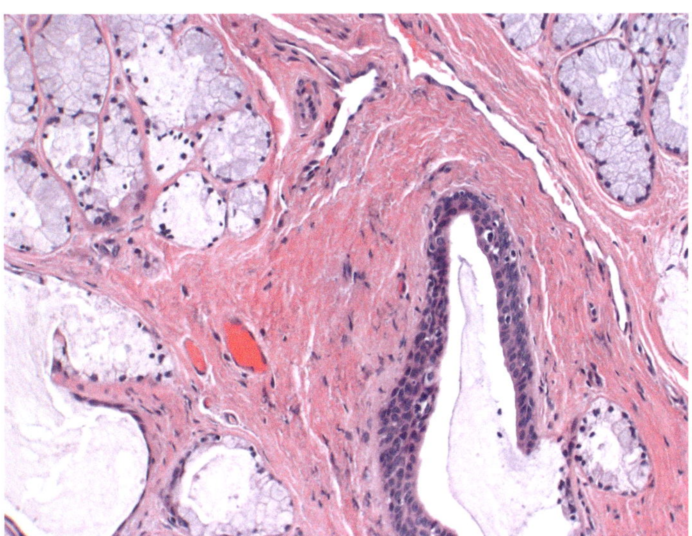

Fig. 2.9 Bartholin's glands show mucinous acini. A transitional epithelial-lined duct is seen at the bottom right

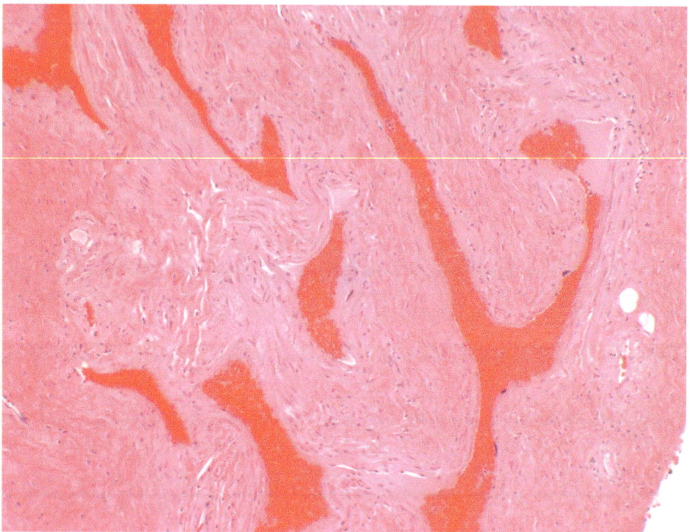

Fig. 2.10 Erectile tissue of the clitoris, containing numerous vascular spaces

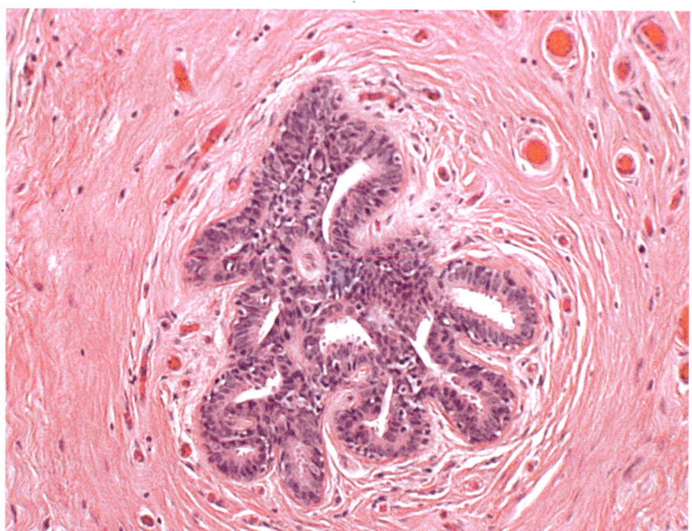

Fig. 2.11 Mammary-like tissue of the vulva showing a ductal structure similar to breast

2.3 Histology of the Vagina

The vagina is lined by non-keratinized stratified squamous epithelium. During reproductive life, the epithelium is highly glycogenated due to the effect of estrogen (Fig. 2.12).

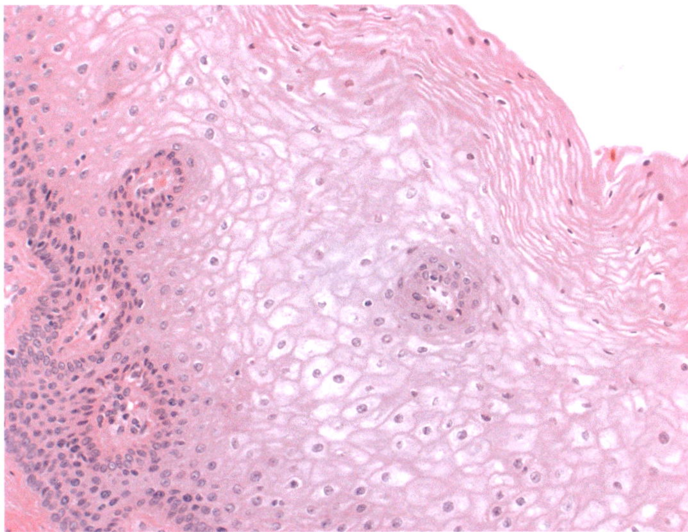

Fig. 2.12 The vagina is lined by non-keratized stratified squamous epithelium containing abundant glycogen during reproductive life

2.4 Histology of the Cervix

2.4.1 Exocervix

The exocervix is lined by non-keratinized stratified squamous epithelium. The cells show an orderly maturation from the basal layer up to the surface, which shows impaired maturation when intraepithelial neoplasia is present. During reproductive life, the presence of estrogen leads to abundant glycogenation of the cells, which should not be mistaken for koilocytes in the absence of nuclear atypia (Fig. 2.13). Persistence of maternal hormones leads to similar glycogenated cervical epithelium in the neonate; however, in the child and menopausal woman, lack of estrogen leads to a more atrophic epithelium. With atrophy there is decreased glycogen in the cells, and the maturation from basal layer to surface is much decreased. This lack of maturation (Fig. 2.14) should not be confused with intraepithelial neoplasia. A Ki-67 immunostain (Fig. 2.15) can be used in difficult cases, because normal epithelium, including atrophic epithelium, will stain only in the parabasal layer, while neoplastic epithelium will stain up to the surface with this proliferation marker.

The epithelium overlies a stroma which is predominantly fibroconnective tissue, with small amounts of smooth muscle and elastin, which transitions into the myometrium in the lower uterine segment. Chronic inflammatory cells are common, and as this does not in most cases indicate a disease state, a diagnosis of "chronic cervicitis" is not appropriate (but used somewhat too liberally at times) unless the inflammation is severe with numerous lymphoid follicles or contains abundant plasma cells [5].

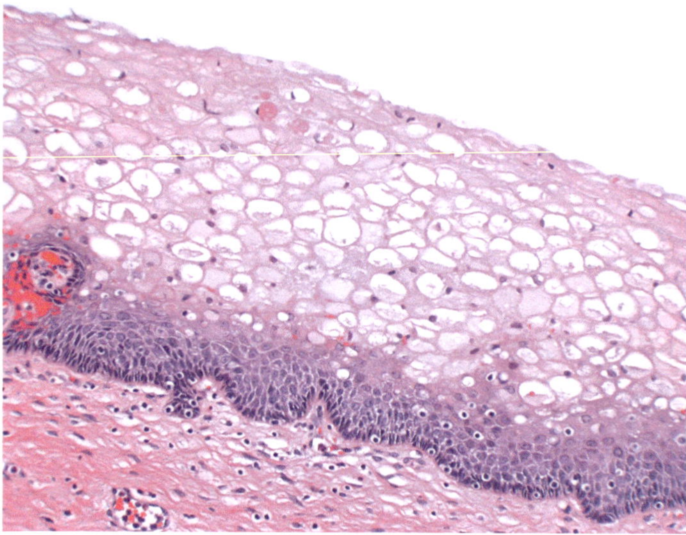

Fig. 2.13 Exocervix showing non-keratinized stratified squamous epithelium with abundant glycogen. Lack of nuclear atypia and orderly maturation rule out koilocytosis and intraepithelial neoplasia, respectively

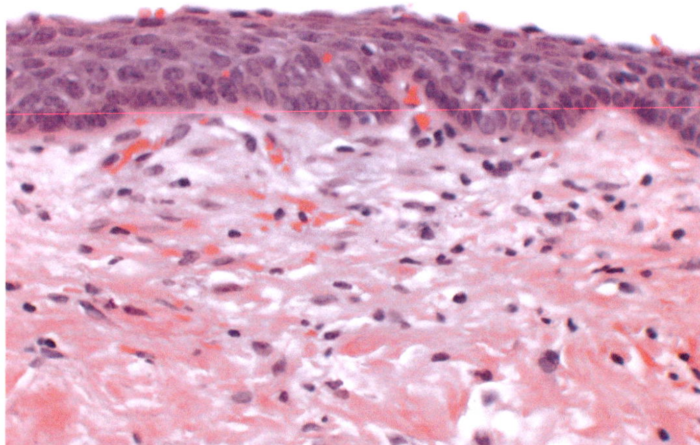

Fig. 2.14 Atrophic exocervix. Maturation and glycogen are decreased, but the cells are orderly

Remnants of the Wolffian ducts (mesonephric remnants) may frequently be seen in the lateral cervical stroma. These are recognizable by location (lateral, present about half way into the depth of the cervix) and by the epithelium, which is usually a flat cuboidal lining without cilia, with prominent eosinophilic lumenal secretions frequent (Fig. 2.16).

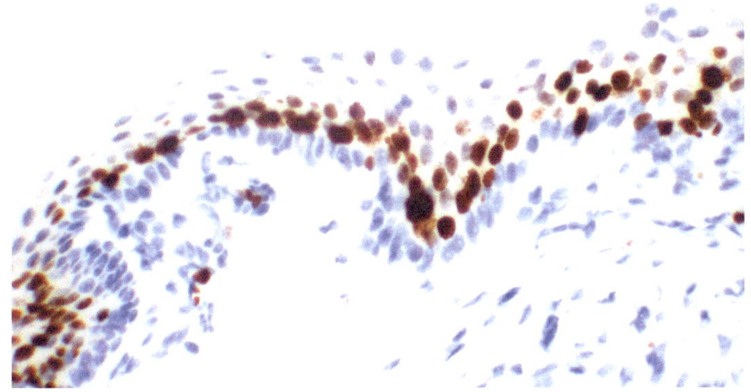

Fig. 2.15 Ki-67 immunostain in atrophy shows staining confined to the parabasal region

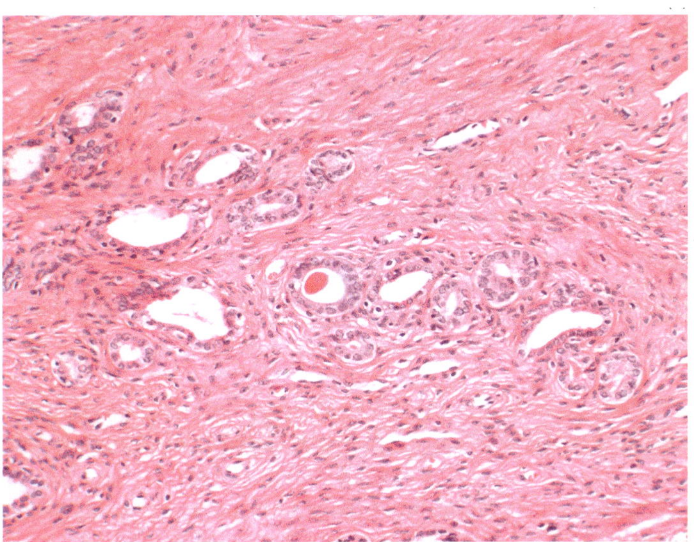

Fig. 2.16 Mesonephric remnants lined by cuboidal epithelium often show eosinophilic luminal secretions, as seen in the center

2.4.2 Endocervix

The endocervical crypts are branching crypts lined by mucinous columnar epithelium. On cross-section, they may appear as circular glands beneath the surface, but they communicate with the surface and produce cervical mucus (Fig. 2.17).

Fig. 2.17 Endocervical crypts may appear as glands, due to the orientation of the section, but communicate with the surface. Note the mucinous columnar epithelium with basal nuclei

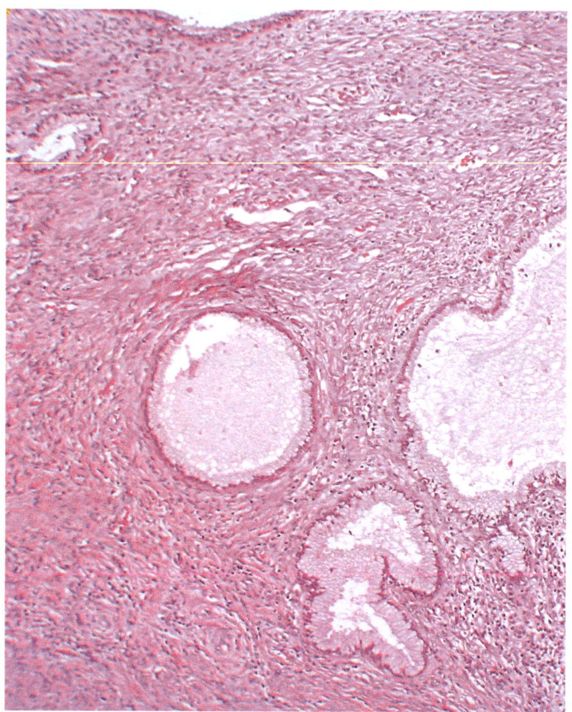

2.4.3   Transformation Zone

The transformation zone is an area of interest as the zone where cervical neoplasia arises. It is the area between the original squamocolumnar junction and the current squamocolumnar junction. The squamocolumnar junction moves over the course of a woman's life. The original squamocolumnar junction is usually located on the exocervix in early reproductive life. The endocervix may then be seen on speculum examination, and in the past beefy pink tissue of the normal endocervix has been mistaken for "erosion." Squamous metaplasia occurs over time and goes up into the endocervical canal, establishing the woman's current squamocolumnar junction, which can be high up the canal in the older woman, making adequate colposcopy challenging. The area in between the original and current squamocolumnar junctions is the transformation zone. Metaplasia is the conversion of one benign epithelial type to another. Metaplastic squamous epithelium appears immature, and lacking in glycogen, but matures and acquires glycogen over time. Histology of the transformation zone may demonstrate an abrupt shift from squamous to columnar epithelium, or the squamous metaplasia may extend over a length. If endocervical crypts are blocked by squamous metaplasia and the secretions get inspissated, Nabothian cysts occur (Figs. 2.18, 2.19, and 2.20).

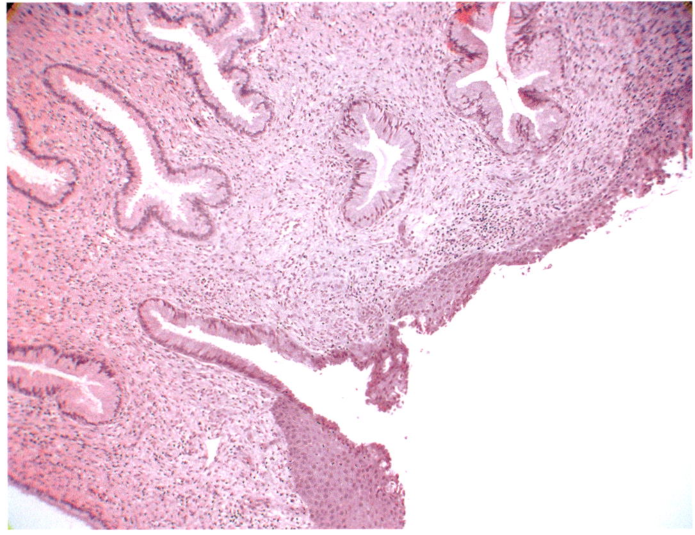

Fig. 2.18 The transformation zone shows squamous metaplasia overlying endocervical crypts

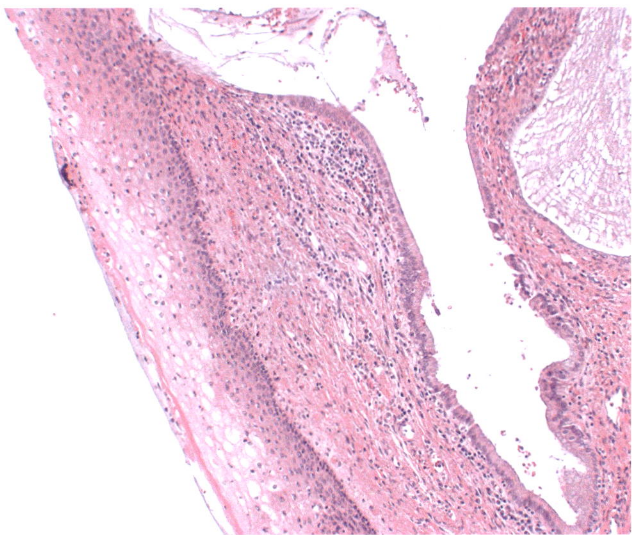

Fig. 2.19 Transformation zone. Blocked endocervical crypts due to overlying squamous metaplasia can form Nabothian cysts, as seen to the right

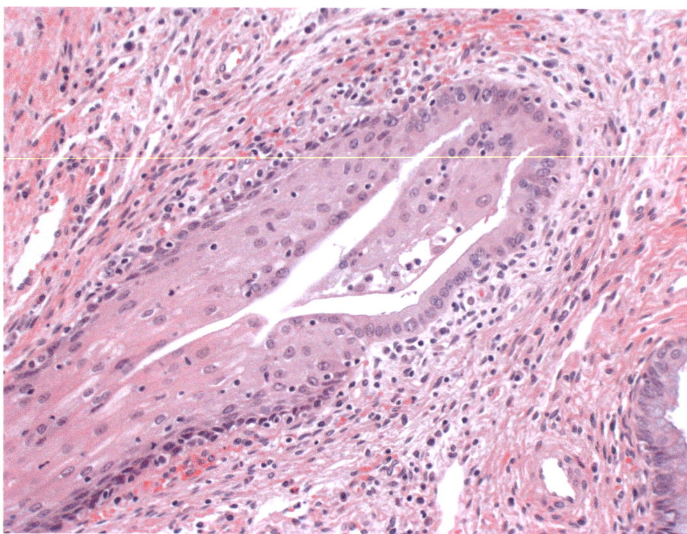

Fig. 2.20 Immature squamous metaplasia replacing an endocervical gland in the transformation zone

2.5 Histology of the Uterus

2.5.1 Endometrium

The endometrium is composed of a basalis layer, which remains behind after menses to regenerate, and a functional layer, which cycles with the ovarian cycle and sloughs at the end of each cycle that doesn't result in a pregnancy. In describing cycling endometrium histopathologically, the assumption is made that the cycle is 28 days, with days 1–5 being menses, as well as the initiation of the new cycle, day 14 is ovulation, and day 28 is the beginning of the next menses (i.e., day 1 again). This is of course not true for all women, and endometrial dating does not always correspond to fertility.

2.5.2 Proliferative Endometrium

Proliferative endometrium is present pre-ovulation (cycle days 1–14), due to the effect of estrogen alone. Proliferative endometrium (Figs. 2.21 and 2.22) is characterized by pseudostratification of the glandular epithelium. Although the glandular nuclei appear to be at different levels, all cells touch the basement membrane, hence the term "pseudo." Mitotic figures are seen in the glands and stroma. The stroma is cellular, with

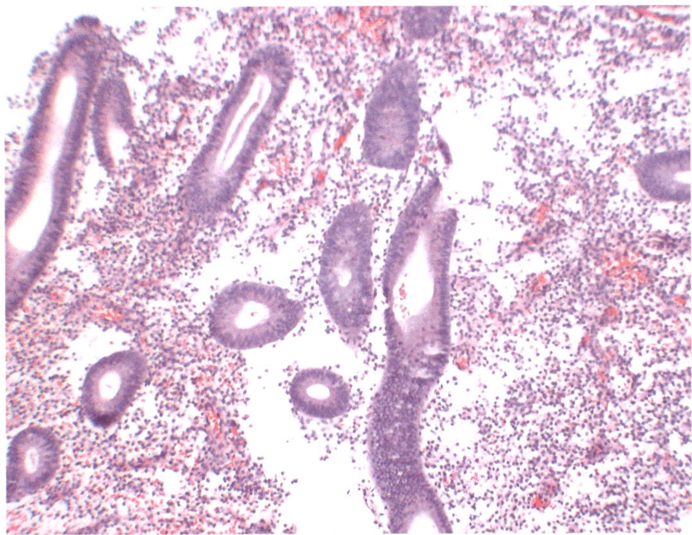

Fig. 2.21 Proliferative endometrium showing fairly straight tubular glands lined by a pseudostratified epithelium with mitotic activity (*inset*)

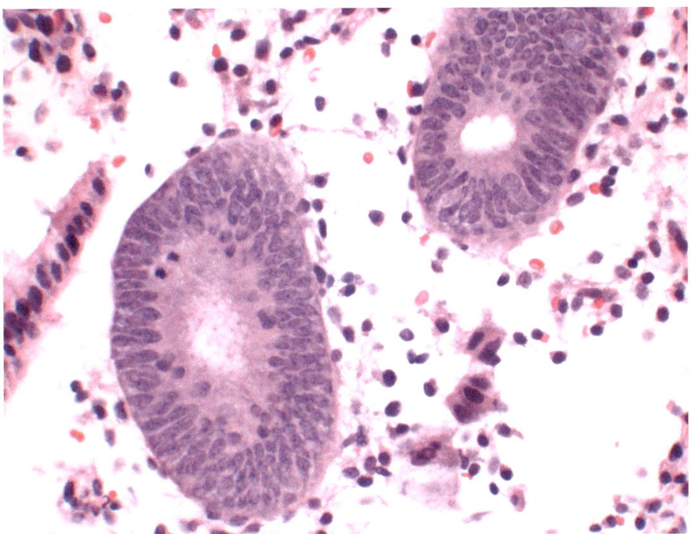

Fig. 2.22 Proliferative endometrium. At higher power, the pseudostratification and mitotic activity (11 o'clock in the gland on the left) can be appreciated

small spindled nuclei. The glands are simple tubular glands in the early proliferative phase, becoming more complex in mid- and late proliferative phases. The stroma shows some edema mid-proliferative, but otherwise is not notably different during this time period.

Table 2.1 Dating the endometrium[a]

Cycle day	Post-ovulatory day	Main distinguishing features
15	1	A few subnuclear vacuoles in a proliferative type endometrium
16	2	Subnuclear vacuoles in about half the glands
17	3	Uniform subnuclear vacuoles. First day ovulation can be confirmed by histopathology
18	4	Half subnuclear, half supranuclear vacuoles
19	5	Supranuclear vacuoles
20	6	Peak secretion
21	7	Early stromal edema
22	8	Peak stromal edema ("naked nuclei")
23	9	Prominent spiral arterioles
24	10	Decidual cuffing around spiral arterioles
25	11	Decidua under surface
26	12	Spreading decidua, not uniform
27	13	Stroma entirely decidualized, inflammatory cells seen
28/1	14	Breakdown, new cycle begins

[a]Based on the criteria of Noyes et al. [6]

2.5.3 Secretory Endometrium and Endometrial Dating

Secretory endometrium (cycle days 14–28) can be dated. The methodology has been around for a long time, as described by Noyes and colleagues in 1950 [6]. As there are more reliable methods of assessing the cycle, histologic dating of the endometrium has become less important in clinical practice. A brief review of the features is shown in Table 2.1. It should be noted that dating is not considered reliable in the presence of chronic endometritis.

The first day that a pathologist can reliably establish ovulation is day 17. The subnuclear vacuoles seen on days 15 and 16 are not uniformly present and may be due to estrogen alone. Changes from day 17 can be reliably interpreted as progestational effect along with estrogen. On day 17, subnuclear vacuoles are uniform, giving a piano key appearance. The glands are no longer pseudostratified, and mitoses are few, decreasing to almost none over the secretory phase (Fig. 2.23). The vacuoles migrate to the lumen, with half above and half below on day 18, and all above on day 19. Day 20 is peak secretion. At this point, the remainder of the changes seen are in the stroma. There is stromal edema beginning on day 21, peaking on day 22, giving a "naked nuclei" appearance. Stromal decidualization occurs for the rest of the cycle, spreading outwards. On day 23, spiral arterioles become prominent, with a thin layer of decidua around them (Fig. 2.24). This expands on day 24, and on day 25, decidua is seen under the surface epithelium. It continues to coalesce on day 26,

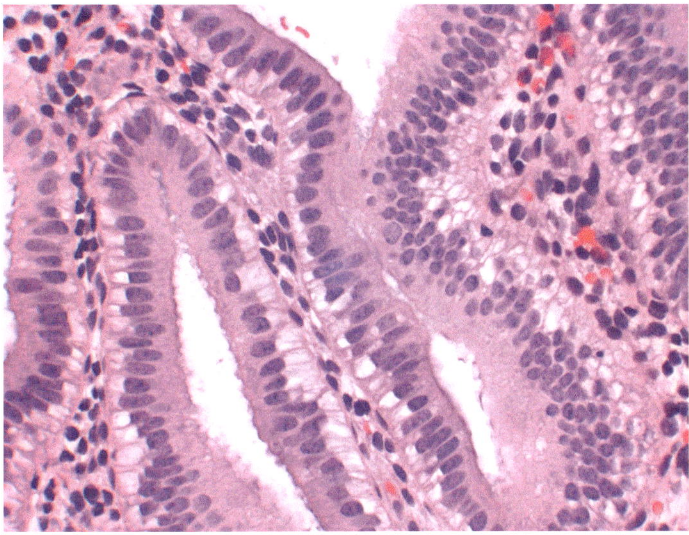

Fig. 2.23 Day 17 endometrium showing uniform subnuclear vacuoles in a "piano-key" configuration

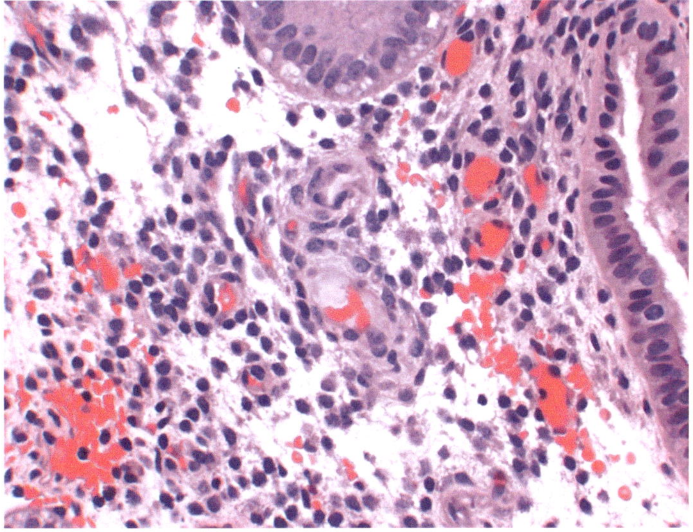

Fig. 2.24 Day 23 endometrium—Prominent spiral arterioles are seen in the center of the image

and by day 27 (Fig. 2.25), the stroma is entirely decidualized. Inflammatory cells, comprised of lymphocytes and neutrophils influx at the end of the cycle, and on day 28, breakdown begins, with thrombi in vessels, and gland-stromal dissociation (Fig. 2.26). If pregnancy doesn't ensue, there is repair, and a new cycle begins.

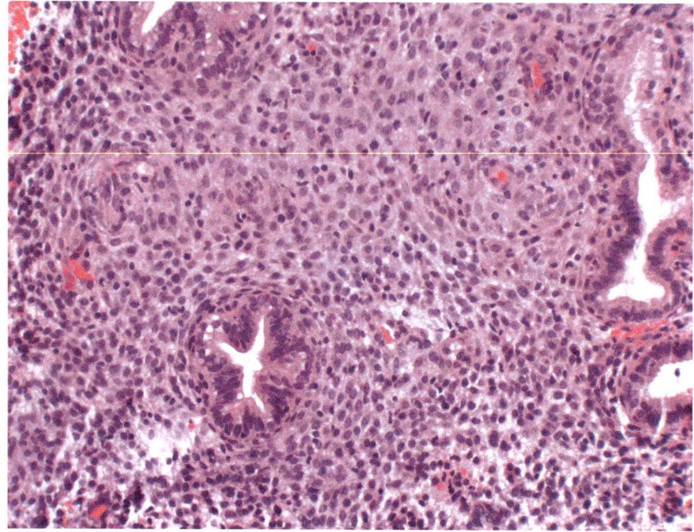

Fig. 2.25 Day 27 endometrium. Decidualization of stroma and secretory exhaustion of glands is present. Influx of inflammatory cells begins

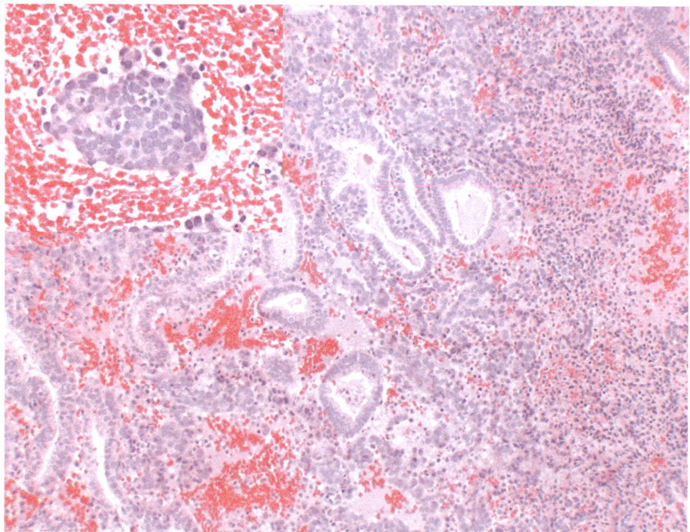

Fig. 2.26 Menstrual endometrium. Gland-stromal dissociation leads to formation of stromal "blue balls" (*inset*). With crumbling of the architecture, the establishment of whether ovulation occurred or determination of hyperplasia may not be possible

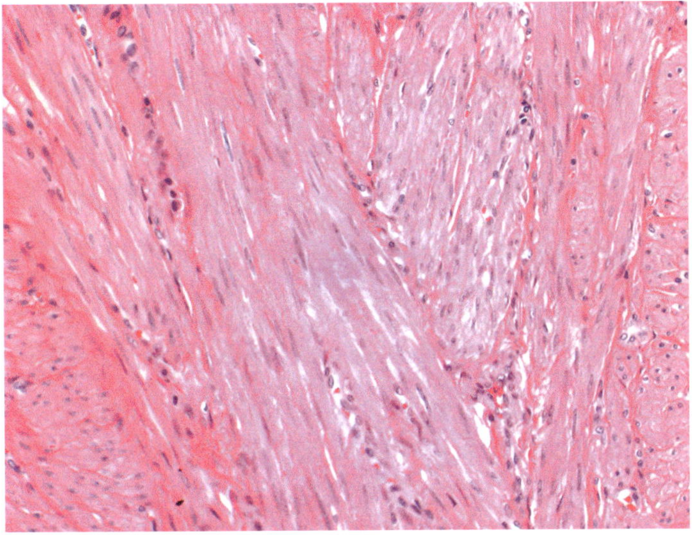

Fig. 2.27 Myometrium. Smooth muscle bundles extend in various directions

2.5.4 Myometrium

Myometrium is composed of predominantly smooth muscle, which is aggregated in bundles going in various directions (Fig. 2.27), along with some collagen and elastin. The cells have elongated cigar-shaped nuclei. Histologically, normal myometrium looks very much like leiomyomata on high power.

2.6   Histology of the Fallopian Tubes

The epithelium of the fallopian tube is mixed ciliated columnar, secretory nonciliated columnar cells with intercalated cells, which may represent a developmental stage of the secretory cells [5] (Figs. 2.28 and 2.29). The complexity of the infoldings of the fallopian tube varies by region, being prominent in the ampullary region. The individual folds are thin and delicate in the normal tube. The folds rest on two layers of smooth muscle, the inner circular and outer longitudinal. The cilia and muscle both work to transport the fertilized ovum to the uterine cavity.

2.7   Histology of the Ovaries

The lining of the ovaries, the surface epithelium, is derived embryologically from the same coelomic epithelium that forms the peritoneum. At ovulation, this surface becomes disrupted and may heal by invagination, forming small epithelial inclusion cysts.

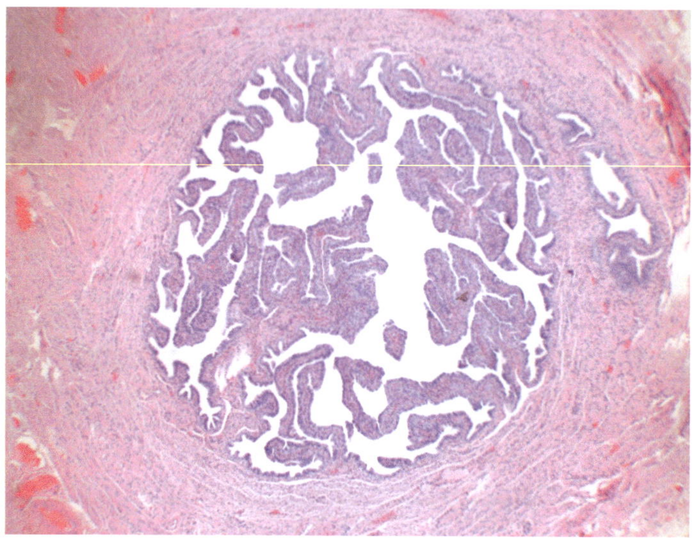

Fig. 2.28 Fallopian tube showing the delicate mucosal folds resting on a two layer muscular wall

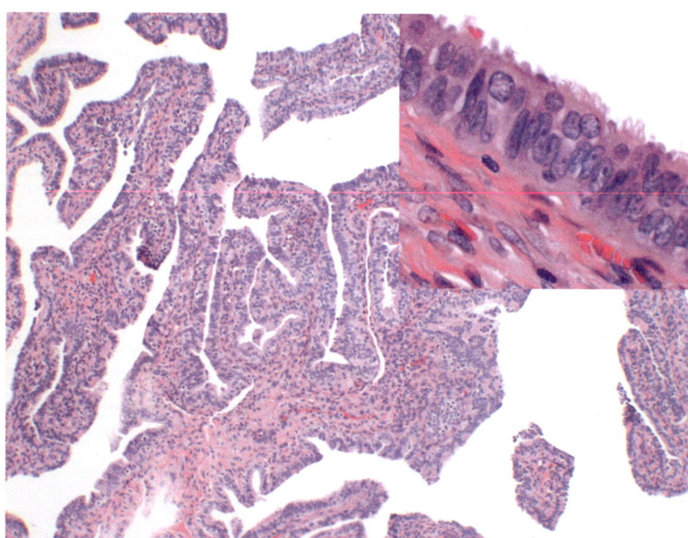

Fig. 2.29 Fallopian tube. At higher power, the delicate folds are seen to be lined by epithelium over a fibrovascular core. The epithelium is a combination of ciliated, secretory, and occasional intercalated cells (*inset right*)

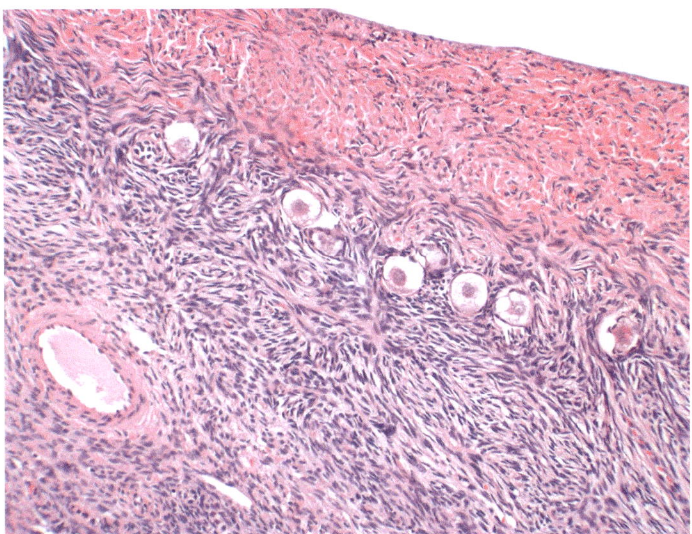

Fig. 2.30 Ovary showing primordial follicles in the spindle cell stroma of the cortex

These were previously thought to be related to the formation of epithelial ovarian carcinomas, particularly serous; however, malignant serous neoplasms are currently thought to arise from the fallopian tube fimbria [7]. The non-specialized ovarian stroma is a spindle cell stroma containing nerves and blood vessels. The specialized stroma, the granulosa cells and theca cells, surround the ova, forming the follicles. Normally, by adult life, the primordial follicles are much reduced and reside in the cortex (Fig. 2.30). A number of follicles are recruited each month; however, usually only one is destined to ovulate, although more than one may develop into an antral follicle (Fig. 2.31). After ovulation, the corpus luteum is formed. Grossly, this is yellow-orange in color, a reflection of the endocrine function. Histologically, the configuration is said to be cerebriform, mimicking the brain convolutions, and is composed of larger luteinized granulosa cells and smaller luteinized theca interna cells (Fig. 2.32) with central hemorrhage. Rarely, the corpus luteum may rupture and the hematoperitoneum may mimic a ruptured ectopic. If pregnancy does not occur, the corpus luteum regresses to become a corpus albicans, the name reflecting the gross white appearance. The corpus albicans retains the cerebriform configuration, but as these accumulate, they shrink down to small fibrous scars (Fig. 2.33). If pregnancy occurs, the corpus luteum of pregnancy, a somewhat larger structure, is formed.

2.8 Anatomy and Histology of the Placenta

The placental disk is comprised of a fetal surface and a maternal surface (Figs. 2.34 and 2.35). The fetal surface amnion and chorion extend in continuity with the fetal membranes of the gestational sac. The umbilical cord is usually inserted

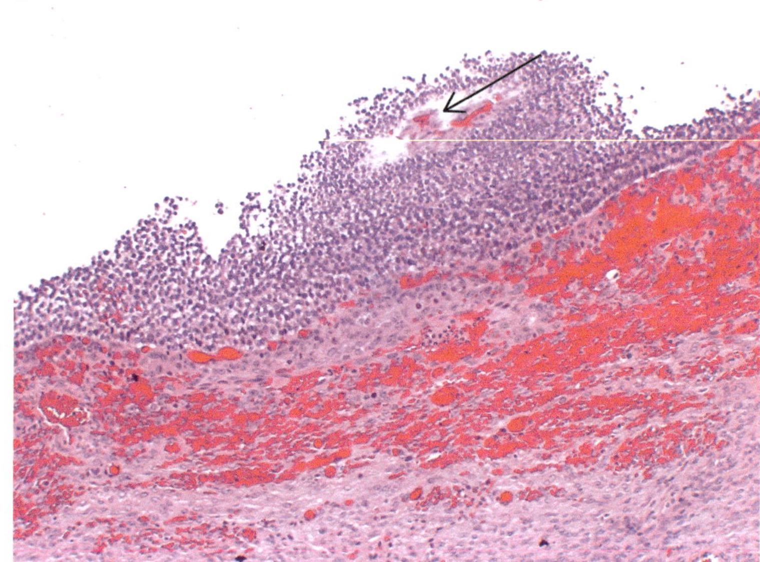

Fig. 2.31 Antral follicle. The antral space is above. The granulosa cells surround the ovum (*arrow* points to location of ovum, not well-visualized on this level) and form the inner lining of the antrum. The next layer is the vascular theca interna. The theca externa blends with ovarian stroma and is not well-delineated as a separate layer on sections

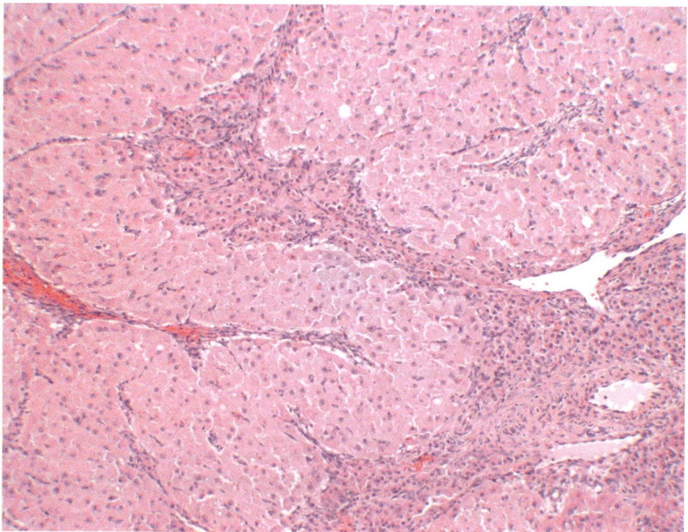

Fig. 2.32 Corpus luteum. The larger luteinized granulosa cells and smaller luteinized theca interna cells are arranged in a cerebriform configuration

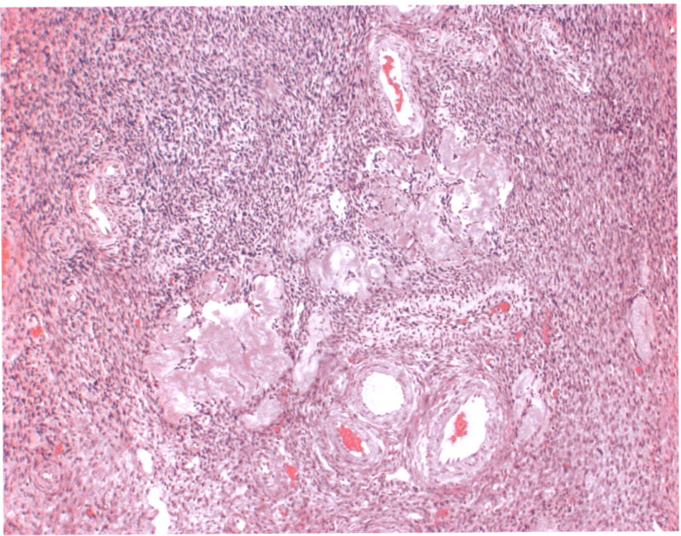

Fig. 2.33 Corpora albicantia retain the cerebriform configuration of the corpora lutea initially, eventually shrinking into small scars

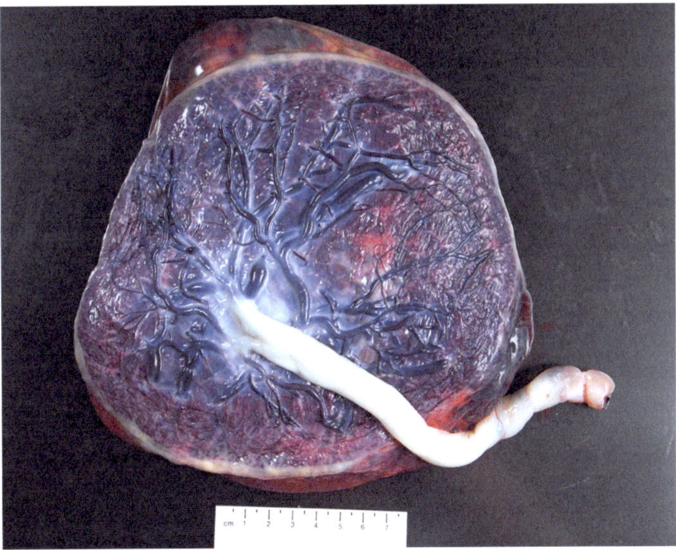

Fig. 2.34 Fetal surface of the placenta. The paracentral cord is seen inserting into the membranes of the chorionic plate

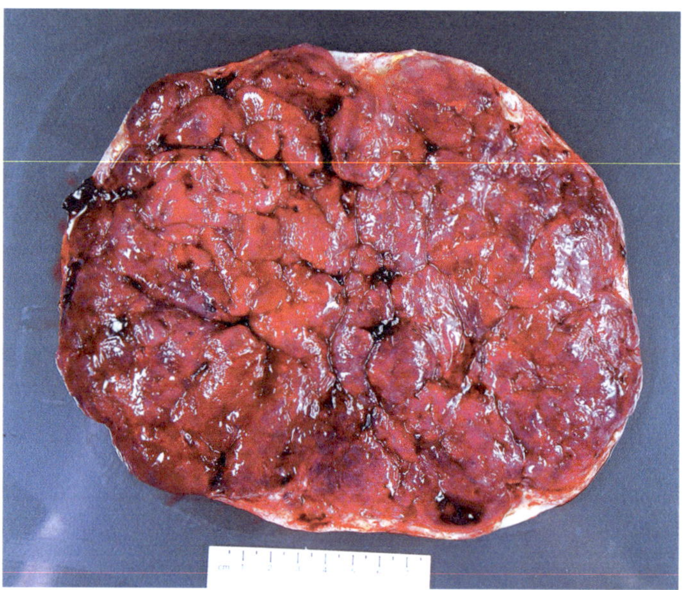

Fig. 2.35 Maternal surface of the placenta showing intact cotyledons

paracentrally and arises from the fetal surface. On cross-section, the two arteries and single umbilical vein can be seen embedded in the protective Wharton's jelly. The parenchyma of the placenta is made up of chorionic villi. The space between the villi, the intervillous space, contains the maternal blood which provides oxygen and nutrients to the fetus. The maternal surface of the placenta is composed of cotyledons of placental tissue which implant into the maternal decidua. The decidua splits at birth, with a layer adherent to the maternal surface of the placenta. The decidua remaining in the uterus gives rise to the regenerating endometrium. During early placentation, physiologic conversion occurs, with the cells from the invading implantational intermediate trophoblast replacing the endothelium of the maternal spiral arterioles in the placental bed. This serves to convert the arterioles into passively patent venous channels. It is the absence of this physiologic conversion which is thought to be associated with later development of preeclampsia [8].

First trimester chorionic villi (Fig. 2.36) are larger than third trimester villi, which have continued to branch (Fig. 2.37). First trimester villi show a two cell layer, inner cytotrophoblast, and outer syncytiotrophoblast. Nucleated red blood cells may be seen in fetal vessels. These are most prominent at 8–12 weeks gestational age. Second trimester villi are intermediate in size, and the inner cytotrophoblast is mostly unapparent. Third trimester villi are smaller, and although still present, the cytotrophoblast is no longer seen on routine histology, leaving only the syncytiotrophoblast visible in histologic sections. Part of normal maturation is the formation of syncytial knots, which are the syncytiotrophoblast nuclei piling up as

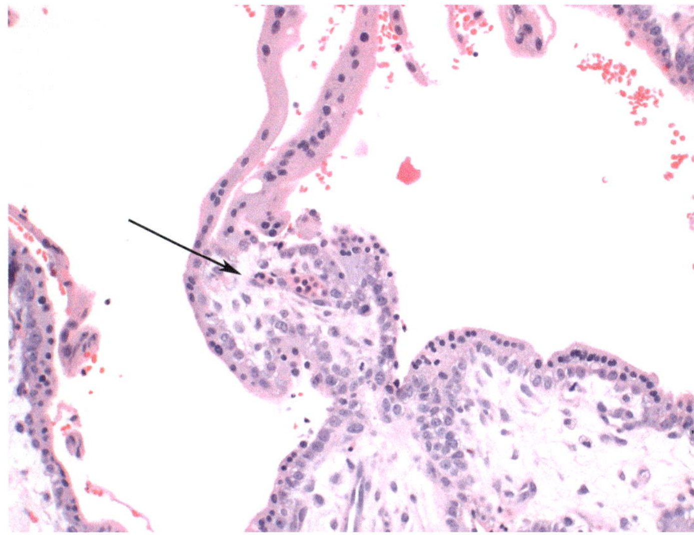

Fig. 2.36 First trimester chorionic villi show a two cell layer, inner cytotrophoblast, and outer syncytiotrophoblast. Nucleated red cells may be seen in a fetal vessel (*arrow*)

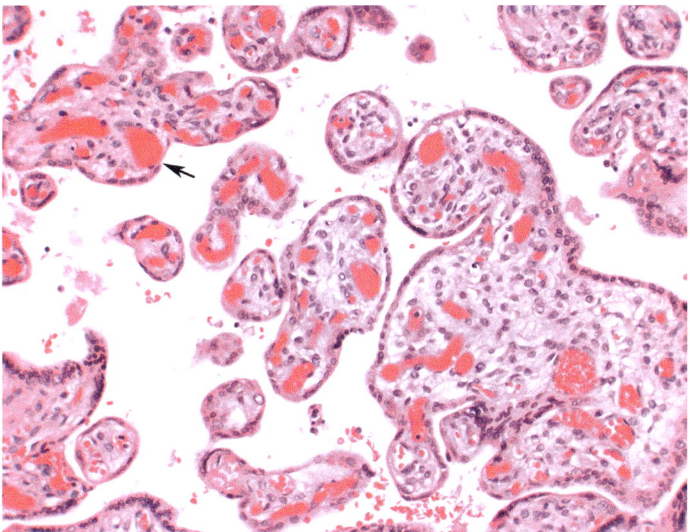

Fig. 2.37 Third trimester chorionic villi are smaller due to branching. A single syncytiotrophoblast layer is seen on sections. Villous capillaries are oriented peripherally in the villi, as close as possible to the maternal blood. The capillary, basement membrane of the villus, and attenuated syncytiotrophoblast cytoplasm form the "vasculosyncytial membrane" (*arrow*)

the cytoplasm of the syncytiotrophoblasts becomes attenuated over fetal capillaries of the villous stroma. These capillaries, which were more central earlier in pregnancy, are located more peripherally in the third trimester, to be closer to the maternal blood. The vessels, along with the attenuated syncytiotrophoblast cytoplasm, form the "vasculosyncytial membranes." These are not true membranes, but the smallest interface between the fetal and maternal circulations, functioning analogously to alveolar septa.

References

1. Yin Y, Ma L. Development of the mammalian female reproductive tract. J Biochem. 2005; 137:677–83.
2. Moore KL. Development of the genital system. In: Moore KL, Persaud RVN, Torchia MG, editors. The developing human. 9th ed. Philadelphia: Saunders; 2011. p. 265–86.
3. Gondos B. Development of the reproductive organs. Ann Clin Lab Sci. 1985;15:363–73.
4. Chung AF, Lewis WJM, Jr JL. Malignant melanoma of the vulva: a report of 44 cases. Obstet Gynecol. 1975;45:638–46.
5. Atkins KA, Hendrickson MR, Kempson RL. Normal histology of the uterus and fallopian tubes. In: Mills SE, editor. Histology for pathologists. 4th ed. Philadelphia: Lippincott Williams & Wilkins; 2012. p. 1071–117.
6. Noyes R, Hertig A, Rock J. Dating the endometrial biopsy. Fertil Steril. 1950;1:3–25.
7. Crum CP, Drapkin R, Miron A, et al. The distal fallopian tube: a new model for pelvic serous carcinogenesis. Curr Opin Obstet Gynecol. 2007;19:3–9.
8. Goldman-Wohl D, Yagel S. Regulation of trophoblast invasion: from normal implantation to pre-eclampsia. Mol Cell Endocrinol. 2002;187:233–8.

3.1 Diseases of the Vulva

The vulva is both a dermatologic and gynecologic organ, and thus prone to conditions affecting both. Clinical history is important, and orientation of excisions is critical if marginal assessment is required (Tables 3.1 and 3.2). There are limitations specific to the interpretation of vulvar biopsies (Table 3.3). Some conditions do not have a specific diagnosis, and a descriptive diagnosis may be received. Common dermatologic terms used in the vulva are listed in Table 3.4.

3.2 Congenital Anomalies of the Vulva

3.2.1 Ambiguous Genitalia

A discussion of the complex subject of intersex disorders is beyond the scope of this text. In an XX individual, the most common cause of newborn ambiguous genitalia is in utero exposure to androgens, either due to congenital adrenal hyperplasia, or maternal endogenous or exogenous androgens, resulting in female pseudohermaphroditism. Here the term "female" corresponds to the presence of an ovary. Clitoromegaly and labial fusion of various degrees may be seen in such cases.

3.2.2 Imperforate Hymen

Imperforate hymen, due to persistence of the urogenital membrane, may not present until after puberty, with hematocolpos, or difficulty with first intercourse. Rarely, accumulation of secretions may make this condition present as a congenital or newborn condition, presenting as an abdominal cyst [1].

© Springer International Publishing Switzerland 2015

D.S. Heller, *OB-GYN Pathology for the Clinician*,

DOI 10.1007/978-3-319-15422-0_3

Table 3.1 What to tell the pathologist about a vulvar lesion

Clinical history
Exact location of lesion
Orientation of specimen, particularly if marginal evaluation is needed

Table 3.2 History provided affects the diagnosis

Case 1
Clinical history A provided: vulvar cyst
Pathology report: benign mucinous cyst
Clinical history B provided: vulvar cyst, clinically Bartholin's cyst
Pathology report: benign mucinous cyst consistent with Bartholin's duct cyst
Case 2
Clinical history A provided: vulvar cyst
Pathology report: squamous mucosa containing a thin-walled squamous epithelial-lined cyst
Clinical history B provided: cystic mass at lateral introitus
Pathology report: squamous epithelial-lined cyst consistent with Bartholin's duct cyst

Table 3.3 Limitations of vulvar biopsy

May not be able to provide location of positive margin without prior orientation
Superficial biopsy may be nondiagnostic in thick lesions such as verrucous carcinoma
Lack of provided location may decrease accuracy of diagnosis of type of cyst

Table 3.4 Glossary of vulvar dermatology terms

Hyperkeratosis—increased thickness of the keratin layer without nuclei
Parakeratosis—increased thickness of the keratin layer. Nuclei are present
Acanthosis—thickening and fusing of the rete pegs
Rete peg—epithelial extension into dermis
Dermal papillae—dermal projections up into epidermis
Granular cell layer—the layer just below the keratin, containing keratohyaline granules
Koilocytosis—cells containing atypical nuclei with a perinuclear halo. Cytopathic effect of HPV
Papillomatosis—skin surface elevations
Metaplasia—change from one benign tissue type to another
Desmoplasia—fibrosis

3.3 Pediatric and Adolescent Lesions of the Vulva

3.3.1 Infantile Perianal Pyramidal Protrusion

This lesion of unknown etiology is characterized by a small fleshy protuberance anterior to the anus (Fig. 3.1). Reported cases have been almost entirely in females [2]. The lesion may be constitutional, acquired, most often in association with

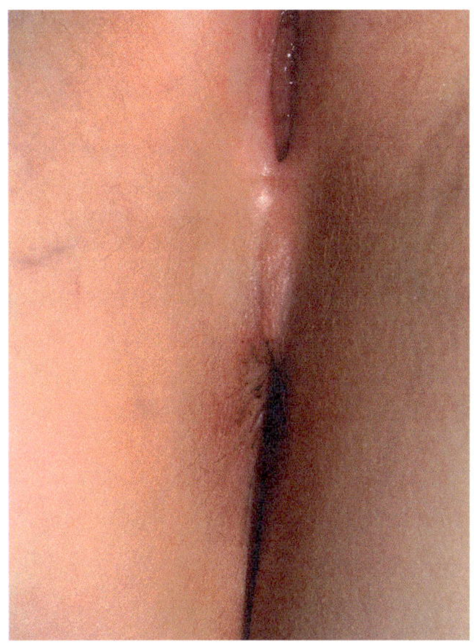

Fig. 3.1 Infantile perianal pyramidal protrusion*. A small fleshy protuberance is seen anterior to the anus. *Copyright Libby Edwards, MD. Used with permission. All permission requests for this image should be made to the copyright holder

constipation, or associated with lichen sclerosus [2]. It may regress spontaneously. Associated conditions should be treated appropriately.

3.3.2   Vulvar Ulcers in Adolescents

Vulvar ulcers in young girls may represent apthae, or Epstein–Barr virus infection, in addition to possible sexually transmitted diseases. Apthae are painful ulcers of unknown etiology associated with systemic symptoms [3]. They may be associated with oral apthae (canker sores), and if associated with systemic symptoms, particularly uveitis, this constitutes Behçet's disease [4]. Epstein–Barr vulvar ulcers are also painful and present with flu-like symptoms [5]. A systematic history and workup is helpful, as the differential diagnosis of vulvar ulcers is broad, with the most common etiology in North America being Herpes Simplex [6]

3.3.3   Vestibular Adenosis

Adenosis is the persistence of glands in areas where there is usually only squamous epithelium, such as the vestibule or vagina. Adenosis is thought to be due to a disturbance in embryogenesis during the urogenital sinus meeting up with the fused Müllerian ducts. The most common location is upper vagina, but adenosis can rarely occur on the vulva or vestibule. In those locations, some have occurred secondary to

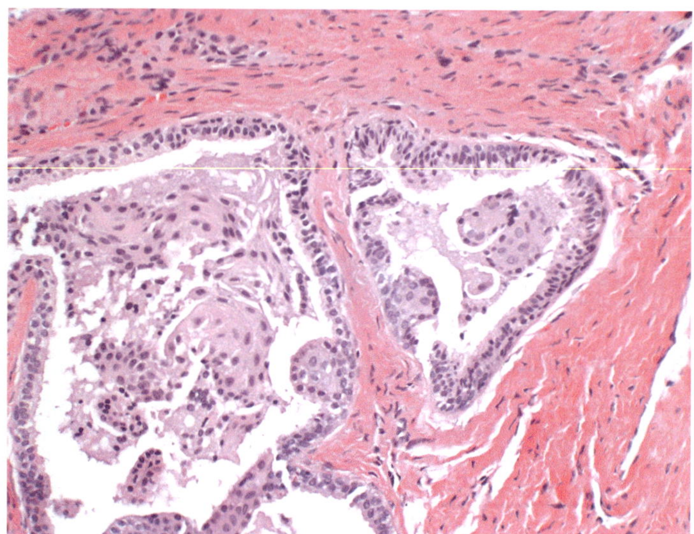

Fig. 3.2 Adenosis-subepithelial glands are seen repairing by squamous metaplasia

prior Stevens–Johnson syndrome or CO_2 laser therapy [7]. While there has histori-
cally been an association of adenosis with in utero exposure to diethylstilbestrol
(DES), the condition can arise spontaneously. In the vestibule, the lesion may present as red friable tissue that resembles granulation tissue and is tender. Histologically,
glands of endocervical, endometrial, or tubal type epithelium are seen under the
surface squamous epithelium, often repairing by squamous metaplasia (Fig. 3.2).

3.3.4 Lichen Sclerosus

There are two age peaks to vulvar lichen sclerosus, childhood and in postmenopausal women. Children who have lichen sclerosus may appear to have significant
improvement or even regression in adolescence, but must be followed indefinitely,
to evaluate for architectural disturbances, and due to the increased risk of vulvar
squamous cell carcinoma [8]. The pathologic features of lichen sclerosus are
discussed with the noninfectious dermatoses.

3.4 Cysts of the Vulva

A variety of benign cysts may occur on the vulva or in the vagina. Attention to the
location may provide the origin of the cyst; however, even with that information, it
may not be possible to determine the exact origin of some of these cysts. Clinicians
should provide the pathologist with the location of the cyst, as this will lead to more
precision in the pathology report (see Table 3.2).

3.4.1 Epidermal Inclusion Cyst

Epidermal inclusion cysts of the vulva are very common. They may be due to prior surgical intervention such as episiotomy, but can arise de novo. Clitoral epidermal inclusion cysts can arise in association with female genital cutting/circumcision [9]. Epidermal inclusion cysts may also arise on hair-bearing portions of the vulva. The keratinaceous debris produces the contents of the cyst, which grossly appear cheesy (Fig. 3.3a). Histologically, these cysts are lined by keratinizing stratified squamous epithelium (Fig. 3.3b).

3.4.2 Endometriosis/Endometrioma

Endometriosis may present as a cystic or nodular mass on the vulva, most often in a prior episiotomy site, supporting implantation as the origin [10]. It may cycle with the menstrual cycle, swelling and bleeding and causing pain. Grossly, it may appear blue tinged. Histologically, as in endometriosis elsewhere, endometrial glandular epithelium and stroma, not just old hemorrhage, must be present to confirm the diagnosis histopathologically (Fig. 3.4).

3.4.3 Mucinous Cyst/Ciliated Cyst of Vestibule

Cysts lined by mucinous or ciliated epithelium (Fig. 3.5a, b) may arise in the vestibule. The origin of these cysts is controversial. They may arise from Müllerian remnants, particularly in the vagina; however, in the vestibule may arise from minor vestibular glands. Another possible origin is arising in adenosis.

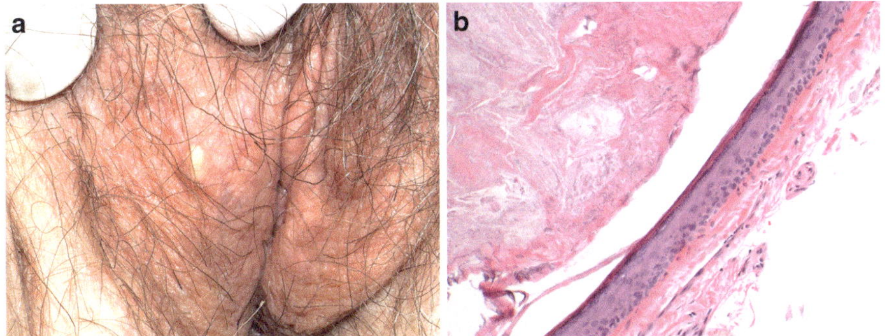

Fig. 3.3 Epidermal inclusion cyst. Grossly, the contents contain yellow cheesy material (**a***). Histologically, the cyst is lined by keratinizing squamous epithelium, with cyst contents comprised of keratinaceous debris (**b**). *Copyright Libby Edwards, MD. Used with permission. All permission requests for this image should be made to the copyright holder

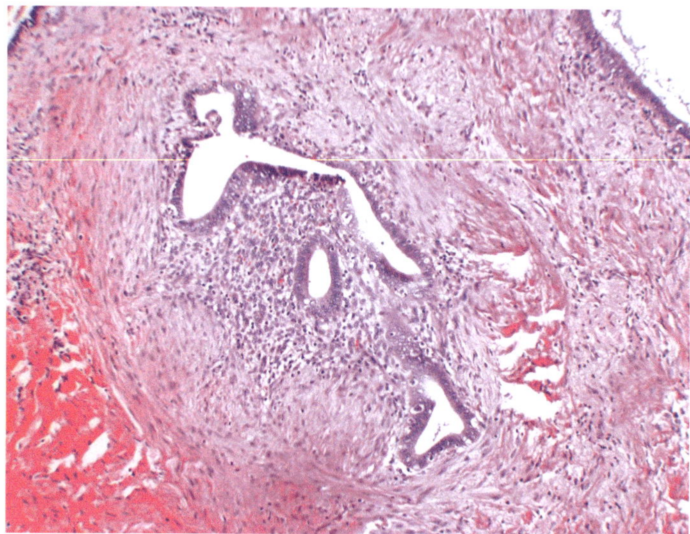

Fig. 3.4 Endometriosis. The lesion is composed of endometrial glands and stroma

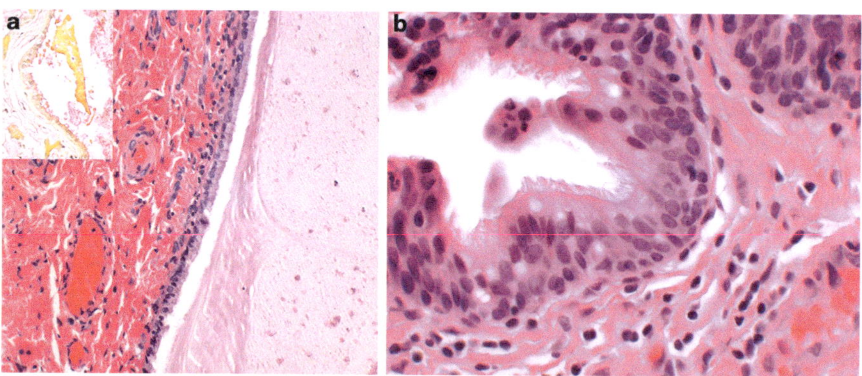

Fig. 3.5 Mucinous/ciliated cysts of the vulva. Mucinous cyst (**a**) is lined by mucinous columnar epithelium. Mucicarmine staining (*inset*) highlights the mucin (fuchsia staining material). Ciliated cyst (**b**) showing ciliated lining

3.4.4 Bartholin's Duct Cyst

Bartholin's duct cysts are often marsupialized, but a surgical excision may be performed for recurrence, or in a woman over 40 to rule out a carcinoma. The cysts may be lined by any of the epithelial types encountered in the gland or duct, or a mixture of glandular, transitional, and squamous epithelium (Fig. 3.6a, b).

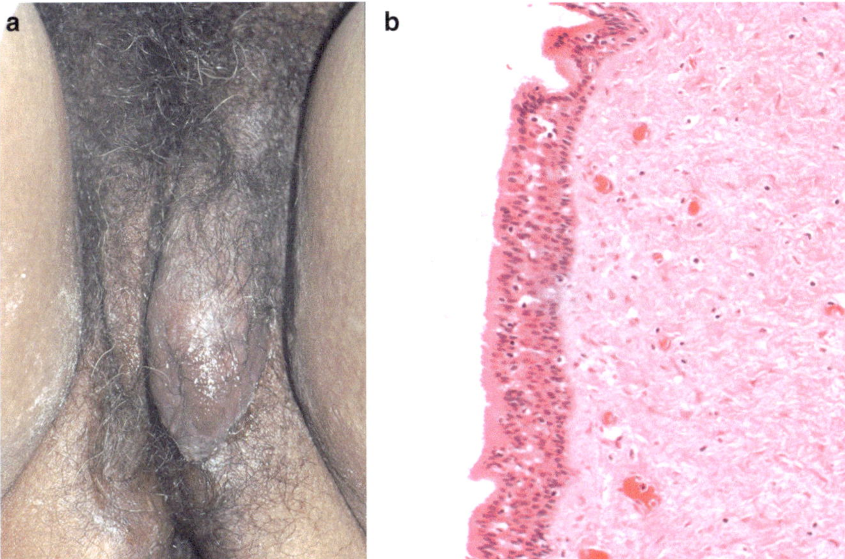

Fig. 3.6 Bartholin's duct cyst at its characteristic location (**a***). This cyst is lined by a mix of transitional and mucinous epithelium consistent with Bartholin's duct (**b**). *Copyright Libby Edwards, MD. Used with permission. All permission requests for this image should be made to the copyright holder

3.4.5   Cyst of Canal of Nuck

The Canal of Nuck is the parietal peritoneum that accompanies the round ligament through the inguinal canal. If it fails to obliterate, a cyst can develop, equivalent to a male hydrocele, and may mimic an inguinal hernia. It is lined by a flattened mesothelium consistent with peritoneum (Fig. 3.7a, b).

3.4.6   Skene's Duct Cyst

Skene's duct cysts are uncommon. They are best suspected by the paraurethral location. It is important to consider other masses that may arise on the anterior vaginal wall, such as ectopic ureterocele, and additional imaging studies may be indicated prior to surgery. Skene's duct cysts may be seen in newborns as well as adults and may resolve spontaneously. Histologically, they may be lined by transitional, ciliated columnar, or squamous epithelium [10].

3.4.7   Lymphangioma Circumscriptum

This lesion may be congenital or acquired. Secondary causes include prior surgery, radiation, or infection [11]. Clinically the lesion is said to resemble frog spawn, but it may be interpreted clinically as condylomata acuminata. It is difficult to treat and

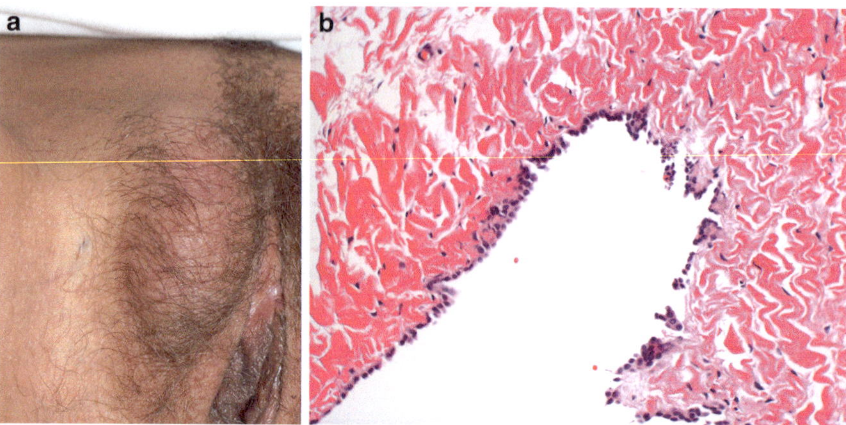

Fig. 3.7 Cyst of the canal of nuck. Clinically, a cyst of the canal of nuck may mimic an inguinal hernia (**a***). It is lined by mesothelium (**b**). *Copyright Libby Edwards, MD. Used with permission. All permission requests for this image should be made to the copyright holder

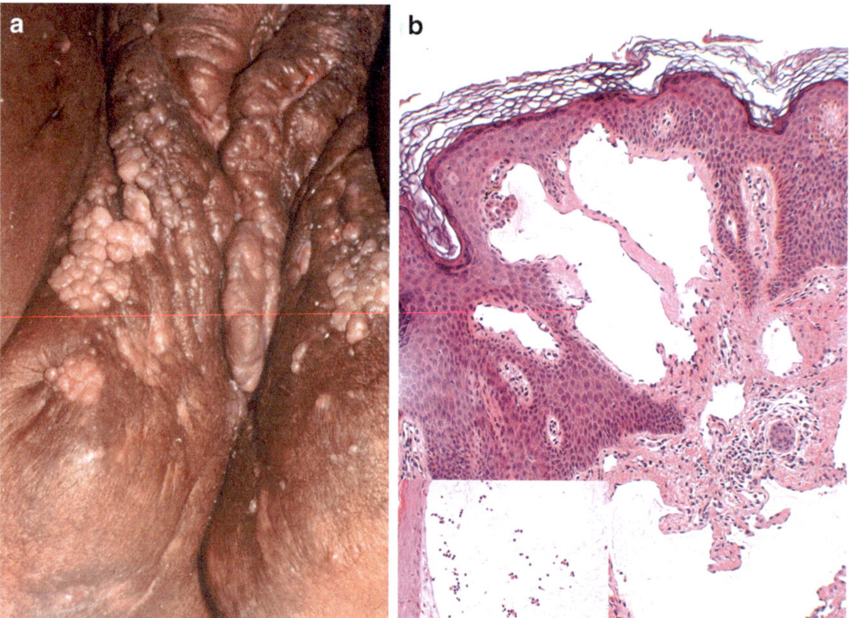

Fig. 3.8 Lymphangioma circumscriptum. Vesicles seen in a patient with hidradenitis suppurativa (**a***). The vesicles are dilated lymphatics (**b**) containing numerous lymphocytes (*inset*). *Copyright Libby Edwards, MD. Used with permission. All permission requests for this image should be made to the copyright holder

is comprised of multiple oozing dilated lymphatic channels that cluster as vesicles (Fig. 3.8a, b). Recurrence can occur after excision, and laser therapy has also been utilized [11].

3.5 Infections and Inflammations of the Vulva

3.5.1 Ulcers

The differential diagnosis for ulcers of the vulva is large, and so a systematic approach is needed. Vulvar specialists have divided vulvar ulcers into infection, dermatoses, tumors, trauma, and miscellaneous [12]. Infection may be sexually transmitted. Clinical history and investigation of possible infectious agents are good first steps. Biopsy may be part of the workup; however, some of the conditions that cause vulvar ulceration do not have pathognomonic findings on histopathology. Syphilis may show increased plasma cells and vasculitis, raising suspicion, but biopsy does not necessarily confirm the diagnosis unless organisms can be identified on special stains. Lymphogranuloma venereum, chancroid, and granuloma inguinale do not have specific histologic findings. Herpes simplex virus can sometimes be confirmed by the presence of the characteristic intranuclear inclusions (Fig. 3.9a, b). Crohn's disease, which presents with characteristic knife-cut ulcerations, or fistulas, may show granulomatous inflammation, with multinucleated giant cells, but clinical confirmation is necessary (Fig. 3.10).

3.5.2 Condyloma Acuminatum

Most vulvar condylomas are caused by low-risk HPV types 6 or 11 and are sexually transmittable. The histology corresponds to the gross appearance, and there is hyperkeratosis, papillomatosis, and koilocytosis (Fig. 3.11a, b). Koilocytosis derives from the Greek word Koilos, which means empty. The koilocyte is a cell with an abnormally enlarged and irregular nucleus with a perinuclear halo. The koilocyte is the cytopathic manifestation of the human papillomavirus.

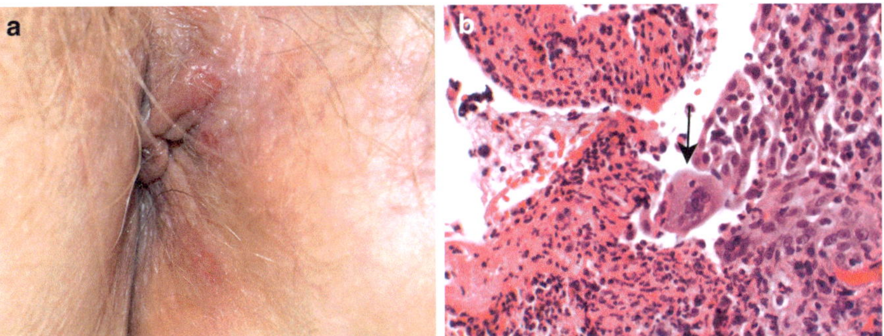

Fig. 3.9 Herpes. Characteristic erosion seen after rupture of the vesicles (**a***). Histologically, herpes (**b**, *arrow*) is characterized by multinucleation with ground glass nuclei. Sometimes Cowdry A intranuclear inclusions may be seen (not shown). *Copyright Libby Edwards, MD. Used with permission. All permission requests for this image should be made to the copyright holder

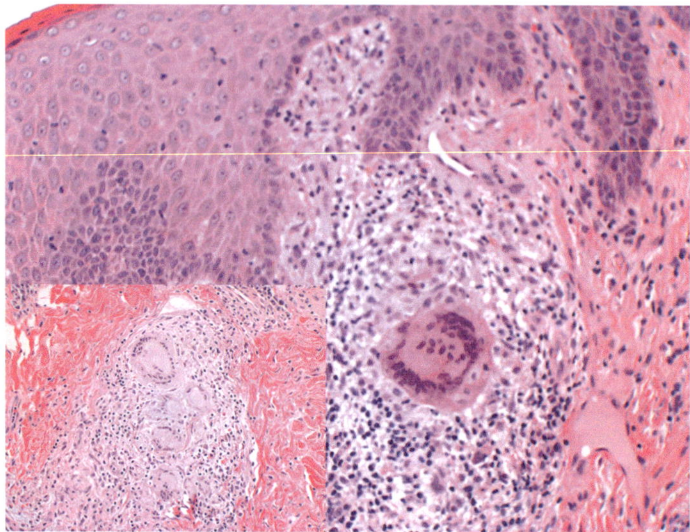

Fig. 3.10 Crohn's disease. Granulomatous vulvitis in a patient with a history of gastrointestinal Crohn's disease. Note well-formed granuloma (*inset*) with multinucleated giant cells

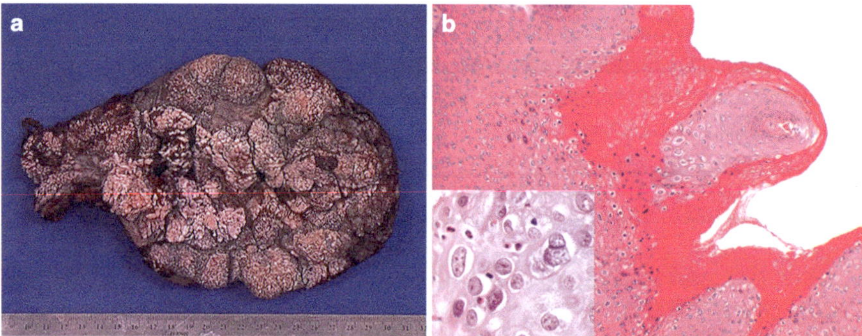

Fig. 3.11 Condyloma acuminatum. This excision (**a**) shows the features that correspond to the histologic finding of papillomatosis (**b**). *Inset* shows koilocytosis and multinucleation

Condylomas may be overdiagnosed both by clinicians and pathologists. Normal vulvar glycogenated epithelium is not koilocytosis, which requires the presence of nuclear atypia to make the diagnosis. A variety of papillary lesions may clinically be considered as condyloma. A very common one is micropapillomatosis labialis (Fig. 3.12). Uniform finger-like projections are seen in the vestibule. Histologically, they lack koilocytosis. Micropapillomatosis is considered a normal anatomic variant and is not caused by Human papillomavirus.

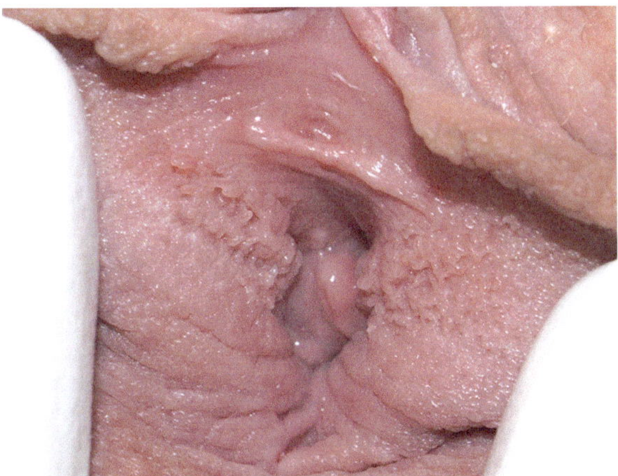

Fig. 3.12 *Micropapillomatosis labialis showing more uniform finger-like projections than is seen with condyloma acuminatum. Micropapillomatosis is a normal variant. *Copyright Libby Edwards, MD. Used with permission. All permission requests for this image should be made to the copyright holder

3.5.3   Molluscum Contagiosum

Molluscum contagiosum is caused by a pox virus infection and most commonly seen in children, with characteristic pruritic umbilicated papules over the body (Fig. 3.13a). Occasionally they can occur on the vulva of adults, either singly or in groups. They will eventually regress, however may be excised when the diagnosis is unknown, or the lesions may be scraped as therapy. Histologically, the characteristic intracytoplasmic viral inclusions may be seen (Fig. 3.13b)

3.5.4   Hidradenitis Suppurativa

Hidradenitis is a potentially debilitating condition that occurs in sites with abundant apocrine glands, including the groin and axilla. It is more common in women. The cause is unknown, but it is associated with obesity [13]. Clinically it presents as numerous draining boils and sinuses with scarring (Fig. 3.14). Although medical management may be attempted, severe cases may come to surgery. Histology is nonspecific, with severe inflammation, often near apocrine glands.

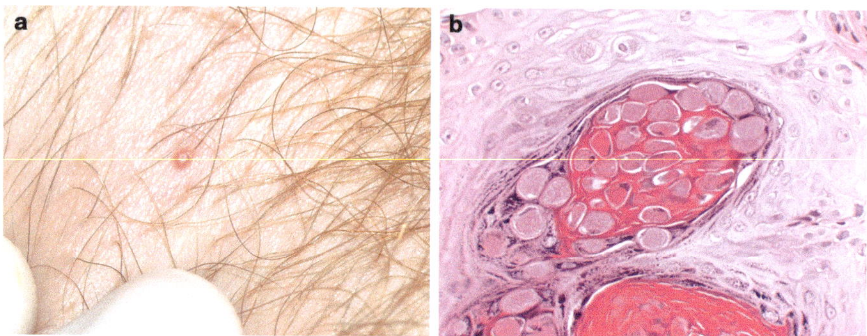

Fig. 3.13 Molluscum contagiosum. Typical umbilicated lesion (**a***). Histology shows the characteristic intracytoplasmic eosinophilic viral inclusions (**b**). *Copyright Libby Edwards, MD. Used with permission. All permission requests for this image should be made to the copyright holder

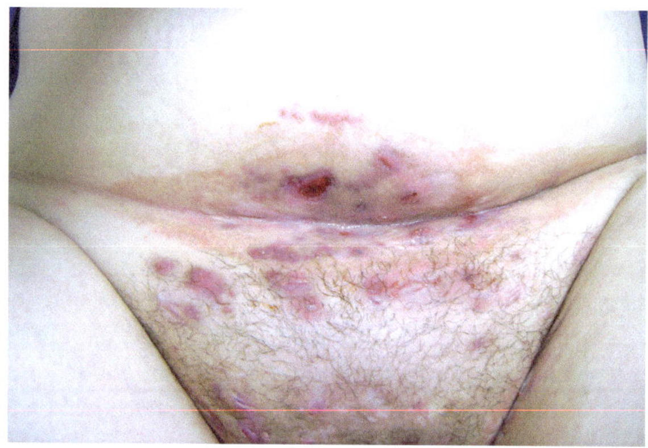

Fig. 3.14 *Hidradenitis suppurativa showing draining sinuses and scarring. *Copyright Libby Edwards, MD. Used with permission. All permission requests for this image should be made to the copyright holder

3.5.5   Noninfectious Inflammatory Diseases of the Vulva

The International Society for the Study of Vulvovaginal Diseases (ISSVD) has established a classification for dermatologic diseases of the vulva to assist in clinical diagnosis [14]. The authors recognize that biopsy will often be necessary to finalize a diagnosis. The approach divides lesions first into a descriptive noun, i.e., "papule," "fissure," "erosion," etc., further modifying the noun by color, circumscription, surface, and configuration, with the goal to help narrow and develop differential diagnoses. A few of the more common inflammatory dermatoses of the vulva will be considered here.

3.5.6   Lichen Planus

Lichen planus (LP) may present with itching, soreness, and/or dyspareunia. It is most commonly erosive in the vulvar area, with a characteristic lacy white edge (Wickham's striae (Fig. 3.15a). Less commonly, the classic type of lichen planus with purple papules may be seen. The least common type on the vulva is hypertrophic [15]. Unlike lichen sclerosus, lichen planus can extend into the vagina, where strictures can occur. The oral cavity should always be examined for the characteristic lacy white lesions as well in patients with suspected vulvar lichen planus. Histologically, LP shows hyperkeratosis, sawtooth acanthosis, apoptotic basal cells (colloid bodies), and a band-like chronic inflammatory infiltrate (Fig. 3.15b). Therapy can be difficult, with first-line therapy usually ultra-potent topical steroids.

3.5.7   Lichen Sclerosus

As mentioned previously, vulvar lichen sclerosus shows a bimodal age peak, affecting children and postmenopausal women. Patients may complain of severe pruritis. Grossly, there is whitening of the vulva, which may show wrinkling and a "cigarette

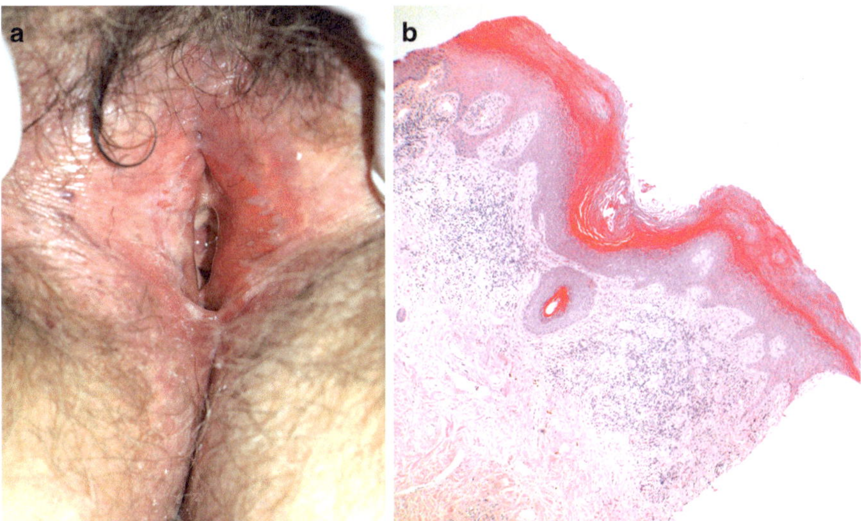

Fig. 3.15 Lichen planus. Typical erosive lichen planus (**a***). Histologically (**b**) there is sawtooth acanthosis with hyperkeratosis and a band-like dermal inflammatory infiltrate. *Copyright Libby Edwards, MD. Used with permission. All permission requests for this image should be made to the copyright holder

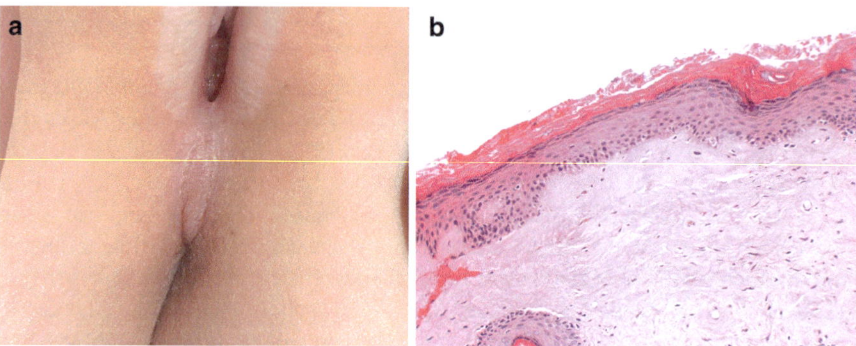

Fig. 3.16 Lichen sclerosus. Clinically, the lesion is white in appearance and shows a characteristic "keyhole" distribution around the introitus and anus. This child also has a perianal pyramidal protrusion (**a***). Histologically lichen sclerosus shows hyperkeratosis, loss of rete pegs, dermal homogenization, and a variable dermal inflammatory infiltrate, here minimal (**b**).* Copyright Libby Edwards, MD. Used with permission. All permission requests for this image should be made to the copyright holder

paper" appearance (Fig. 3.16a). There may be loss of architecture, with narrowing of the introitus. Histologically, the lesion is characterized by hyperkeratosis, loss of rete pegs, a band of dermal homogenization, and a variable dermal chronic inflammatory infiltrate (Fig. 3.16b). Patients need to be followed long term, due to the association with invasive squamous cell carcinoma. Therapy is usually with ultrapotent topical steroids.

3.5.8 Squamous Cell Hyperplasia

Squamous cell hyperplasia, or lichen simplex chronicus, is due to an uninterrupted itch/scratch cycle, which leads to thickening of the vulvar skin with increased skin markings. Histologically there is hyperkeratosis, acanthosis, and variable chronic dermal inflammation (Fig. 3.17). Topical steroids are frequently used.

3.6 Benign Pigmented Lesions of the Vulva

A variety of benign pigmented lesions can occur on the vulva [28]. They may be biopsied out of concern for melanoma, but most don't need excision except for concern of malignancy, symptoms, or patient preference.

3.6.1 Lentigo

Lentigo is basically a freckle, although the pigmentation may spread into broader areas, i.e., lentigenosis (Fig. 3.18a, b). It tends to involve the non-keratinized areas

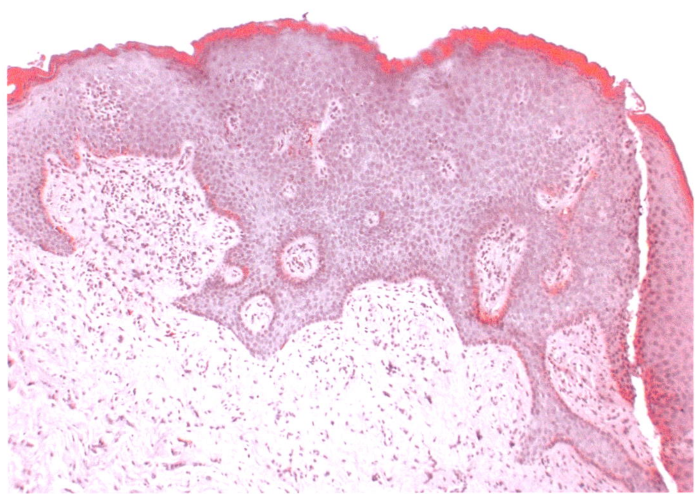

Fig. 3.17 Squamous cell hyperplasia showing hyperkeratosis and acanthosis. Dermal inflammation and pigment incontinence are sometimes seen

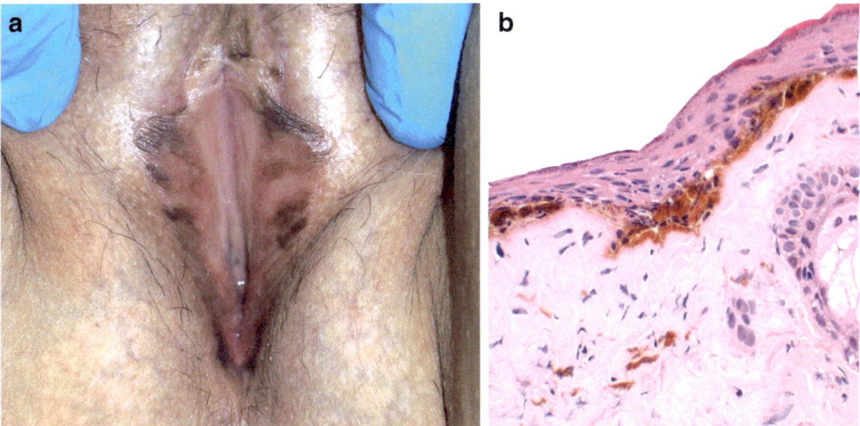

Fig. 3.18 Lentigenes. Multiple pigmented areas on the vulva (**a***). Histologically, lentigo shows increased pigment in the basal layer of the epidermis and dermis, but no atypia (**b**). *Copyright Libby Edwards, MD. Used with permission. All permission requests for this image should be made to the copyright holder

of the vulva, the inner labia minora and introitus [17]. This may result in biopsy over concern to rule out melanoma. Histologically there is increased pigmentation of the basal keratinocytes, as well as possible increase in melanocytes. Melanophages may be present in the upper dermis [16].

3.6.2 Nevus

Nevi are common on the skin, and occasionally arise on the vulva. They are composed of benign melanocytes which may be intradermal (intradermal nevus), at the dermal-epidermal junction (junctional nevus), or in the dermis and junction (compound nevus) (Fig. 3.19a, b). A rare but characteristic site-specific lesion, atypical genital nevus, can arise on the vulva and is clinically and histologically different from usual dysplastic nevi [17]. Atypical genital nevi occur in premenopausal women, and while they can recur if not completely excised, have not shown malignant behavior.

3.6.3 Pigmented Seborrheic Keratosis

Seborrheic keratosis (SK) may show prominent pigmentation. They can occur anywhere on the skin and increase with age. Clinically, they appear as greasy-looking stuck on papules. Histologically, they show hyperkeratosis, acanthosis, and characteristic pseudohorned cysts (Fig. 3.20a, b). Scattered intraepithelial dendritic melanocytes and pigment incontinence contribute to the pigmented appearance [16].

3.6.4 Angiokeratoma

Angiokeratomas are composed of dilated vascular spaces just under a hyperkeratotic dermis, giving a blue/red appearance. These are not melanotic lesion but the dark purple color may raise concern (Fig. 3.21a, b)

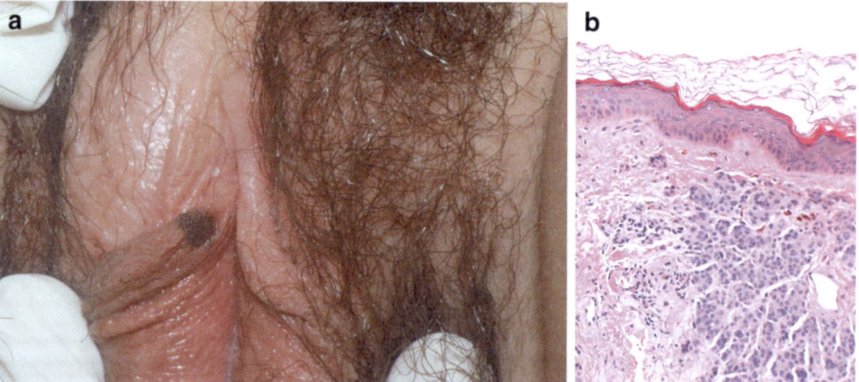

Fig. 3.19 Nevus. While not requiring removal, nevi may be excised for patient preference or when the color raises concern of a more serious lesion (**a***). This intradermal nevus shows nests of nevus cells, a type of melanocyte, without atypia. Pigmentation is seen (**b**). *Copyright Libby Edwards, MD. Used with permission. All permission requests for this image should be made to the copyright holder

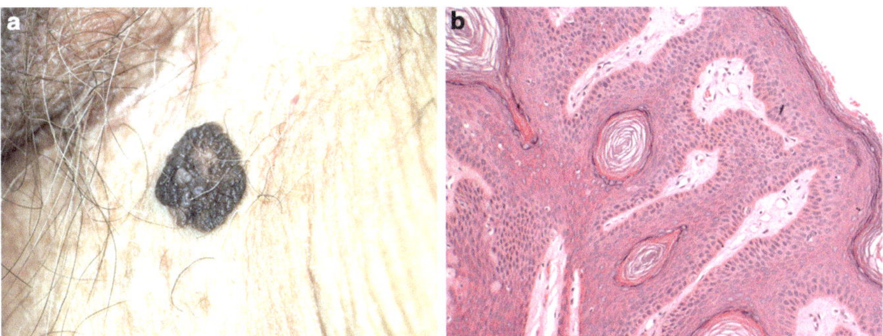

Fig. 3.20 Seborrheic keratosis. Some of these lesions are highly pigmented, raising concern of a melanoma (**a***). Histologically, there is hyperkeratosis, acanthosis, and characteristic pseudohorn cysts containing lamellated keratin (**b**). *Copyright Libby Edwards, MD. Used with permission. All permission requests for this image should be made to the copyright holder

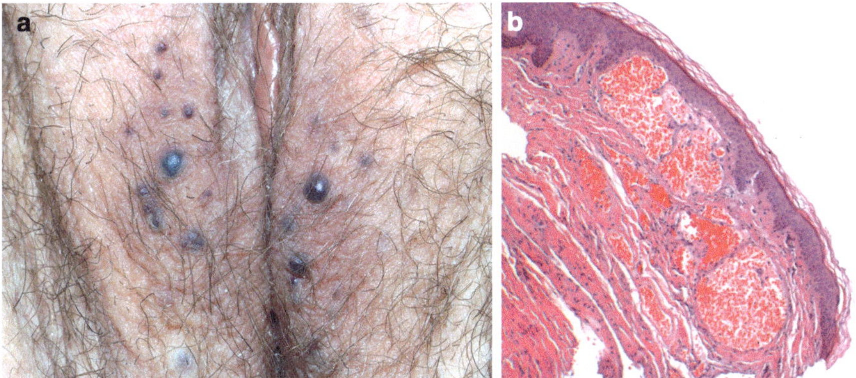

Fig. 3.21 Angiokeratoma. Multiple purple papules are seen (**a***), composed of dilated vessels under the surface (**b**), sometimes associated with hyperkeratosis (not shown). *Copyright Libby Edwards, MD. Used with permission. All permission requests for this image should be made to the copyright holder

3.6.5 Acanthosis Nigricans

Acanthosis nigricans occurs along flexural areas, and hence may be seen in the groin. It is associated with insulin resistance and obesity [16]. Clinically, it appears as darkened, velvety skin plaques. Histologically, there is hyperkeratosis and papillomatosis. There is no significant increase in melanin.

3.6.6 Post-inflammatory Hyperpigmentation

Post-inflammatory hyperpigmentation can occur anywhere on the skin and is characterized by melanin pigment incontinence in the dermis (Fig 3.22).

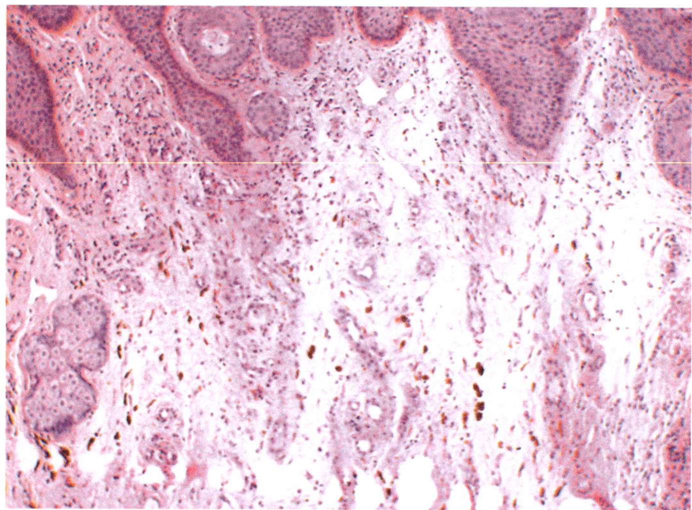

Fig. 3.22 Post-inflammatory hyperpigmentation shows pigment incontinence in the dermis with no increase in melanocytes

3.7 Benign Neoplasms of the Vulva

3.7.1 Acrochordon (Fibroepithelial Polyp, Skin Tag)

Skin tags of the vulva are fairly common and require no action unless troublesome to the patient. They are occasionally large and may be pedunculated [18]. They should not be mistaken for condyloma acuminatum, and the lack of HPV-related histologic changes should rule that out. They are lined by stratified squamous epithelium overlying a fibroconnective tissue core (Fig. 3.23a, b).

3.7.2 Syringoma

Syringomas often occur on the head and neck, but can present on the vulva as multiple small pruritic skin-colored papules (Fig. 3.24a). They are benign lesions of eccrine sweat ducts. Histologically, the duct-like structures have a very characteristic comma or tadpole shape (Fig. 3.24b). Therapeutic modalities have included excision, electro-desiccation, laser, and cryotherapy [19].

3.7.3 Granular Cell Tumor

Granular cell tumors can occur anywhere on the body, but occasionally arise on the vulva. While the majority are benign, rare cases have exhibited malignant behavior.

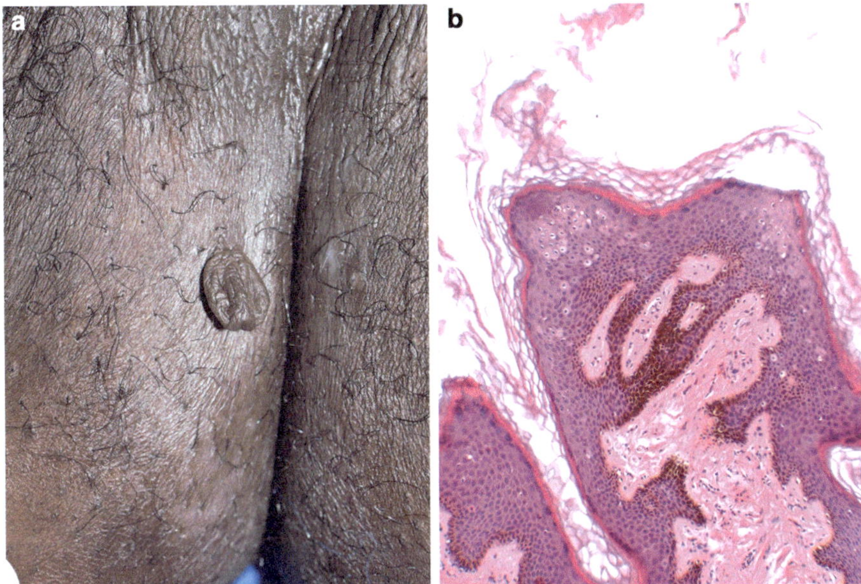

Fig. 3.23 Skin tags may be large and pedunculated (**a***). Histology shows hyperkeratosis and acanthosis of the squamous epithelium over a fibrovascular core. Basal pigmentation corresponds to pigmented skin in this case (**b**). *Copyright Libby Edwards, MD. Used with permission. All permission requests for this image should be made to the copyright holder

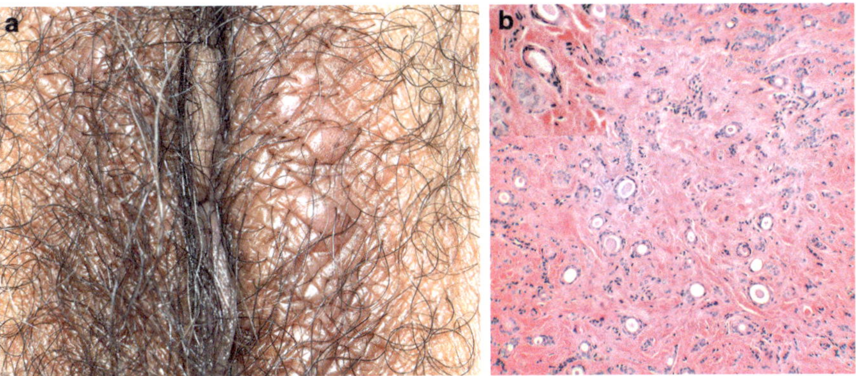

Fig. 3.24 Syringoma. Grossly syringoma appears as multiple flesh-colored papules (**a***). Histologically, characteristic tubules are seen, often comma-shaped (*inset upper left*) (**b**). *Copyright Libby Edwards, MD. Used with permission. All permission requests for this image should be made to the copyright holder

Clinically granular cell tumors present as subcutaneous nodules and may mimic an epidermal inclusion cyst. Histologically, they are characterized by an unusual granular appearing cytoplasm, hence the name (Fig. 3.25). They are thought to be of Schwann cell origin. Older age, lesion recurrence, and larger size may be predictive

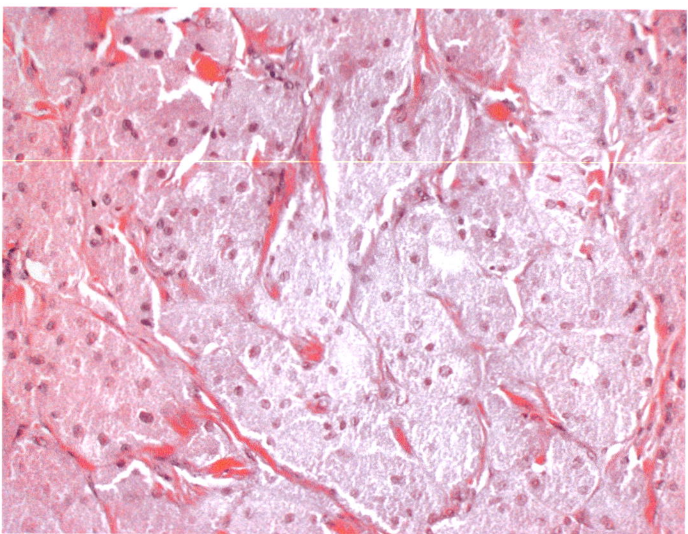

Fig. 3.25 Granular cell tumor, so named for the granular cytoplasm

of malignant behavior [20]. Recurrences are more common if the lesion is incompletely excised, and individual tumor cells may extend beyond the visible nodule, making a wider excision prudent [20]. Detailed histologic criteria have been put forth for benign, atypical, and malignant granular cell tumors [21].

3.7.4   Fibroma

Fibromas of the vulva are uncommon. They may become large and pedunculated. They are composed of fibroblasts and dense collagen with overlying squamous epithelium (Fig. 3.26).

3.7.5   Leiomyoma

Leiomyomas of the vulva are rare, and similar in appearance to the uterine counterpart. The criteria for malignancy is more stringent than the uterine lesions, with evaluation of the following criteria:: $\geq$5 cm in greatest dimension, infiltrative margins, $\geq$5 mitoses per 10 high power fields, and moderate to severe cytologic atypia. If three or more are present, the lesion is a leiomyosarcoma, if two, atypical, and if one or less, benign. Recommendations have been suggested for follow-up of all groups, with wider excision for the leiomyosarcomas [22].

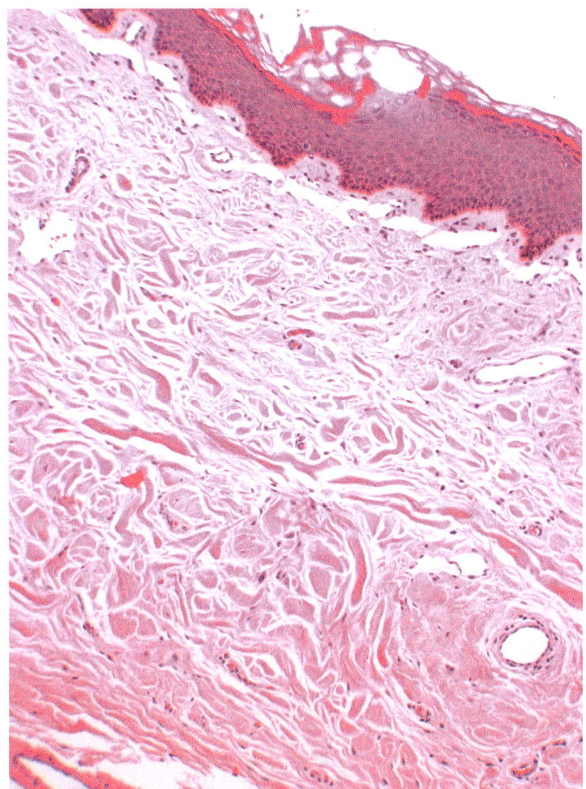

Fig. 3.26 Fibroma. Squamous epithelium overlies densely collagenous tissue

3.7.6 Hemangioma

Most hemangiomas on the vulva are small incidental capillary hemangiomas, composed of a dermal proliferation of capillaries. Rarely, cavernous hemangiomas can occur and may be clinically suspected to be varicosities [23].

3.7.7 Hidradenoma Papilliferum

Hidradenoma papilliferum is a benign lesion of either apocrine or anogenital mammary-like gland origin. It may present as a small nodule (Fig. 3.27a), but may raise clinical concern of malignancy due to a tendency to ulcerate. Hidradenoma may raise concern of malignancy for the inexperienced pathologist due to the crowded glands; however, the characteristic two cell layer (Fig. 3.27b) demonstrates that it is a benign lesion.

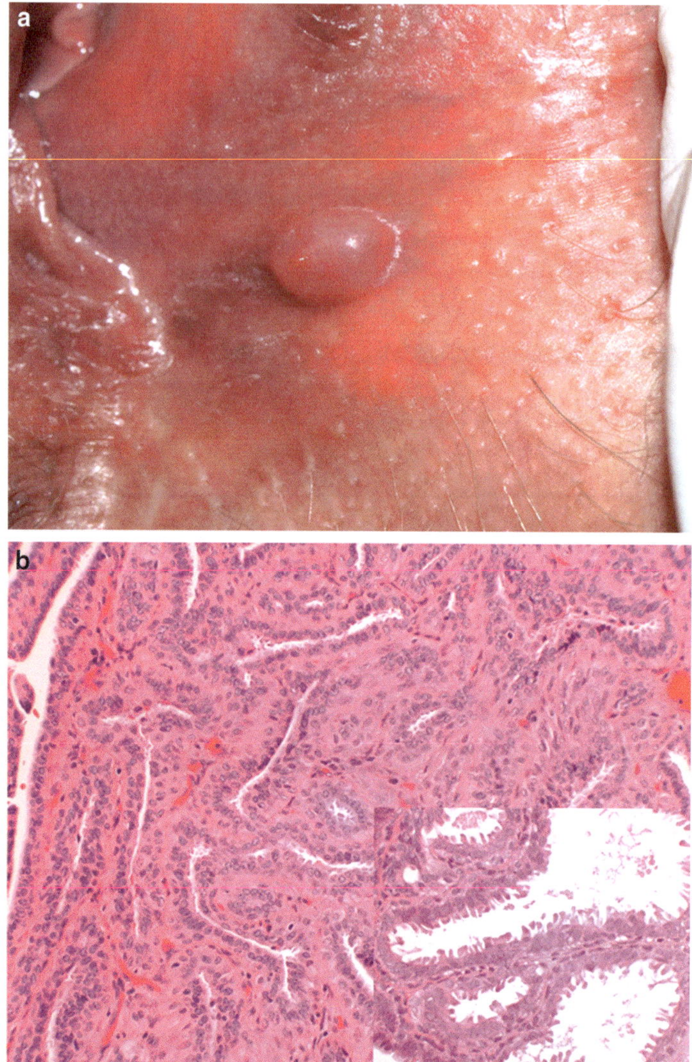

Fig. 3.27 Hidradenoma papilliferum presents as a small nodule (**a***), which may ulcerate. Histologically, crowded glands lined by a 2-cell layer are seen (**b**). The inset lower right shows apocrine snouts on the luminal cells. *Copyright Libby Edwards, MD. Used with permission. All permission requests for this image should be made to the copyright holder

3.7.8 Aggressive Angiomyxoma

A rare neoplasm, aggressive angiomyxoma often extends beyond the clinically apparent lesion and may extend up into the pelvis, making complete excision sometimes difficult. Hence, imaging is an important modality in preoperative evaluation. Incomplete excision may explain some of the tendency for local recurrence of this

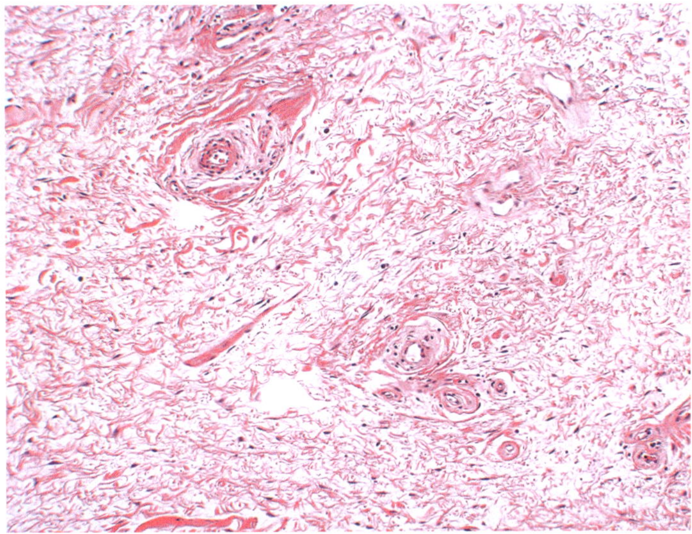

Fig. 3.28 Aggressive angiomyoma A deceptively bland hypocellular lesion with spindle cells and blood vessels. Sometimes histology shows a myxoid background (not demonstrated in image)

benign lesion. Grossly, the cut surface is gelatinous, and although the lesion may grossly appear circumscribed, it actually may have extended beyond the visible circumscription. Histologically, the lesion is a low cellularity lesion composed of spindle cells and vessels in a myxoid background (Fig. 3.28).

3.7.9   Other Soft Tissue Benign Lesions

A variety of soft tissue lesions that can occur anywhere on the body may occasionally arise on the vulva, including lipoma, schwannoma, and neurofibroma.

3.8   Preinvasive Neoplasia of the Vulva

3.8.1   Usual Vulvar Intraepithelial Neoplasia

Usual squamous intraepithelial neoplasia of the lower genital tract is associated with HPV. The terminology has evolved over time. The two most commonly encountered terminologies are the one that is analogous to the Bethesda pap smear grading, i.e., LSIL and HSIL (low-grade squamous intraepithelial lesion and high-grade squamous intrapithelial lesion), or vulvar intraepithelial neoplasia (VIN) 1, 2, or 3 analogous to cervical tissue terminology. The two-tiered system is the recommended terminology of the Lower Anogenital Squamous Terminology (LAST) group, with a proviso that including the other terminology in use, in 1, 2, 3, in this case VIN 1, 2, or 3 in parentheses, is acceptable [24]. VIN 1 is analogous to LSIL,

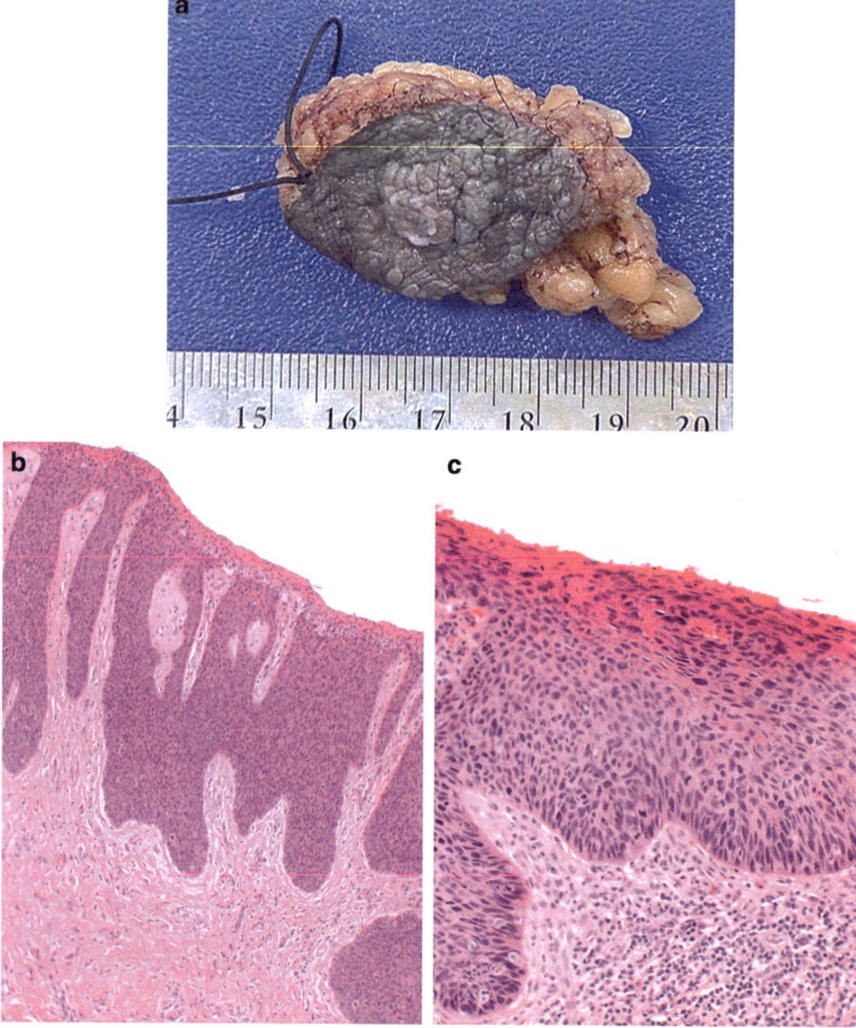

Fig. 3.29 Vulvar intraepithelial neoplasia. This excision for VIN shows a grey raised lesion arising in a background of vulvar skin with increased markings. Note the orienting suture, placed in case re-excision is needed for a positive margin (**a**). Low power histology shows acanthosis, and even at this power, there seems to be a lack of maturation (**b**). At higher power, full thickness maturation abnormality is present (**c**)

and VIN 2 and 3 both are analogous to HSIL. The terminology reflects the degree of maturation abnormality of the squamous epithelium. In low-grade lesions (which are essentially flat condylomas, and in fact not recognized as premalignant), the maturation abnormality is confined to the lower 1/3. As VIN2 (up to 2/3) and VIN 3 (over 2/3) are difficult to tell apart, and treated similarly, many pathologists lump them into HSIL, or VIN2-3. Clinically, HGSIL can have a variety of appearances, pigmented, red, white, unifocal, or multifocal (Fig. 3.29a–c), and may be asymptomatic, or sometimes cause pruritis. The rest of the lower genital tract should be evaluated for HPV disease in patients with VIN. Treatment is often surgical, although immune modulators and laser have also been utilized. For a surgical excision meant to be curative, it is important to provide specimen orientation to the pathologist, so that the provision of marginal status can be made, to help guide potential future re-excision.

3.8.2 Differentiated VIN

Differentiated VIN is not thought to be related to HPV. It is thought to be associated with a greater risk of progression to squamous cell carcinoma than usual HPV-related VIN. It is often seen adjacent to invasive squamous cell carcinomas unrelated to HPV (see section on invasive carcinoma to follow), but occasionally occurs in the absence of invasive disease. Clinically, it is less obvious than usual VIN and is more likely to be a single plaque. Differentiated VIN can be a difficult histopathologic diagnosis. Atypia is predominantly confined to the basal epithelium, and therefore biopsies must be deep enough to see the basal portion of the epithelium and stroma, which may be difficult due to the hyperkeratosis and acanthosis (Fig. 3.30a–c).

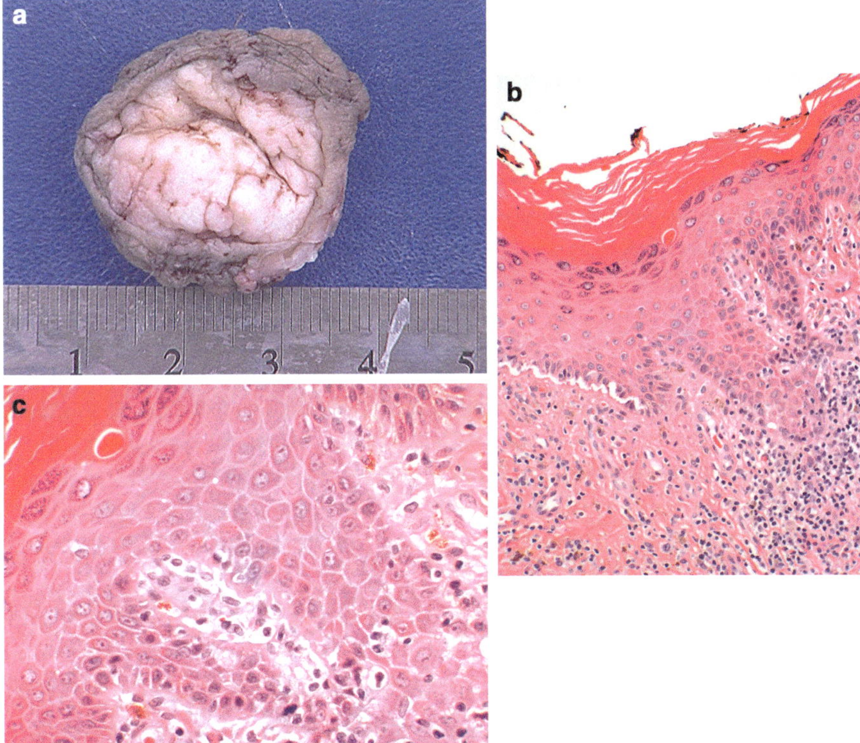

Fig. 3.30 Differentiated VIN. A white plaque-like lesion is seen in this excision (**a**). Histology shows hyperkeratosis, acanthosis, dyskeratosis, and atypia confined to the basal epithelium (**b**). Higher power shows a dyskeratotic cell near the surface, exaggerated cell markings, nucleoli, and basal atypia (**c**)

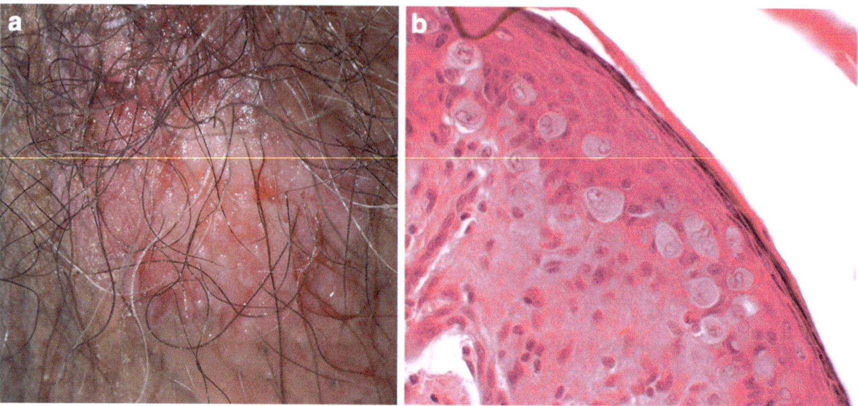

Fig. 3.31 Paget's disease. The lesion is velvety red with white areas (**a***). Histologically, the individual Paget cells percolate up to the surface (**b**). *Copyright Libby Edwards, MD. Used with permission. All permission requests for this image should be made to the copyright holder

3.8.3   Paget's Disease of the Vulva

Paget's disease of the vulva is thought to arise from an aberrant stem cell. Clinically, it presents with pruritis and appears as red velvety skin with white overlying plaques (Fig. 3.31a). Histologically, the individual and clustered Paget cells are seen at the dermal-epidermal interface and percolating up the epithelium (so-called Pagetoid spread (Fig. 3.31b). Paget's disease is usually an in situ lesion, but invasive Paget's can occur. Paget's is treated commonly by surgical excision. Vulvar Paget's disease tends to extend beyond the grossly visible lesion, and hence positive margins may be part of why the disease is often associated with local recurrence. Paget's disease of the vulva is associated with an underlying carcinoma in about 25–30 % of cases, much less frequently than the breast lesion, a totally different disease, although histologically similar. Underlying cancers associated with vulvar Paget's disease may include invasive Paget's, skin appendage carcinomas, or even distal carcinoma of unrelated organs. In addition, histologically, spread of urothelial or anorectal carcinoma can be by pagetoid spread (individual cells percolating up the epithelium). Immunohistochemistry can assist in making the distinction.

3.9   Malignant Neoplasms of the Vulva

3.9.1   Squamous Cell Carcinoma

Squamous cell carcinoma of the vulva may be HPV-related or unrelated. The HPV-related lesions are associated with usual VIN and seen in a slightly younger

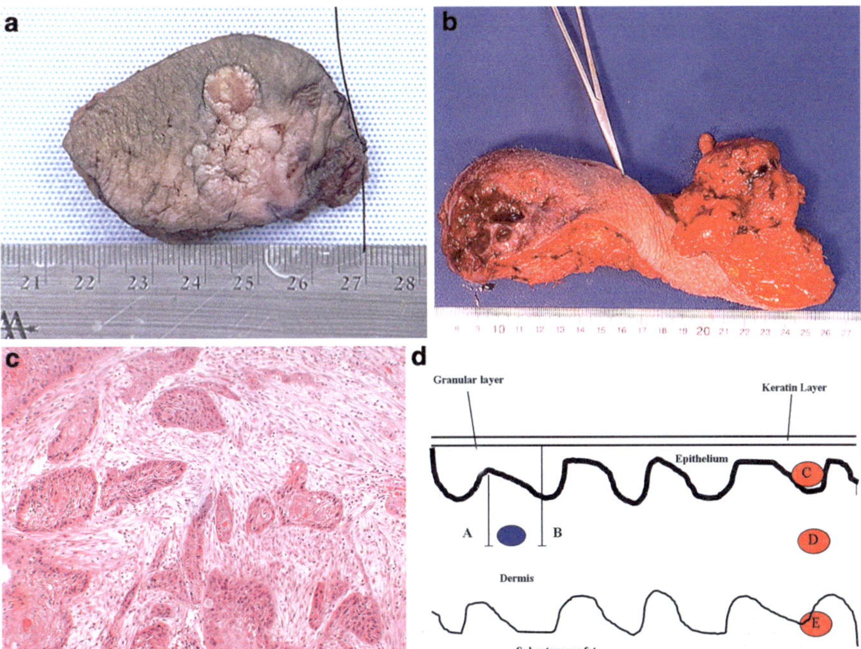

Fig. 3.32 Different appearances of squamous cell carcinoma of the vulva include plaque-like (**a**) and ulcerated lesions (**b**). Note that (**b**) isn't oriented, and grossly the lesion extends to a resection margin. Histologically, irregular nests of well-differentiated keratinized squamous cell carcinoma are seen eliciting a desmoplastic stromal reaction (**c**). Depth of invasion is measured from the nearest dermal papilla to the deepest portion of the lesion "A," in distinction to Breslow thickness "B," or Chung levels I "C," II–IV "D" or V "E" used for melanoma (**d**)

population than the HPV unrelated lesions, associated with lichen sclerosus and differentiated VIN. As surgical excisions are now tailored to the specific patient, aiming to avoid the butterfly excision of the past, it is important for the clinician to orient an excision, in case re-excision is needed. Grossly, invasive squamous cell carcinoma can have a variety of appearances and may be endophytic or exophytic (Fig. 3.32a, b). Histologically, squamous cell carcinoma may be well (Fig. 3.32c), moderately, or poorly differentiated. Well-differentiated lesions are usually keratinizing and may show keratin pearls. Poorly differentiated lesions are barely recognizable as squamous. Moderate is in between. The lesion's size in two dimensions is generally measured clinically for staging purposes; however, the depth is assessed by histopathology. Depth is measured from the most adjacent dermal papillae to the bottom of the deepest invasive focus (Fig. 3.32d). Sentinel lymph node sampling may also be part of the surgical procedure, and immunohistochemistry is an ancillary technique helpful for identifying small metastatic deposits.

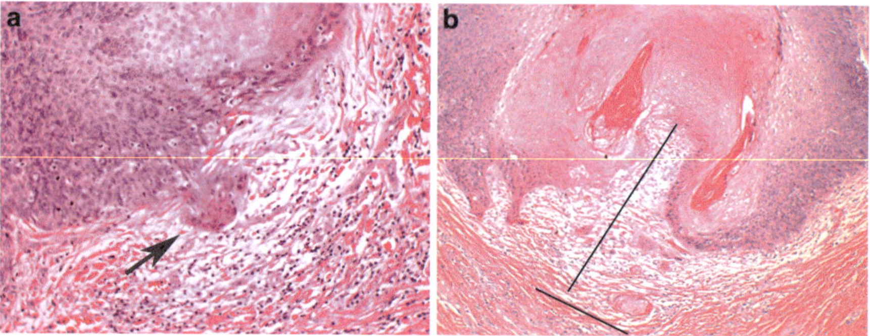

Fig. 3.33 Superficial invasion. A small finger-like invasive focus (*arrow*) elicits an inflammatory stromal reaction (**a**). The depth from the adjacent dermal papilla and the width (**b**) are shown. Measurement of width is more critical in the staging of cervical lesions

3.9.2 Superficial Invasion

The term "microinvasion" should not be used in diagnosis of lower genital tract lesions. Staging and criteria are different at different sites. The term "Superficially invasive squamous cell carcinoma" (SISSCA in LAST terminology) and a depth measurement should be provided. For vulvar squamous cell carcinoma, LAST defines SISSCA as a lesion meeting the FIGO T1a criteria, i.e., 2 cm or less in size, and 1 mm stromal invasion or less (Fig. 3.33a, b). The goal of defining SISSCA is to separate out a subset of lesions with a significantly low enough risk of lymph node metastases to justify less radical surgery and avoid lymph node dissection.

3.9.3 Verrucous Carcinoma

Verrucous carcinoma is an uncommon variant of squamous cell carcinoma. The relationship to HPV is uncertain. Grossly, the lesion appears as a giant condyloma (Fig. 3.34). (Hence the old term "Giant condyloma of Bushke-Lowenstein.") It invades the underlying tissue in a pushing front, rather than the invasive finger-like projections of usual squamous cell carcinoma. Atypia is minimal. Hence, it is important to get a deep enough biopsy to be diagnostic, but sometimes difficult due to thickness of the lesion. It can recur locally, but doesn't tend to go to regional lymph nodes.

3.9.4 Melanoma

Although rare, vulvar melanoma represents about 10 % of vulvar malignancies. The prognosis continues to be poor, particularly for lesions extending beyond

Fig. 3.34 Verrucous
carcinoma. The *inset* shows
the "warty" configuration
which may be confused with
condyloma, particularly on a
superficial biopsy. Note the
deeper pushing front. This
demonstrates the necessity
for a deep enough biopsy to
confirm this diagnosis. The
pushing front is an important
diagnostic feature, as atypia
may be minimal

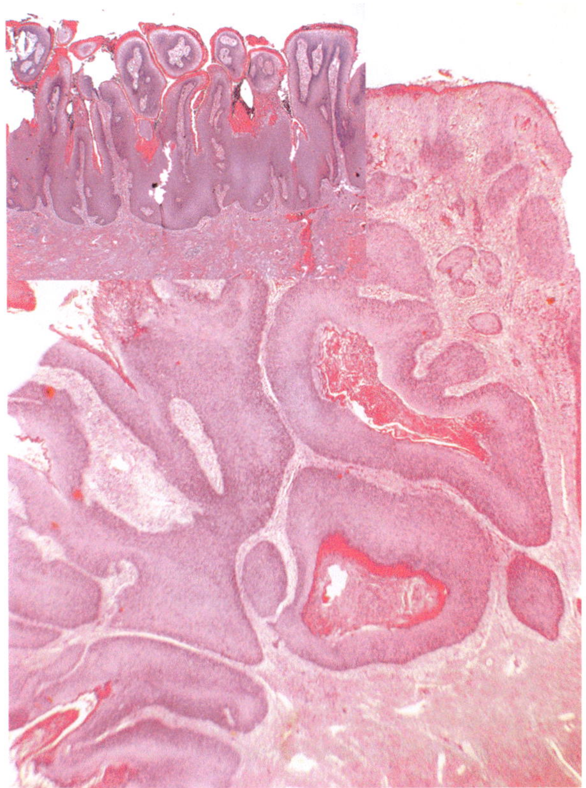

extremely superficial invasion. As such, liberal biopsy of pigmented lesions is
prudent (Fig. 3.35). Melanoma is measured by Breslow thickness of tumor
rather than depth, or sometimes Chung levels are used [25, 26]. Breslow thickness measurement extends from the top of the epithelium (beneath acellular
keratin) to the deepest point of invasion (Fig. 3.32d). Chung's levels are a modification of Clark levels used in skin melanoma, devised because of the less
clear-cut papillary and reticular dermis in the vulva. Chung levels are I—
intraepidermal, II—less than or equal to 1 mm, III—1–2 mm, IV—over 2 mm,
V—subcutaneous fat [26]. Histologically, pigmentation may be present or
absent in vulvar melanoma. The cells are often sheets of atypical melanocytes
with prominent nucleoli (Fig. 3.35). Wide local excision with sentinel node
mapping is currently being suggested as therapy [27].

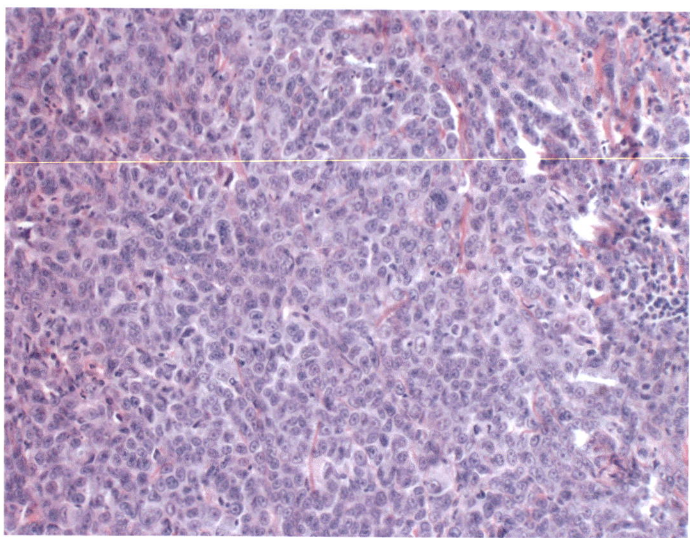

Fig. 3.35 Melanoma. Sheets of amelanotic melanoma cells, showing prominent nucleoli. Pigmented melanomas may show prominent amounts of melanin in addition, sometimes obscuring cellular features

3.9.5   Basal Cell Carcinoma

Basal cell carcinomas can occur anywhere on the skin. They may be pigmented. They can occasionally arise on the vulva. Histologically, the lesion shows characteristic palisading of nuclei at the periphery of the basal nests (Fig. 3.36). Excision is the treatment of choice.

3.9.6   Leiomyosarcoma

Vulvar leiomyosarcoma is very rare. However, it is important to note that the criteria separating benign from malignant smooth muscle tumors is more stringent in the vulva than the uterus (see discussion above, leiomyoma) [22].

3.10   HPV-Related Neoplasia of the Anus

HPV-related disease of the lower genital tract is thought to be via field effect. Although our knowledge of HPV-related intraepithelial and invasive neoplasms of the anus is not as advanced as our knowledge of vulva and cervix, clinicians providing care to women are seeing more of these diseases. Immunosuppression markedly increases the risk of anal squamous neoplasia; however, neither immunosuppression nor anal-receptive intercourse are necessary for disease to occur. Clinicians are

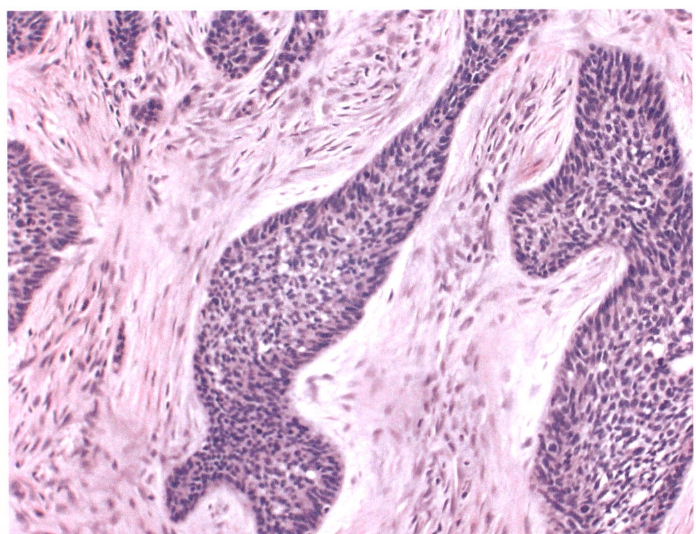

Fig. 3.36 Basal cell carcinoma showing characteristic palisading of cells around the periphery of the tumor islands

performing more anal pap smears in high-risk women, and some gynecologists are starting to perform anoscopy, while others refer these patients. A brief review of the pathology of HPV-related anal disease follows.

3.10.1 Anal Pap Smears

The anus has a transformation zone, much as the cervix does. The perianal area is composed of keratinized squamous epithelium. The upper anus is lined by the same columnar epithelium as the colon. The transformation zone is often a mixture of squamous and glandular epithelium and may contain transitional epithelium. It can extend above the dentate line. Anal pap smears should ideally sample this area, and while obtaining glandular cells is not a requisite for adequacy, it is preferable (Fig. 3.37a). An anal pap smear containing only anucleate squames and fecal material (Fig. 3.37b) is not adequate. Interpretation of paps is similar otherwise to cervical paps, and both lgsil (Fig. 3.36c) and hgsil (Fig. 3.37d) may be seen.

3.10.2 Anal Carcinoma

The majority of anal carcinomas are squamous cell carcinomas, and these are similar histologically to squamous cell carcinoma elsewhere. The LAST project [24] has proposed that superficially invasive squamous cell carcinoma of the anus (SISSCA) be defined as squamous carcinoma with an invasive depth of ≤ 3 mm from the

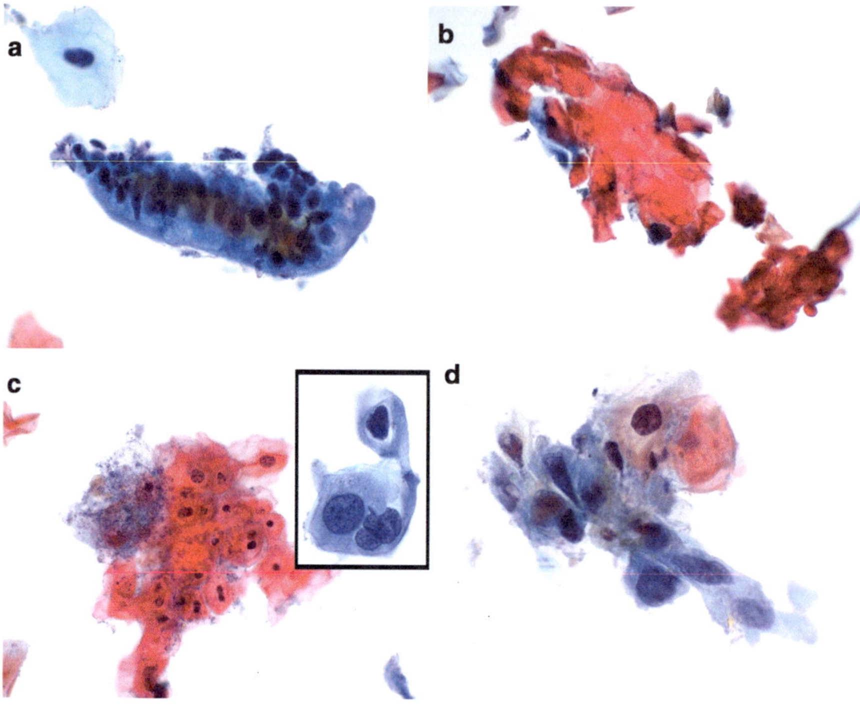

Fig. 3.37 Anal pap smears. Obtaining glandular cells indicates sampling of the transition zone (**a**). Anucleate squames alone constitute an inadequate specimen (**b**). Lgsil (**c**) shows multinucleation and koilocytosis (*inset*). Hgsil (**d**) shows small cells relative to normal squamous cells; however, they have a high nuclear to cytoplasmic ratio and may be hyperchromatic

basement membrane of the point of origin, has a horizontal spread of ≤ 7 mm in greatest extent, and has been completely excised; however, literature is scarce in this area, and future studies are needed.

3.11 Anal Paget's Disease

Paget's disease arising in the perianal area may represent the vulvar disease discussed previously, but may also reflect Pagetoid spread of a colonic-type adenocarcinoma. Immunohistochemistry can be utilized to distinguish these entities.

3.12 Anal Melanoma

Anal melanoma is rare and is a type of mucosal melanoma. It may be mistaken for thrombosed hemorrhoids and is often diagnosed late, when metastatic disease has already occurred.

References

1. Vitale V, Cigliano B, Vallone G. Imperforate hymen causing congenital hydrometrocolpos. J Ultrasound. 2013;16(1):37–9.
2. Zavras N, Christianakis E, Tsamoudaki S, Velaoras K. Infantile perianal pyramidal protrusion: a report of 8 new cases and a review of the literature. Case Rep Dermatol. 2012;4(3):202–6.
3. Huppert JS, Gerber MA, Deitch HR, Mortensen JE, Staat MA, Adams Hillard PJ. Vulvar ulcers in young females: a manifestation of aphthosis. J Pediatr Adolesc Gynecol. 2006;19:195–204.
4. Rosen T, Brown TJ. Ulcers. In: Edwards L, editor. Genital dermatology atlas. Philadelphia: Lippincott Williams & Wilkins; 2004. p. 117–30.
5. Halvorsen JA, Brevig T, Aas T, Skar AG, Slevolden EM, Moi H. Genital ulcers as initial manifestation of Epstein-Barr virus infection: two new cases and a review of the literature. Acta Derm Venereol. 2006;86:439–42.
6. Cheng SX, Chapman MS, Margesson LJ, Birenbaum D. Genital ulcers caused by Epstein-Barr virus. J Am Acad Dermatol. 2004;51:824–6.
7. Noël JC, Buxant F, Fayt I, Bebusschere G, Parent D. Vulval adenosis associated with toxic epidermal necrolysis. Br J Dermatol. 2005;153:457–8.
8. Dendrinos ML, Quint EH. Lichen sclerosus in children and adolescents. Curr Opin Obstet Gynecol. 2013;25:370–4.
9. Heller DS. Lesions of the clitoris: a review. J Low Genit Tract Dis. 2014;19(1):68–75.
10. Ds H. Vaginal cysts: a pathology review. J Low Genit Tract Dis. 2012;16:140–4.
11. Shetty V, Venkatesh S. Acquired lymphangioma circumscriptum of the vulva. Int J Gynaecol Obstet. 2012;117:190.
12. Julian TM, Haefner HK, Margesson LJ, Kaufman RH, Wilkinson EJ, Edwards L. Clinical question: ask the experts. J Low Genit Tract Dis. 2005;9:188–92.
13. Collier F, Smith RC, Morton CA. Diagnosis and management of hidradenitis suppurativa. BMJ. 2013;346:f2121.
14. Lynch PJ, Moyal-Barracco M, Scurry J, Stockdale C. 2011 ISSVD terminology and classification of vulvar dermatological disorders: an approach to clinical diagnosis. J Low Genit Tract Dis. 2012;16:339–44.
15. Lewis FM, Bogliatto F. Erosive vulval lichen planus: a diagnosis not to be missed—a clinical review. Eur J Obstet Gynecol Reprod Biol. 2013;171:214–9.
16. Murphy R. Lichen sclerosus. Dermatol Clin. 2010;28(4):707–15.
17. Brenn T. Atypical genital nevus. Arch Pathol Lab Med. 2011;135:317–20.
18. Kassinove A, Raam R. Acrochordon of the labia. J Emerg Med. 2013;44:e361–2.
19. Kavala M, Can B, Zindanci I, Kocatürk E, Türkoğlu Z, Büyükbabani N, et al. Vulvar pruritus caused by syringoma of the vulva. Int J Dermatol. 2008;47:831–2.
20. Rivlin ME, Meeks GR, Ghafar MA, Lewin JR. Vulvar granular cell tumor. World J Clin Cases. 2013;1:149–51.
21. Fanburg-Smith JC, Meis-Kindblom JM. Malignant granular cell tumor of soft tissue: diagnostic criteria and clinicopathologic correlation. Am J Surg Pathol. 1998;22:779–94.
22. Nielsen GP, Rosenberg AE, Koerner FC, Young RH, Scully RE. Smooth-muscle tumors of the vulva. A clinicopathological study of 25 cases and review of the literature. Am J Surg Pathol. 1996;20:779–93.
23. Cebesoy FB, Kutlar I, Aydin A. A rare mass formation of the vulva: giant cavernous hemangioma. J Low Genit Tract Dis. 2008;12:35–7.
24. Darragh TM, Colgan TJ, Cox JT, Heller DS, Henry MR, Luff RD, et al. The lower anogenital squamous terminology standardization project for HPV-associated lesions: background and consensus recommendations from the college of american pathologists and the american society for colposcopy and cervical pathology. Int J Gynecol Pathol. 2013;32(1):76–115.
25. Heller DS. The lower female genital tract: a clinicopathologic approach. Baltimore: Lippincott Williams & Wilkins; 1998. p. 159.
26. Chung AF, Woodruff JM, Lewis Jr JL. Malignant melanoma of the vulva: a report of 44 cases. Obstet Gynecol. 1975;45:635–46.
27. Leitao Jr MM. Management of vulvar and vaginal melanomas: current and future strategies. Am Soc Clin Oncol Educ Book. 2014;2014:e277–81.
28. Heller DS. Pigmented vulvar lesions: a pathology review of lesions that are not melanoma. J Low Genit Tract Dis. 2013;17:320–5.

Diseases of the Vagina and Urethra

4

4.1 Diseases of the Vagina

"The vagina … seems almost an afterthought in the minds of most pathologists, a structure serving only to connect other far more interesting reproductive organs which harbor more curious and challenging diseases" [1]. Pathologists receive many fewer vaginal specimens than from other areas of the female reproductive tract. This is probably due to the lower rates of primary vaginal malignancies. This chapter serves to review vaginal pathology. An appropriate history supplied with these specimens will assist pathologists in providing a more useful diagnosis, and perhaps recognizing that the vagina is more than a conduit between the vulva and cervix (Table 4.1).

4.2 Congenital Anomalies of the Vagina

The vagina is formed embryologically by two different structures. The lower 1/3 is formed by the urogenital sinus, which meets up with the upper 2/3 of the vagina, which is formed after fusion of the two Müllerian ducts. Anomalies of the vagina are subsequent to abnormalities of this process. A proposed classification based on embryology has been set forth [2]. The more common are touched on briefly here.

4.2.1 Vaginal Agenesis

Vaginal agenesis may be isolated, or may be part of the Mayer–Rokitansky–Küster–Hauser syndrome in association with uterine agenesis.

© Springer International Publishing Switzerland 2015
D.S. Heller, *OB-GYN Pathology for the Clinician*,
DOI 10.1007/978-3-319-15422-0_4

Table 4.1 Key points about vaginal pathology

History and location of vaginal cysts may assist in evaluating the origin of these lesions
Superficial biopsies may impede diagnosis of processes requiring evaluation of subepithelial tissue
Metastatic squamous cell carcinoma from cervix or vulva, including a prior history of these neoplasms, should be ruled out before primary vaginal squamous cell carcinoma is diagnosed

4.2.2   Vaginal Duplication

Failure of fusion of the two Müllerian ducts leads to vaginal duplication, which may occur in isolation, or with duplication of the uterus as well.

4.2.3   Longitudinal Vaginal Septum

If fusion occurs, but the septum is not resorbed, longitudinal vaginal septum is present.

4.2.4   Transverse Vaginal Septum

Transverse vaginal septum occurs due to failure of resorption of the Müllerian septum at the interface of the urogenital sinus and fused Müllerian ducts [1]. A specimen from an excision of a transverse vaginal septum may show squamous epithelium on the more caudal aspect and columnar epithelium on the more rostral.

4.2.5   Imperforate Hymen

Imperforate hymen may present in childhood as mucocolpos, or not show up until menarche as hematocolpos. Hymenal tissue is lined by nonkeratinizing squamous epithelium.

4.2.6   Adenosis

During embryogenesis, the urogenital sinus meets up with the fused Müllerian ducts. At birth, the lower genital tract is lined by squamous epithelium extending up the vagina to the squamo-columnar junction of the cervix. While it had been believed that this was urogenital squamous epithelium replacing any glandular epithelium that had been present in the upper vagina, more recently, some investigators have put forth that the upper vaginal squamous epithelium is derived from Müllerian epithelium [3]. Either spontaneously, or due to an exogenous interference with

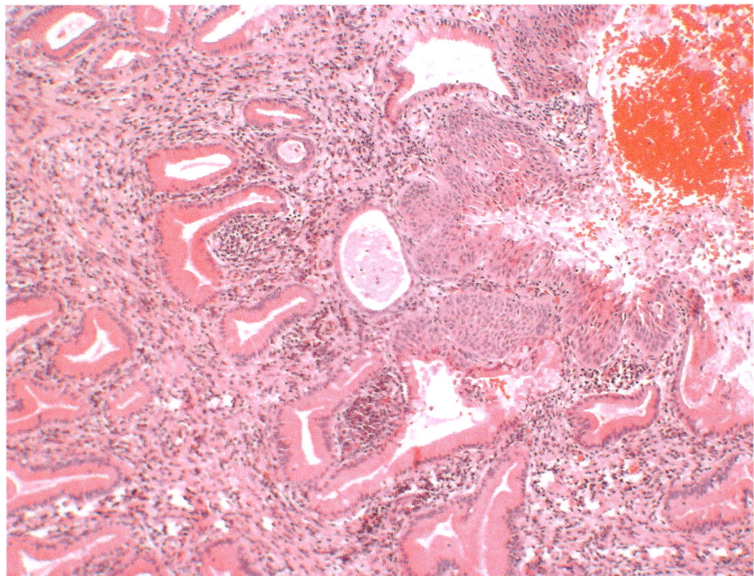

Fig. 4.1 Adenosis. Submucosal glands are being replaced by squamous metaplasia (*center*)

embryogenesis such as diethylstilbestrol (DES) exposure, remnants of glands may remain in the vaginal submucosa (adenosis), and over time, are replaced by metaplastic squamous epithelium (Fig. 4.1).

4.3 Cysts of the Vagina

Vaginal cysts are fairly common and may be either congenital or acquired. Congenital cysts may raise consideration of a genitourinary anomaly and require investigation including imaging. Acquired cysts are often at the site of prior surgery such as episiotomy [4]. The location in the vagina as well as how long the cyst has been present may be helpful to the pathologist in determining a cyst's origin, although this can't always be confirmed.

4.3.1 Müllerian Cyst

Müllerian cysts may arise from foci of adenosis. They are the most common vaginal cysts and may be symptomatic owing to their larger size, with symptoms including sensation of mass, pain, dyspareunia, discharge, and urinary symptoms [4]. They can occur anywhere in the vagina. Lining is variable, typical of the multipotential Müllerian epithelium, and hence mucinous, tubal, endometrioid or squamous epithelium may be seen (Fig. 4.2a).

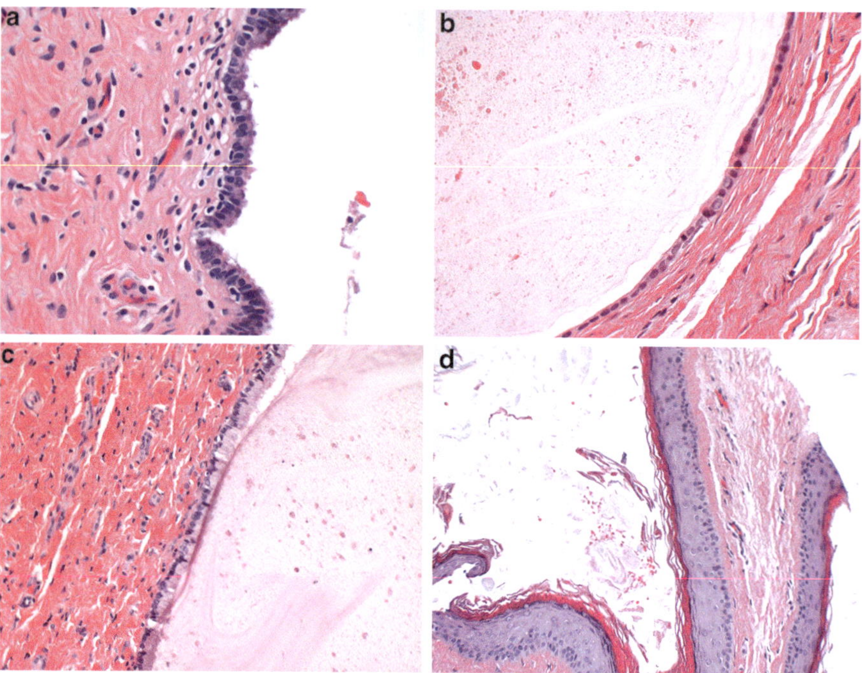

Fig. 4.2 (**a**) Müllerian cyst lined with a fallopian tube type lining. (**b**) Gartner's (Wolffian) duct cyst with a flat cuboidal lining. (**c**) Mucinous cyst, lined with a single layer of mucinous columnar epithelium. (**d**) Epidermal inclusion cyst, lined by squamous epithelium and containing keratinaceous debris

4.3.2   Gartner (Mesonephric, Wolffian) Cyst

The mesonephric ducts regress during embryogenesis of a female. Remnants can form cysts. These cysts are generally located along the lateral vagina, in the location of the mesonephric ducts. They tend to be smaller and less symptomatic than Müllerian cysts [4]. They are lined by a cuboidal non-mucinous epithelium and may contain eosinophilic secretions (Fig. 4.2b).

4.3.3   Mucinous Cyst

Mucinous cysts are often located in the vestibule. They may be either congenital or acquired and are thought to arise from minor vestibular glands (Fig. 4.2c).

4.3.4   Epidermal Inclusion Cyst

Squamous inclusion cysts are usually localized to prior surgery such as episiotomy, but can occur in any vaginal location. Histologically, they are lined by squamous epithelium, and the cheesy contents are histologically seen to be keratinaceous debris (Fig. 4.2d).

4.3.5 Endometriosis

Endometriosis may be cystic or solid and tends to occur in sites of prior surgery such as episiotomy, or trauma, lending credence to the implantation theory. Symptoms may be cyclic. Histologically, endometrial glandular epithelium and stroma must be present to confirm the diagnosis for the pathologist (Fig. 4.3).

4.3.6 Vaginitis Emphysematosa

This is a rare self-limiting condition where multiple vaginal blebs are formed. Symptoms may include pressure, with relief if the blebs rupture during intercourse or examination [4]. The condition is thought to be related to trichomonas or bacterial vaginosis [5]. The lesions are rarely biopsied, but consistent of empty gas-filled subepithelial spaces [6].

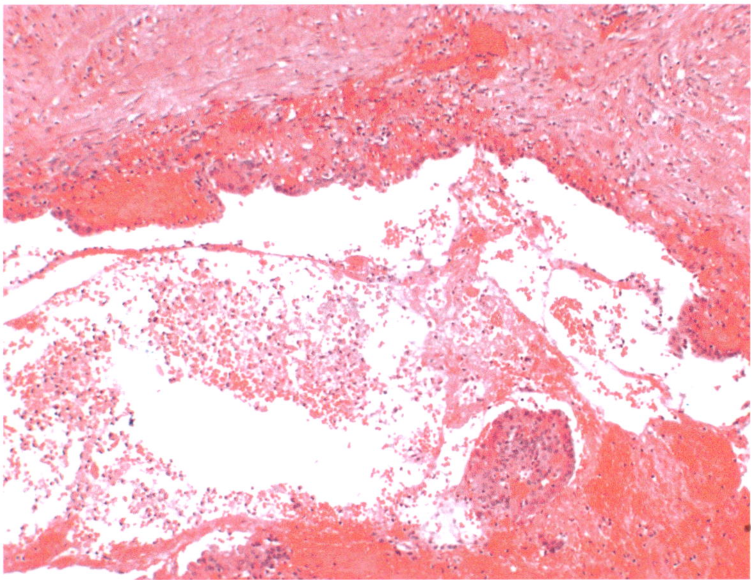

Fig. 4.3 Endometriosis. Abundant hemorrhage makes appreciation of the compressed stroma under the endometrial glandular type epithelium difficult

4.4　Infections and Inflammations of the Vagina

4.4.1　Vaginitis

Pap smear findings associated with trichomonas, bacterial vaginosis, candida, and herpes are covered in the chapter on cytology.

4.4.2　Condyloma Acuminatum

Condyloma acuminatum in the vagina is histologically similar to the vulva (see discussion, Chap. 3) (Fig. 4.4).

4.4.3　Herpes Simplex

Herpes may appear as erosions after rupture of the vesicles. A smear of the lesion or exudate may show the characteristic inclusions (Fig. 4.5).

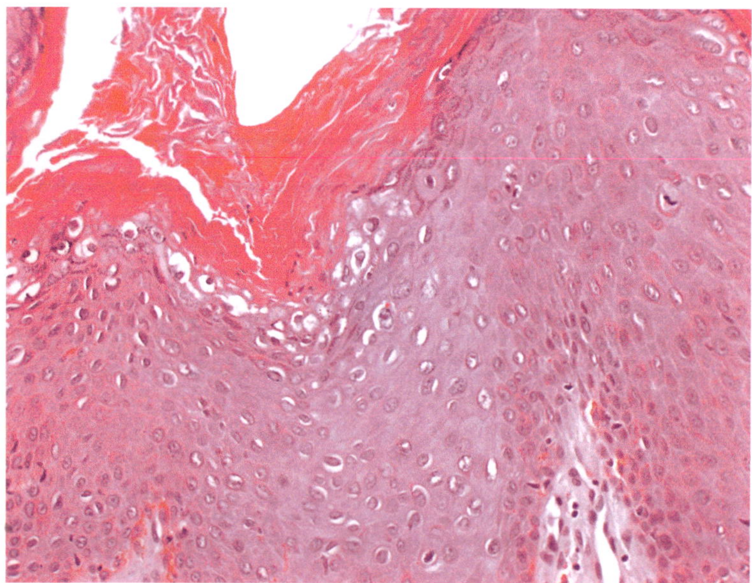

Fig. 4.4 Condyloma acuminatum showing hyperkeratosis and koilocytosis

Fig. 4.5 Herpes simplex showing classic ground glass intranuclear inclusions in a multinucleated cell (*black arrow*) as well as Cowdry type A intranuclear inclusions (*green arrow*)

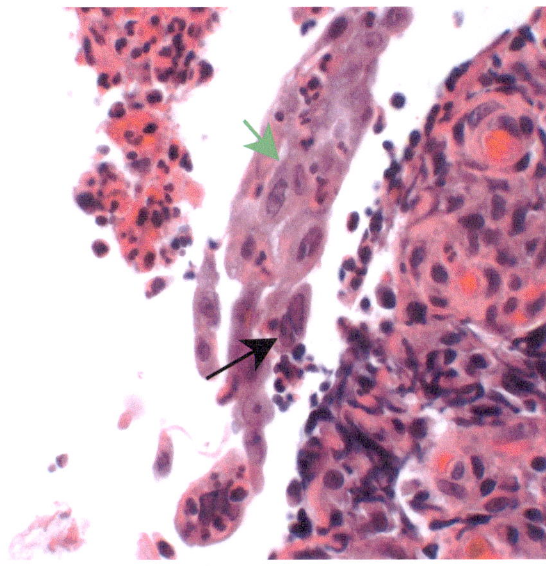

4.5   Benign Lesions of the Vagina

4.5.1   Postsurgical Lesions

Two lesions seen after hysterectomy may clinically appear similar, prolapsed fallopian tube, and granulation tissue. Both appear grossly as reddish polypoid lesions at the vaginal apex. Prolapsed fallopian tube is clinically more tender and may be associated with dyspareunia and pain on touch during examination. It is associated with processes that keep the vaginal vault open longer after hysterectomy, such as hematoma, infection, or heavy drainage [7]. Histologically, inflamed and edematous fallopian tube, usually from the fimbria, is seen. Granulation tissue is an exuberant reparative response composed of new vessels in fibroconnective tissue associated with inflammatory cells (Fig. 4.6).

4.5.2   Ulcers

Ulcers may be seen in association with pessaries or tampons. They are rarely biopsied and show no specific histology, simply loss of surface epithelium, inflammation, and possibly granulation tissue with repair.

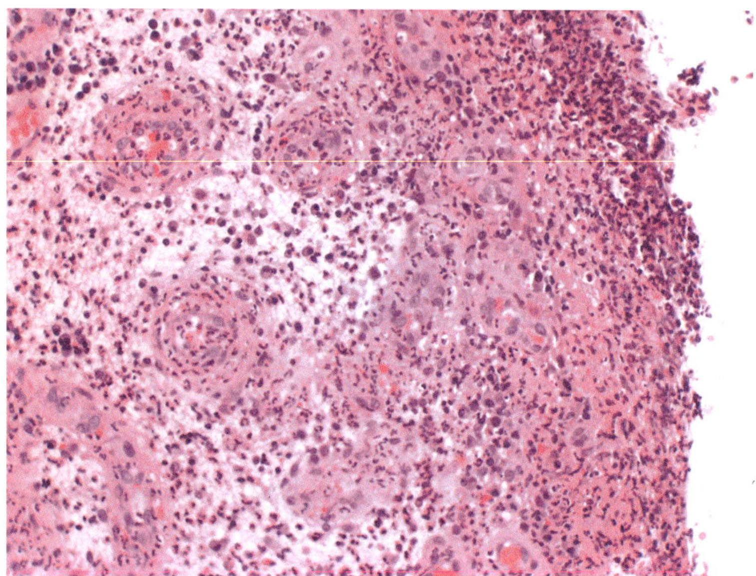

Fig. 4.6 Granulation tissue, composed of new vessels in a background of severe acute and chronic inflammation

4.5.3 Fistulas

Fistulas between the vagina and bladder or rectum are occasionally biopsied. Mucosa of both structures is sometimes seen, but often only inflammation and fibro-connective and granulation tissue is present. If the fistula is from a malignant neoplasm, this may sometimes be seen on biopsy.

4.6   Benign Neoplasms of the Vagina

4.6.1 Fibroepithelial Polyp

Fibroepithelial stromal polyps of the lower genital tract, including vagina, are usually easily recognized benign lesions; however, there are a few histologic pitfalls. The overlying squamous epithelium may be hyperplastic or papillomatous, mimicking condyloma; however, lack of koilocytosis rules out an HPV-related lesion (Fig. 4.7a). Although most of these lesions have a hypocellular stroma containing occasional spindle and stellate cells (Fig. 4.7b), some lesions may be hypercellular, show significant atypia, high mitotic rate, or atypical mitotic features, particularly

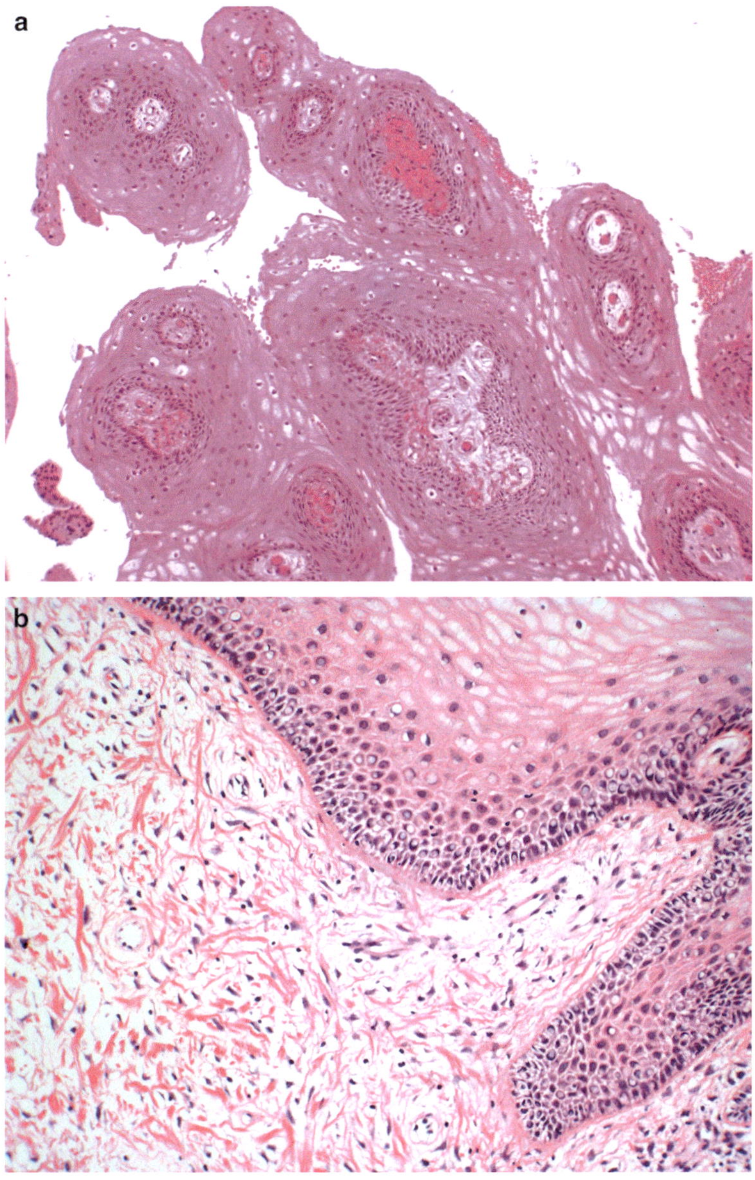

Fig. 4.7 (**a**) Fibroepithelial polyp may show surface papillomatosis, mimicking condyloma. Note the lack of koilocytosis. (**b**) The stroma of the lesion is usually hypocellular, with spindle and stellate cells extending up to the surface, with no delineating normal stroma

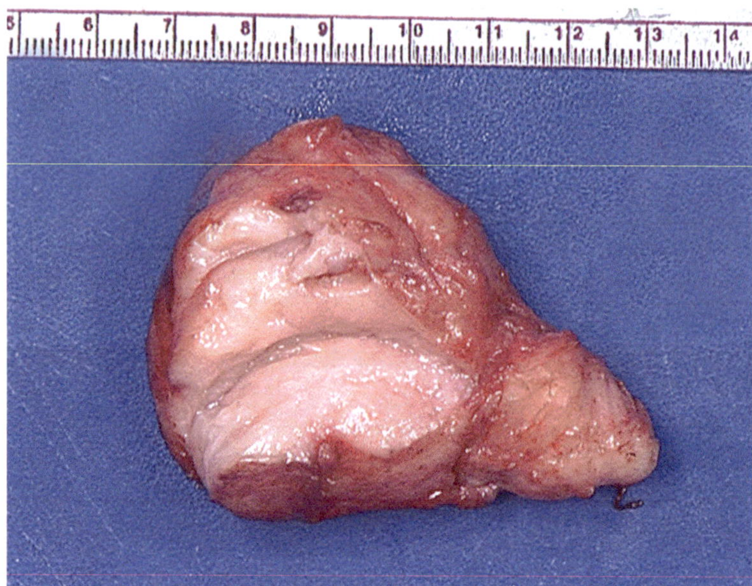

Fig. 4.8 Vaginal leiomyoma (gross). The prominent edema gives this lesion a "fish-flesh" appearance that may raise concern for a sarcoma, but histology was usual leiomyoma

in lesions arising during pregnancy, mimicking a sarcoma [8]. Thus, these lesions may well be hormonally responsive. Lesions with all four histologically worrisome features were more likely to recur [8], but no lesions in Nucci's series showed aggressive malignant behavior. The lack of circumscription of the lesion supports the hyperplastic rather than neoplastic nature, with the stromal lesion extending up to the epithelium, with no "normal" stromal interface.

4.6.2   Leiomyoma

Leiomyomas of the vagina are similar in appearance to their uterine counterpart (Fig. 4.8). Leiomyosarcoma of the vagina is exceptionally rare.

4.7   Preinvasive Neoplasia of the Vagina

4.7.1   Vaginal Intraepithelial Neoplasia

Vaginal intraepithelial neoplasia (VAIN) is associated with human papilloma virus. It is commonly associated with HPV-related disease of other lower genital sites, particularly cervix. It is often detected on a pap smear, as it is not generally symptomatic. This may make finding the origin of an abnormal pap smear challenging if

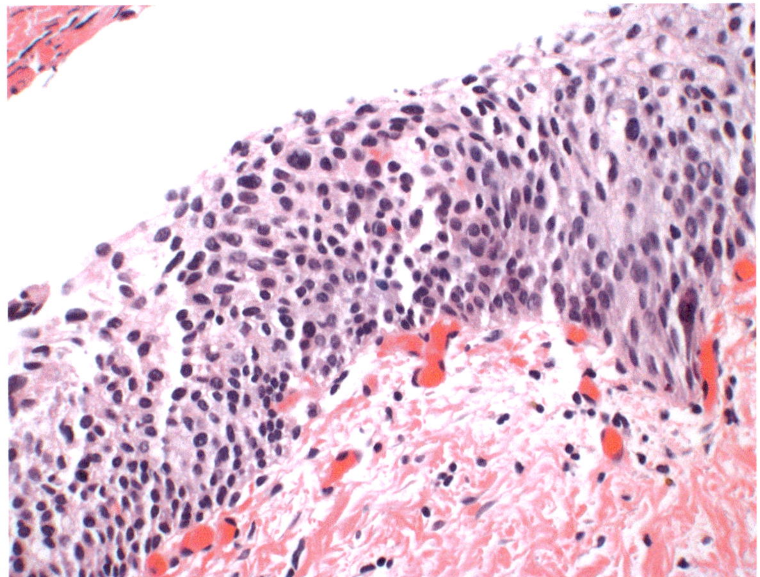

Fig. 4.9 VAIN 3 (HSIL) showing full thickness maturation abnormality

the uterus is in situ, or VAIN may arise after a hysterectomy, and be detected via abnormal pap smear. Histologically, the appearance is the same as intraepithelial neoplasia in other locations. Both VAIN 1, 2, 3 and LSIL/HSIL terminologies are in use (Fig. 4.9).

4.8   Malignant Neoplasms of the Vagina

4.8.1   Squamous Cell Carcinoma

Squamous cell carcinoma that arises as a primary in the vagina is rare and is more likely secondary to concurrent or prior cervical or vulvar carcinoma. Histologically, the appearance is similar to other locations (Fig. 4.10).

4.8.2   Metastatic Carcinoma

A wide variety of carcinomas have spread to the vagina, particularly to the vault after hysterectomy. The most common origins are from endometrial and ovarian primary neoplasms.

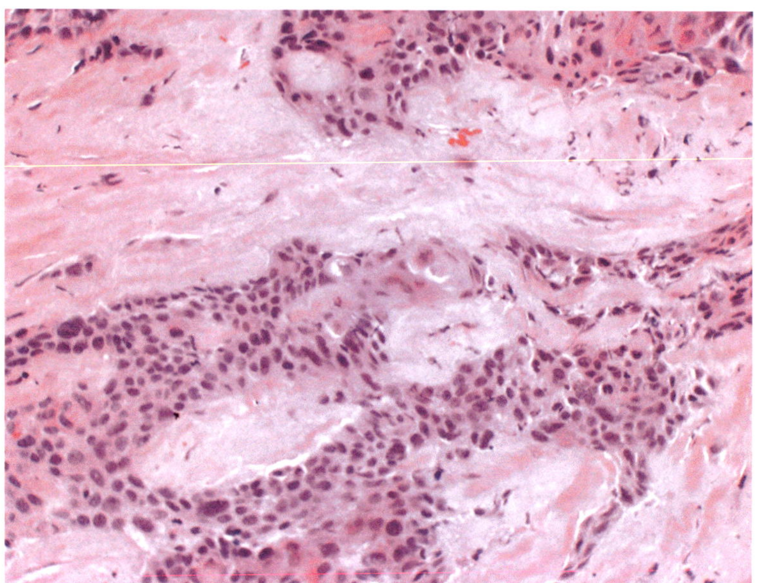

Fig. 4.10 Squamous cell carcinoma, invading in irregular nests

4.8.3   Clear Cell Adenocarcinoma

Most reported cases of the rare clear cell adenocarcinoma of the vagina were seen in association with in utero exposure to DES, but with recognition of this association, this neoplasm is exceptionally rare now. Histologically, the lesion is similar to the somewhat more common clear cell adenocarcinoma arising in endometrium or ovary, with either clear cells, or a tubulopapillary architecture composed of hobnail type cells.

4.8.4   Sarcoma Botryoides

Botryoides refers to the grape-like configuration of the polypoid tumor projections seen protruding from the vagina. This rare neoplasm, an embryonal rhabdomyosarcoma, is mostly seen in girls under the age of 5 (Fig. 4.11a, b). The characteristic finding is of a hypocellular polypoid lesion with condensation of the tumor cells under the surface epithelium, forming the so-called "cambium layer."

4.8.5   Melanoma

Melanoma may rarely arise in the vagina. Diagnosis is usually late, and prognosis tends to be poor.

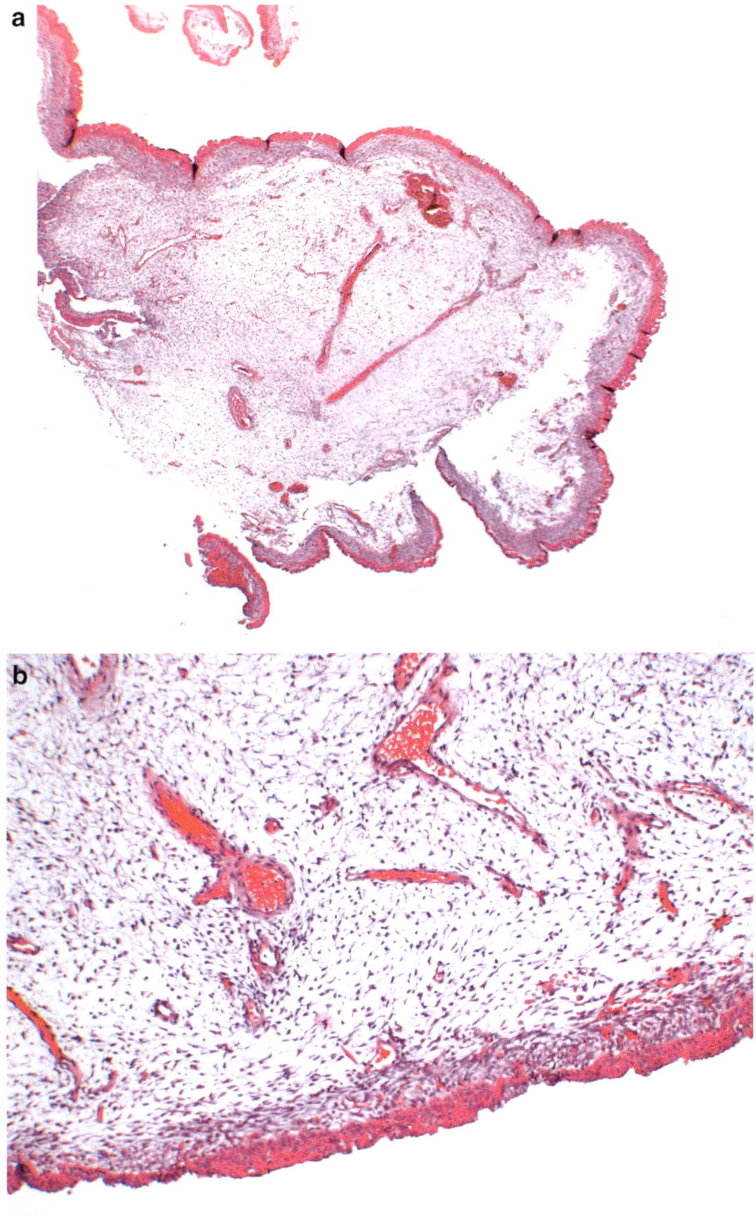

Fig. 4.11 Sarcoma botryoides. On low power (**a**), the polypoid lesion shows condensation of cells under the surface, which on higher power (**b**) is seen to be the same spindle cells as the hypocellular center of the lesion. The condensed area is the characteristic "cambium layer"

4.8.6   Endodermal Sinus Tumor (Yolk Sac Tumor)

Endodermal sinus tumor is a rare pediatric neoplasm more commonly seen in the ovary in adolescents than in the vagina of children. Histology is the same, with a variety of patterns including a lacy one (Fig. 4.12a). Characteristic Schiller–Duval bodies may be seen (Fig. 4.12b). The lesion may contain eosinophilic globules, which stain for alpha-fetoprotein, which is produced by these tumors.

4.9   Lesions of the Urethra

Mass-like lesions of the urethra need to be distinguished from other lesions arising from the anterior (ventral) vagina including genitourinary lesions such as ectopic prolapsed ureterocele or ectopic ureter, cysts (Skene's duct, Gartner's, Müllerian), or vaginal neoplasms. The more common urethral lesions that may be encountered by a gynecologist are described below.

4.9.1   Urethral Prolapse

Urethral prolapse is more common in female children, particularly African-American girls [9], but may occur in postmenopausal women as well. A clinical clue is the donut shape of the protrusion. Topical estrogen and sitz baths have been used as conservative therapy; however, surgery may become necessary. Thrombosis may be seen (Fig. 4.13).

4.9.2   Urethral Diverticulum

Urethral diverticuli are thought to arise secondary to rupture of infected periurethral glands into the urethra [10]. Histologically, urethral diverticuli are comprised of fibro-connective tissue, lined by either squamous, columnar, or transitional epithelium (Fig. 4.14), or devoid of lining. The risk of neoplasia is not inconsequential, particularly adenocarcinoma [11], in distinction to the more common squamous cell carcinoma of the urethra when the carcinoma arises in the absence of a diverticulum [12].

4.9.3   Urethral Caruncle

Most often seen in postmenopausal women, urethral caruncles are red polypoid lesions seen protruding through the urethral meatus, without the characteristic donut shape of prolapse. They are rarely excised unless symptomatic or there is worry for malignancy. They are composed of granulation tissue lined by squamous or transitional epithelium (Fig. 4.15).

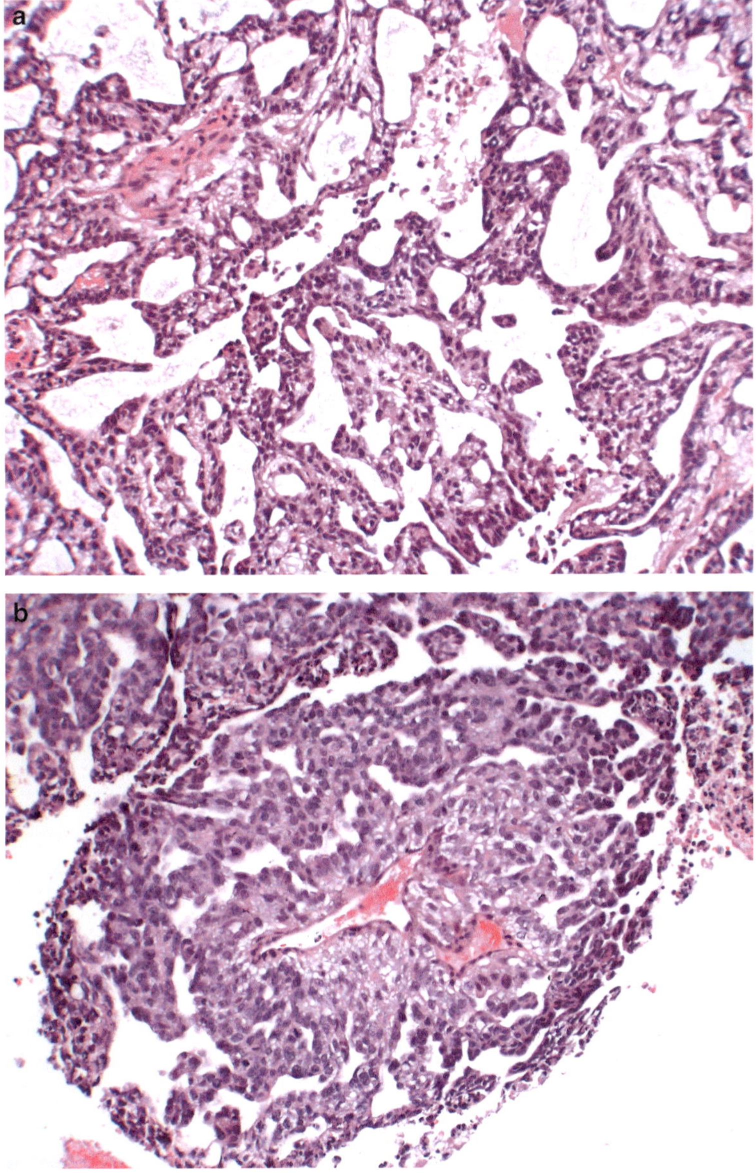

Fig. 4.12 Endodermal sinus tumor (yolk sac tumor) of vagina showing a lacy pattern (**a**). A number of Schiller–Duval bodies, tumor surrounding a vessel residing in a space surrounded by more tumor (**b**), were present. These are not always seen, but are characteristic. Also not shown, but characteristic, are eosinophilic globules that stain for alpha-fetoprotein

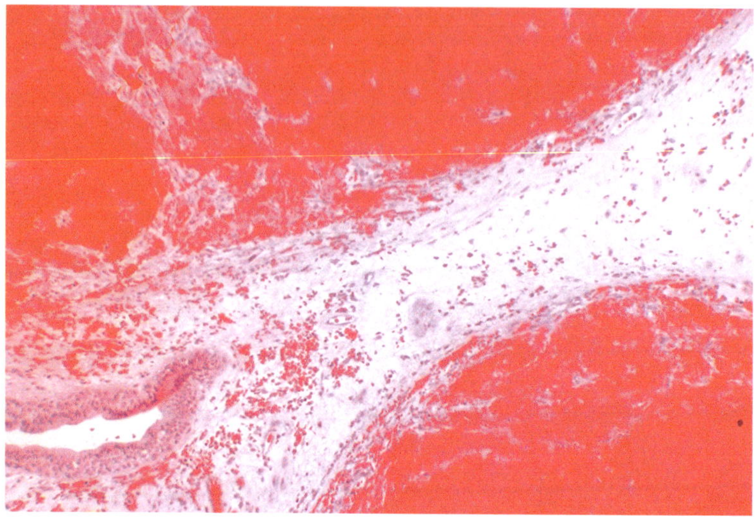

Fig. 4.13 Urethral prolapse. Thrombi are seen adjacent to a suburethral gland

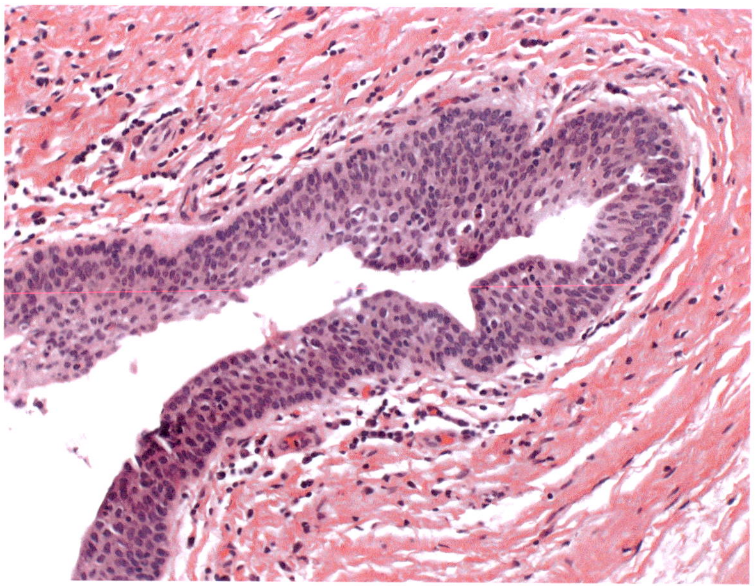

Fig. 4.14 Urethral diverticulum. Transitional epithelium lines fibroconnective tissue

4.9.4 Urethral Carcinoma

These unusual lesions occur in older women. Distal lesions are more common than proximal, and histology may be squamous cell carcinoma (Fig. 4.16), the most common in the absence of a diverticulum [12], adenocarcinoma, transitional cell carcinoma, or a variety of more unusual histologic types.

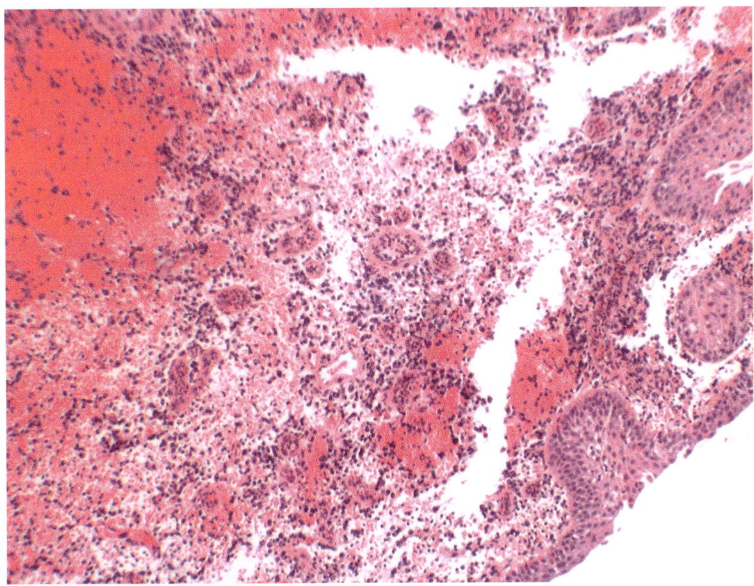

Fig. 4.15 Urethral caruncle. Granulation tissue is seen in the center under the urothelial lining present to the right. Some hemorrhage is also seen

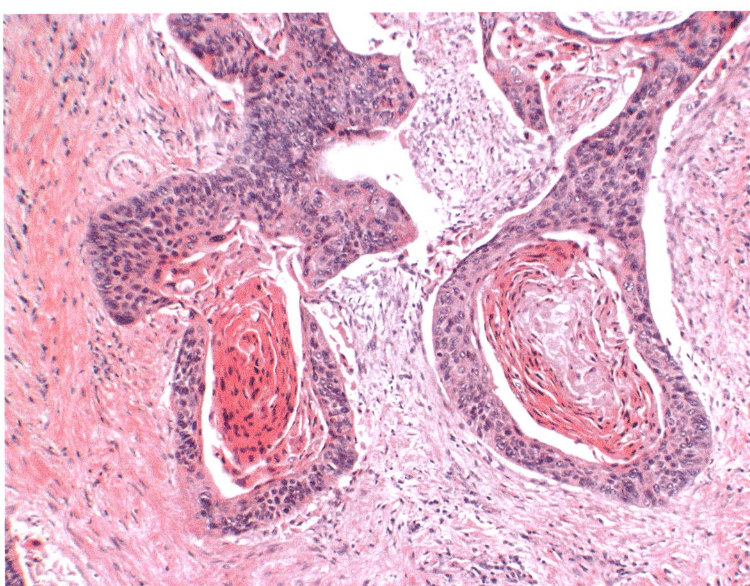

Fig. 4.16 Urethral carcinoma. This neoplasm is a keratinizing squamous cell carcinoma

References

1. Schmidt WA. Pathology of the vagina. In: Fox H, Wells M, editors. Haines and Taylor obstetrical and gynaecological pathology. 5th ed. London: Churchill Livingston; 2003. p. 147.
2. Ruggeri G, Gargano T, Antonellini C, et al. Vaginal malformations: a proposed classification based on embryological, anatomical and clinical criteria and their surgical management (an analysis of 167 cases). Pediatr Surg Int. 2012;28:797–803.
3. Reich O, Fritsch H. The developmental origin of cervical and vaginal epithelium and their clinical consequences: a systematic review. J Low Genit Tract Dis. 2014;18(4):358–60.
4. Heller DS. Vaginal cysts: a pathology review. J Low Gen Tract Dis. 2012;16:140–4.
5. Josey WE, Campbell Jr WG. Vaginitis emphysematosa. A report of four cases. J Reprod Med. 1990;35:974–7.
6. Al Aboud K, Al Hawsawi K, Ramesh V. Vaginitis emphysematosa. Sex Transm Infect. 2002;78:155.
7. Nasir N, Desai M, Marshall J, Gupta N. Prolapsed fallopian tube: cytological findings in a ThinPrep liquid based cytology vaginal vault sample. Diagn Cytopathol. 2013;41:146–9.
8. Nucci MR, Young RH, Fletcher CD. Cellular pseudosarcomatous fibroepithelial stromal polyps of the lower female genital tract: an under recognized lesion often misdiagnosed as sarcoma. Am J Surg Pathol. 2000;24:231–40.
9. Nussbaum AR, Lebowitz RL. Interlabial masses in little girls: review and imaging recommendations. Am J Roentgenol. 1983;141:65–71.
10. Eilber KS, Raz S. Benign cystic lesions of the vagina: a literature review. J Urol. 2003;170:717–22.
11. Cocco AE, MacLennan GT. Unusual female suburethral mass lesions. J Urol. 2005;174:1106.
12. El-Mekresh M. Urethral pathology. Curr Opin Urol. 2000;10:381–90.

Diseases of the Cervix

5

5.1 Lesims of the Cervix

Cervical biopsies and excisions are common specimens in the Pathology laboratory. Management depends heavily on a number of diagnostic features for individual lesions, and there are numerous pitfalls the clinician should be aware of (Table 5.1).

5.2 Congenital Anomalies of the Cervix

The cervix is formed after fusion of the two Müllerian ducts and resorption of the septum. Anomalies are uncommon, but may include agenesis, dysgenesis, or duplication, generally in association with uterine duplication.

5.3 The Transformation Zone

The exocervix is lined by stratified squamous epithelium, normally non-keratinized, although keratinization may be seen with prolapse or HPV-related disease. The endocervix is lined by mucinous columnar epithelium. The meeting point of these two epithelial types is the squamocolumnar junction. This is not a static site, but moves over the course of a woman's life. During early reproductive life, the squamocolumnar junction is easily seen on the portio vaginalis. This led in the past to the mistaken diagnoses of "erosion" or "ectropion," due to the red beefy appearance of the columnar epithelium. The squamocolumnar junction moves cranially over a woman's life, with the location high up in the endocervical canal after menopause, making an adequate colposcopy requiring visualization of the entire transformation zone more difficult. The advancing squamocolumnar junction occurs by advancing squamous metaplasia replacing glandular epithelium. The metaplastic squamous epithelium is an immature squamous epithelium that matures and acquires glycogen over time. This metaplastic squamous epithelium spreads over the surface and into

© Springer International Publishing Switzerland 2015
D.S. Heller, *OB-GYN Pathology for the Clinician*,
DOI 10.1007/978-3-319-15422-0_5

Table 5.1 Key points about cervical pathology

Biopsies obtained below the transformation zone may not detect neoplastic lesions
LEEP introduces artifacts (cautery, fragmentation) that make evaluation of margins more difficult and sometimes not possible
AIS cannot be reliably diagnosed on a punch biopsy, but requires at least a cone type of excision to assess all of the features
Adjunct immunohistochemistry with p16 and Ki-67 is useful in distinguishing SIL from mimics

endocervical crypts. The zone between the original squamocolumnar junction and the woman's current squamocolumnar junction is called the transformation zone (see Chap. 2). This is where cervical neoplasia occurs, and if a biopsy is too low, doesn't sample the transformation zone, as evidenced by the presence of either both epithelial types, or metaplastic squamous epithelium, a neoplastic lesion has not been ruled out.

5.4 Infections and Inflammations of the Cervix

A degree of chronic inflammation is seen in most cervices in hysterectomy specimens and is not pathologic. Gonorrhea and Chlamydia may lead to a mucopurulent cervicitis. Follicular cervicitis, with formation of lymphoid follicular centers, may sometimes be associated with chlamydia [1], but is not a reliable diagnostic finding. The cervix may be involved by other infections such as herpes, or rarely by tuberculosis.

5.5 Benign Lesions of the Cervix

5.5.1 Nabothian Cysts

During the process of squamous metaplasia as the squamocolumnar junction advances, the endocervical crypts may become blocked, with inspissated mucus. Grossly these appear as blue-domed Nabothian cysts. Histologically, they appear as dilated glands lined by mucinous columnar epithelium (Fig. 5.1).

5.5.2 Endocervical Polyps

Endocervical polyps are common. They are polypoid lesions composed of endocervical epithelial-lined glands and crypts lining a fibroconnective tissue polyp containing prominent stalk vessels (Fig. 5.2).

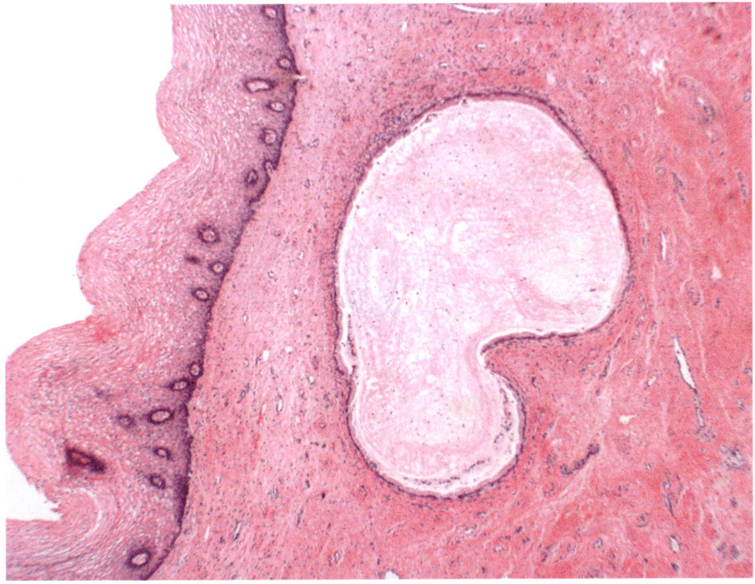

Fig. 5.1 Nabothian cyst. Dilated endocervical gland covered by surface squamous epithelium

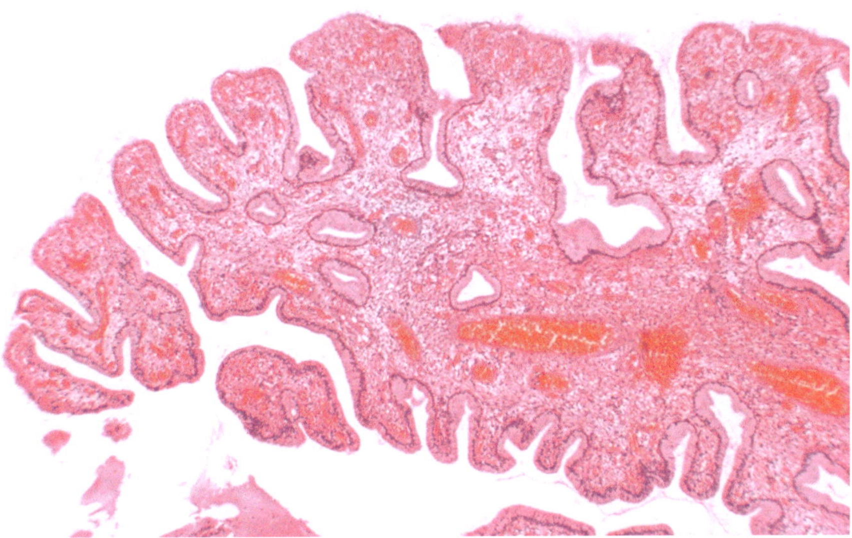

Fig. 5.2 Endocervical polyp. These lesions are lined by mucinous columnar epithelium. Squamous metaplasia is sometimes present. Inflammation is common

5.5.3 Microglandular Hyperplasia

Microglandular hyperplasia is a benign lesion thought to be associated with progestational exposure, such as oral contraceptives or pregnancy. It is of no clinical significance. Histologically, the crowded glands may be mistaken for adenocarcinoma; however, there is no significant atypia, and there is generally a prominent acute inflammatory infiltrate (Fig. 5.3).

5.5.4 Endometriosis

Endometriosis may affect the cervix, where it can appear as purple-blue lesions. Histologically, endometrial glandular epithelium and stroma must be present to confirm the diagnosis, as in other locations.

5.5.5 Leiomyoma

Cervical leiomyomas are histologically similar to the uterine counterpart and are most notable clinically for mechanical issues.

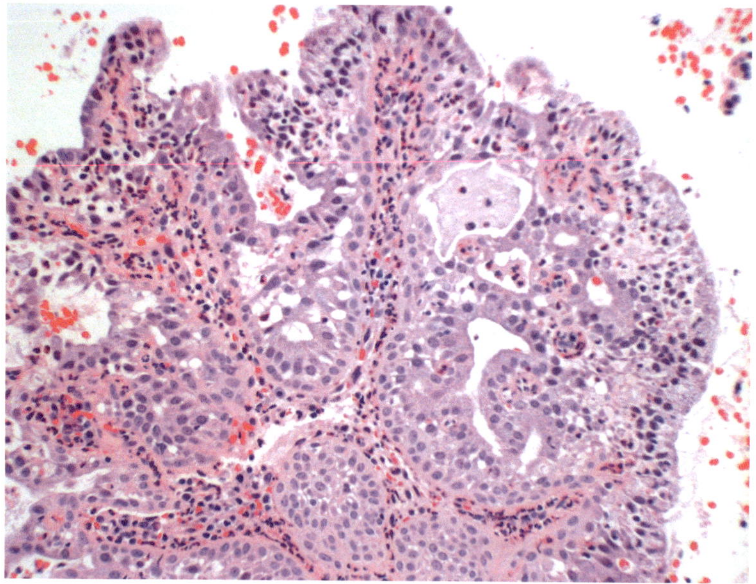

Fig. 5.3 Microglandular hyperplasia characterized by crowded glands without atypia, squamous metaplasia, and acute inflammation with many neutrophils

Fig. 5.4 Mesonephric remnants, lined by cuboidal epithelium and containing eosinophilic secretions

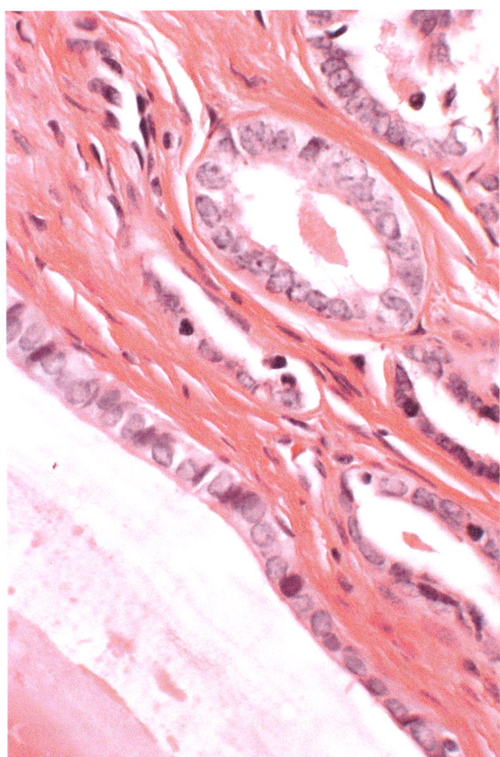

5.5.6   Mesonephric Remnants

Mesonephric remnants are commonly seen in hysterectomy specimens if looked for. These Wolffian duct remnants reside in the lateral aspects of the cervix and are composed of tubules lined by a cuboidal epithelium, often with inspissated eosinophilic secretions (Fig. 5.4). Rarely, these remnants may become hyperplastic or even give rise to carcinoma.

5.6   Preinvasive Neoplasia of the Cervix

5.6.1   Cervical Squamous Intraepithelial Neoplasia

Preinvasive squamous neoplasia is associated with human papillomavirus (HPV). For low-grade lesions, many regress or remain stable. The risk of progression is greater with high-grade lesions. It is important to sample the transformation zone when performing cervical biopsies, in order to obtain the lesion reliably. Positive endocervical curettings may mean that a lesion is up in the canal, but dysplastic squamous epithelium is friable, and fragments from the exocervix can break off during instrumentation and get into the endocervical curetting specimen. For cone biopsies, it is important for clinicians to be aware that LEEP cone biopsies are more difficult to evaluate margins on. This relates to cautery artifact, as well as potentially to tissue fragmentation, particularly if more than one pass is performed. Hence, cold knife cone may be preferable for cases where assessment of the margins is critical.

Two terminologies are currently in use for squamous intraepithelial neoplasia. The Lower Anogenital Squamous Terminology [2] utilizes low-grade and high-grade squamous intraepithelial lesion (LSIL, HSIL), patterned after the Bethesda System pap smear terminology, but permits inclusion secondarily of the older cervical intraepithelial neoplasia (CIN) 1,2,3 terminology (Fig. 5.5a–f). There are times when it is difficult to evaluate these lesions, such as in making the distinction between HSIL and atrophy. Ancillary stains may be helpful. Ki-67, a proliferation marker, shows nuclear staining confined to the basal layers in benign epithelium, but rises above the basal layers in SIL. It does not distinguish the grade of SIL. P16 is a surrogate marker for high-risk HPV and is considered positive when diffusely strongly positive. In combination, these can be used in problematic lesions [3] (Fig. 5.6a–c).

5.6.2   Adenocarcinoma-In-Situ

Unlike squamous neoplasia, which is recognized as being invasive by tongues of tumor breaking through the basement membrane, adenocarcinoma goes from in situ to invasive via whole glands, making the distinction more difficult. Adenocarcinoma-in-situ (AIS) is characterized by nuclear atypia with loss of cytoplasmic mucin, stratification, and mitotic figures in the glands, features also seen in invasive adenocarcinoma. In AIS, these neoplastic glands are admixed with normal glands and do not go deeper than the normal endocervical crypt depth (Fig. 5.7a, b). As such, AIS cannot be reliably diagnosed on a punch biopsy, but requires at least a cone type of excision. AIS is more likely to skip than SIL, an important consideration if a cone biopsy is planned as fertility sparing definitive surgery. If uterine preservation is planned, it is also important to be aware that a LEEP cone may make it more difficult to assess and provide an interpretation of status of margins on than a cold knife cone.

A somewhat different terminology has been utilized in the UK, cervical glandular intraepithelial neoplasia (CGIN), divided into low and high grade. The high grade is analogous to AIS. The low grade is analogous to a controversial diagnosis termed endocervical glandular dysplasia, for lesions that don't quite qualify histologically for a diagnosis of AIS [4].

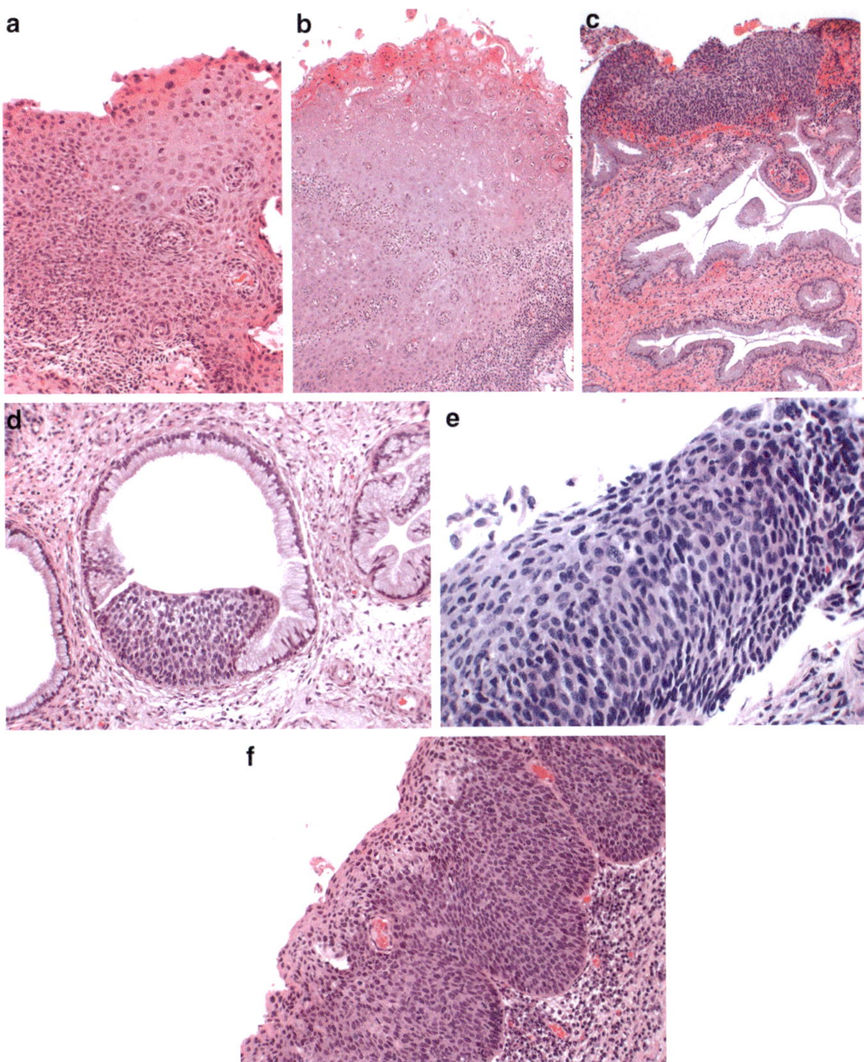

Fig. 5.5 Squamous intraepithelial lesion (SIL). Low-grade SIL shows maturation abnormality confined to the lower third of the tissue with occasional binucleation in the upper epithelium (**a**), or it may resemble condyloma acuminatum (**b**). High-grade SIL involving the transformation zone (**c**), and an endocervical gland (**d**). On higher power, HSIL (CIN3) involves the full thickness of the epithelium (**e**). Lesions where the maturation abnormality extends above two thirds but doesn't reach the surface may be called CIN2 or CIN3 by different reviewers, but this lesion is HSIL in either case (**f**)

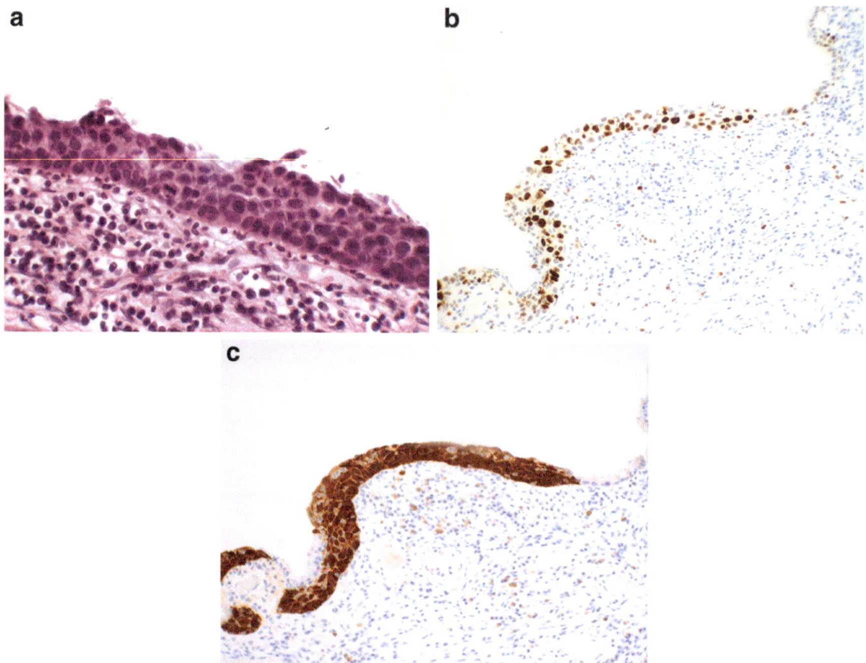

Fig. 5.6 HSIL versus atrophy. Cells are slightly disarrayed, and of parabasal type. A possible mitotic figure is seen (**a**). Ki-67, a nuclear stain, extends above the basal cells (**b**), and p16 is diffusely positive in the cytoplasm (**c**), confirming the diagnosis of HSIL

5.7 Malignant Neoplasms of the Cervix

5.7.1 Squamous Cell Carcinoma

Cervical squamous cell carcinoma may be exophytic or endophytic (Fig. 5.8a, b). Squamous cell carcinoma of the cervix is histologically the same as in other locations. Identification of invasion histologically is based on irregular nests of neoplastic squamous epithelium, which paradoxically look more mature than the SIL often adjacent, eliciting a stromal response. The stromal response means that the basement membrane has been breached, and metastatic potential now exists. The stromal response may be either inflammatory or desmoplastic (fibrotic) (Fig. 5.8c). When a radical hysterectomy specimen is received, it is important to handle the uterus as little as possible before removal of the parametria (Fig. 5.8d), lest artifactual tumor be squeezed into lymphatic spaces. Identification of lymphvascular space invasion is part of the assessment of the lesion (Fig. 5.8e). As tumors make artifactual spaces around nests of tumor cells due to shrinkage with fixation, the space must be lined by endothelium and/or contain blood or lymphatic cells to confirm a lymphvascular space.

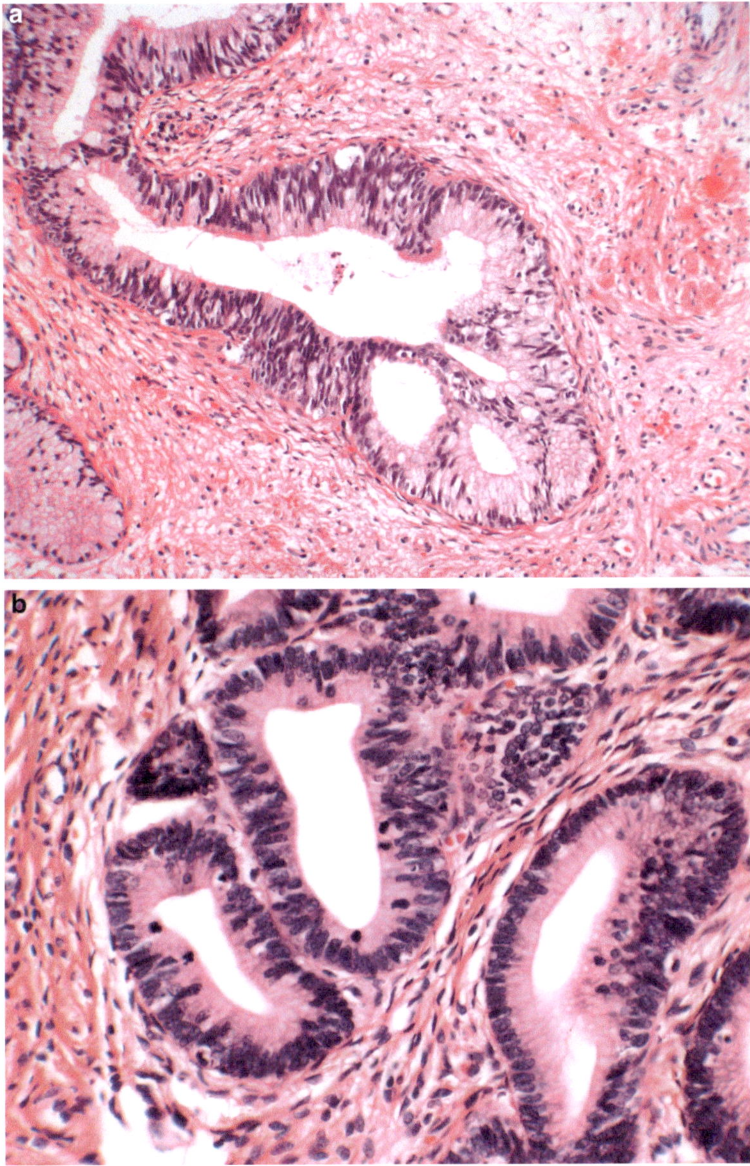

Fig. 5.7 Adenocarcinoma-in-situ involving parts of an endocervical gland (**a**). Note stratification of the epithelium, atypia, and mitotic activity (**b**)

5.7.2 Superficial Invasion (SISSCA)

LAST defines superficial invasion of a cervical squamous cell carcinoma as a FIGO 1a1 lesion [2], one that measures no more than 3 mm in depth and no wider than 7 mm in width. As there is more than one staging system in use, the term

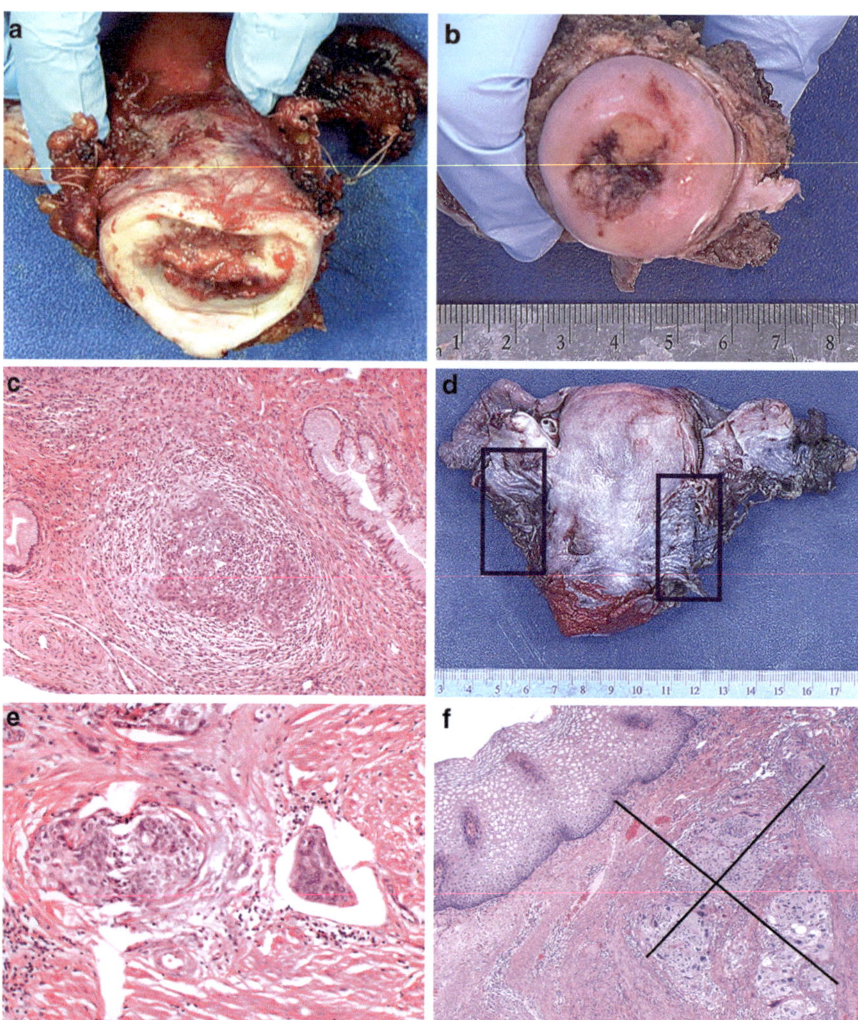

Fig. 5.8 Squamous cell carcinoma of the cervix. The lesion may be exophytic (**a**) or endophytic (**b**). The hallmark of invasion histologically is a stromal reaction around invading nests (**c**). Removal of the parametrium (*boxes*, **d**) from the radical hysterectomy specimen by the pathologist prior to opening the uterus, as well as minimal handling by all involved, will decrease false transport of tumor into lymphvascular spaces. Lymphvascular invasion is a prognostic indicator, and its identification requires an endothelial lining to the tumor-surrounding space (**e**, *right*) or blood or lymphatic cells may be supportive. Retraction artifact mimicking lymphvascular invasion (**e**, *left*) is also seen. Depth of invasion is measured from the basement membrane of the overlying epithelium (or from the basement membrane of the endocervical gland if that is the site of the invasive focus) to the deepest portion of the tumor (line shown on *left*). Width should be provided as well (line under tumor) (**f**)

"microinvasive" is not informative or acceptable. The lesion should be described as superficially invasive, with provision of depth and width. Current staging systems do not address multifocality of superficially invasive foci but it should be reported if present. Superficial invasion is identified to separate lesions that have a low risk of lymph node metastases, and thus may need less radical surgery. Measurement is made from the overlying basement membrane to the deepest point of invasion for depth, and width is reported as well (Fig. 5.8f).

5.7.3 Unusual Squamous Cell Carcinoma Variants (Papillary Squamotransitional Carcinoma, Verrucous Carcinoma)

Unusual variants of squamous cell carcinoma may be more exophytic and require a sufficiently deep biopsy to confirm the diagnosis. These include the rare but potentially aggressive papillary squamotransitional carcinoma and the exceedingly rare verrucous carcinoma (Figs. 5.9 and 5.10a, b).

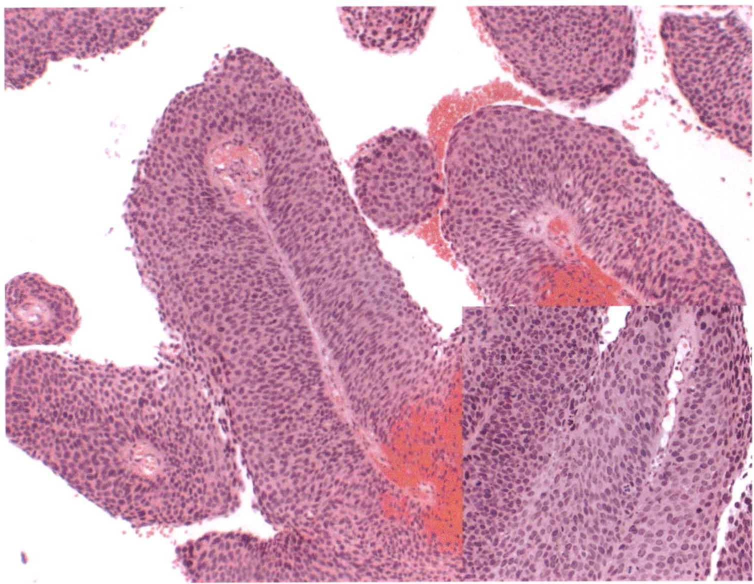

Fig. 5.9 Squamous cell carcinoma variants include lesions where a deep enough biopsy is required to be diagnostic due to the exophytic nature of the tumor. This includes papillary squamotransitional cell carcinoma, with fibrovascular cores lined by squamotransitional epithelium. The epithelium may look more transitional or may more closely resemble the epithelium seen with HSIL (*inset*), hence the need for a deep enough biopsy

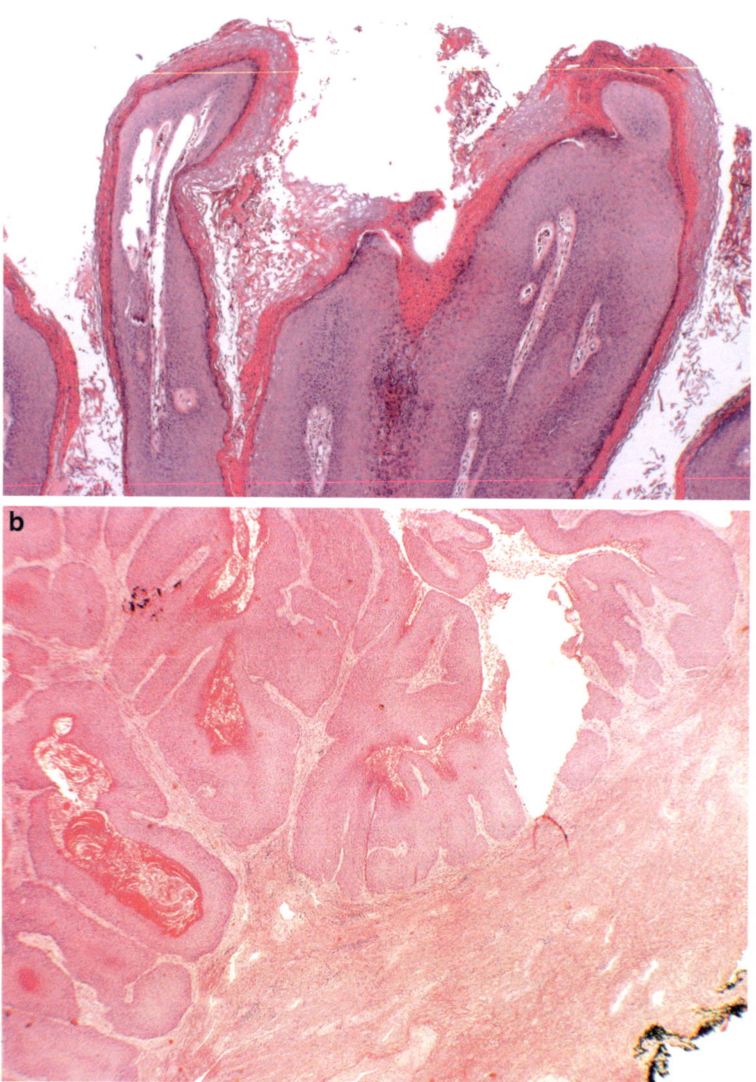

Fig. 5.10 Verrucous carcinoma may appear superficially as a condyloma (**a**), but requires a deep enough biopsy to appreciate the pushing margins of the neoplasm (**b**)

5.7.4 Adenocarcinoma

Like squamous cell carcinoma of the cervix, adenocarcinoma is associated with HPV. Invasive adenocarcinoma of the endocervix is histologically similar to AIS, except now the neoplastic glands have breached the basement membrane. This can

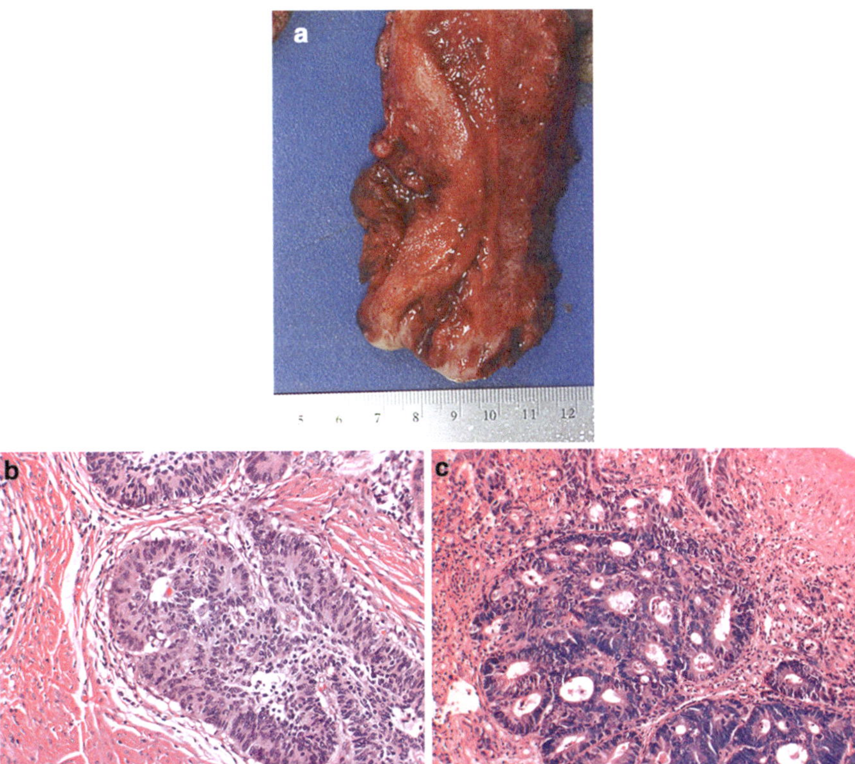

Fig. 5.11 Endocervical adenocarcinoma is seen arising in the endocervical canal (**a**). The invasive neoplastic glands can be seen eliciting a stromal response (**b**), or demonstrating invasion by cribriform pattern (**c**)

be suggested by extension of malignant glands beyond the crypts, or concluded by stromal reaction, or cribriform formation of the glands, which is interpreted as stromal invasion. Endocervical adenocarcinoma may be of endocervical type glandular histology (Fig. 5.11a–c), but may also be endometrioid. Endometrioid histology can create confusion as to whether the tumor arises from cervix or endometrium, particularly on curettings. As the definitive surgical procedures differ for cervical and endometrial primary carcinomas, distinction is important. Immunohistochemistry may be helpful, as endometrial lesions are more likely to stain for estrogen receptor and vimentin, and cervical lesions for HPV, CEA, and p16, a surrogate high-risk HPV marker [5].

5.7.5 Adenoma Malignum

One of the great fears of pathologists is missing the rare diagnosis of adenoma malignum. This is a variant of adenocarcinoma of the endocervix which is histologically deceptively bland, mimicking a benign lesion. Atypia may be limited and

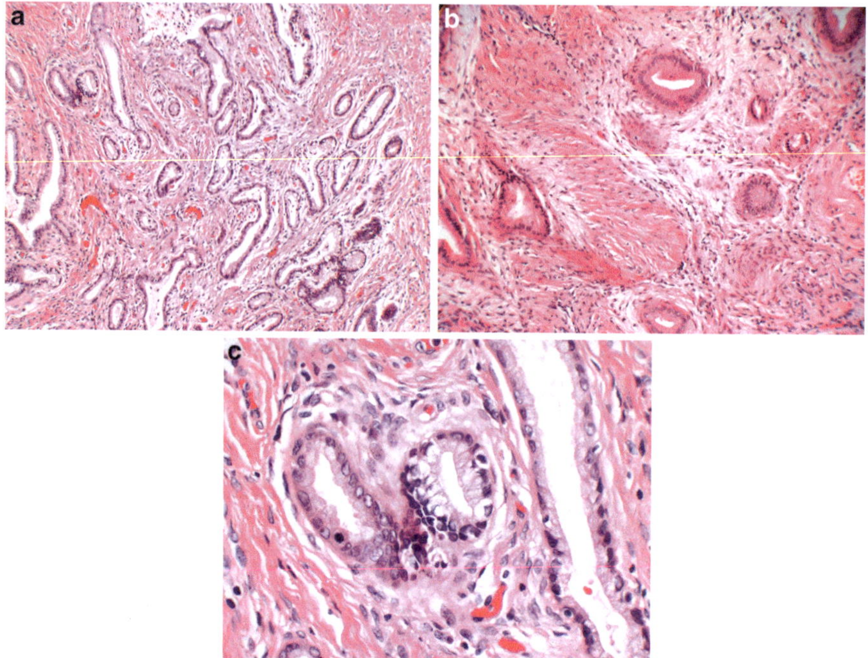

Fig. 5.12 Adenoma malignum. Irregular but minimally atypical glands are deeply invasive (**a**), and elicit a stromal reaction focally (**b**). Atypia and mitoses are sometimes difficult to find, but are present at least focally (**c**)

focal, but must be sought, as it is always at least focally present. Focal stromal reaction, and extension of the glands deeper than the normal crypts are also clues to the correct diagnosis (Fig. 5.12a–c).

5.7.6 Other Variants of Adenocarcinoma

Adenosquamous carcinoma shows features of both squamous cell and adenocarcinoma when well-differentiated. Less differentiated lesions are more solid, suggesting squamous origin, but may have mucin positivity.

Glassy cell carcinoma is an aggressive but uncommon variant of adenocarcinoma where the cytoplasm is prominently glassy (Fig. 5.13).

Adenoid basal carcinoma is rare and tends to be seen in association with SIL. It has not been shown to metastasize, raising the question of whether it actually represents a carcinoma [6] (Fig. 5.14). It must be distinguished from the even rarer aggressive adenoid cystic carcinoma.

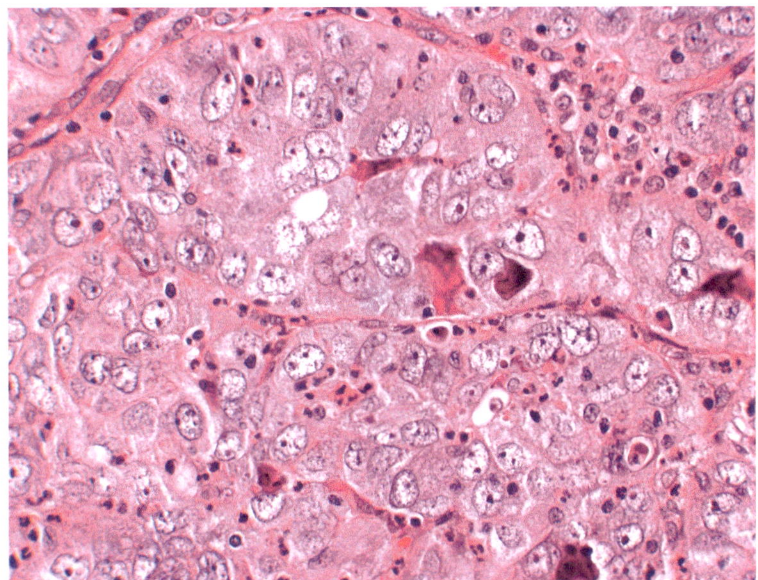

Fig. 5.13 Glassy cell carcinoma. This high-grade adenocarcinoma variant shows prominent nucleoli. Under a microscope, the cytoplasm has a glassy appearance

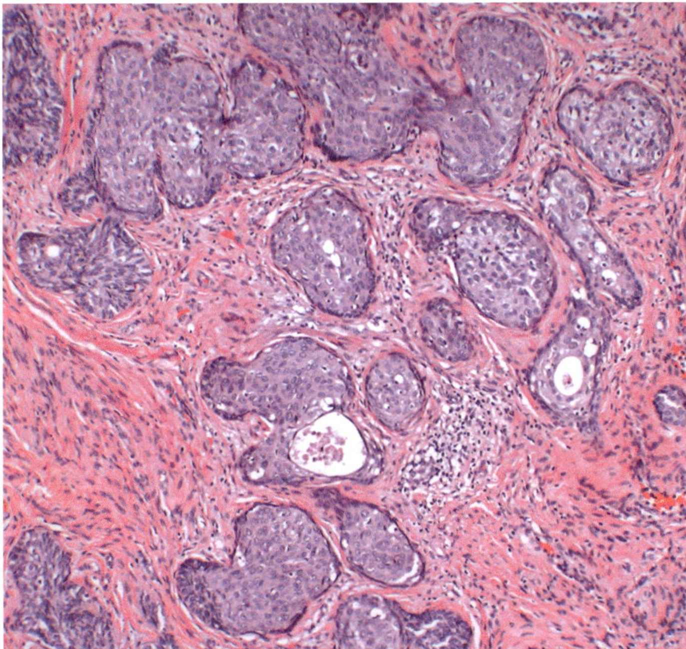

Fig. 5.14 Adenoid basal carcinoma. This lesion is often seen in association with HSIL and consists of nests of cytologically bland cells, some with cystic spaces

5.7.7　Metastatic Carcinoma

The cervix is an uncommon location for a wide variety of metastatic neoplasms, both genital and extragenital. Lymphovascular tumor, tumor only present in the outer portion of the cervix, and lack of an in situ component are important clues, but a good clinical history of prior malignancy, high index of suspicion, and application of immunohistochemistry will be helpful in these cases [7, 8].

References

1. Paavonen J, Vesterinen E, Meyer B, Saksela E. Colposcopic and histologic findings in cervical chlamydial infection. Obstet Gynecol. 1982;59(6):712–5.
2. Darragh TM, Colgan TJ, Cox JT, Heller DS, Henry MR, Luff RD, et al. The lower anogenital squamous terminology standardization project for HPV-associated lesions: background and consensus recommendations from the College of American Pathologists and the American Society for Colposcopy and Cervical Pathology. Int J Gynecol Pathol. 2013;32(1):76–115.
3. Walts AE, Bose S. P16/Ki-67 immunostaining is useful in stratification of atypical metaplastic epithelium of the cervix. Clin Med Pathol. 2008;1:35–42.
4. McCluggage WG. New developments in endocervical glandular lesions. Histopathology. 2013; 62:138–60.
5. Han CP, Lee MY, Tyan YS, Kok LF, Yao CC, Wang PH, Hsu JD. p16 INK4 and CEA can be mutually exchanged with confidence between both relevant three-marker panels (ER/Vim/CEA and ER/Vim/p16 INK4) in distinguishing primary endometrial adenocarcinomas from endocervical adenocarcinomas in a tissue microarray study. Virchows Arch. 2009;455:353–61.
6. Russell MJ, Fadare O. Adenoid basal lesions of the uterine cervix: evolving terminology and clinicopathological concepts. Diagn Pathol. 2006;1:1–14.
7. McCluggage WG, Hurrell DP, Kennedy K. Metastatic carcinomas in the cervix mimicking primary cervical adenocarcinoma and adenocarcinoma in situ. Report of a series of cases. Am J Surg Pathol. 2010;34:735–41.
8. Euscher E, Malpica A. Use of immunohistochemistry in the diagnosis of miscellaneous and metastatic tumors of the uterine corpus and cervix. Semin Diagn Pathol. 2014;31:233–57.

6.1 Lesions of the Endometrium

Endometrial biopsies are among the more common gynecologic specimens received by a pathology laboratory. Most biopsies are performed for abnormal uterine bleeding. Abnormal uterine bleeding can be thought of in categories, including organic (structural abnormalities such as polyps or leiomyomas), dysfunctional (hormonal flux), hyperplastic, or neoplastic. The age and menstrual status of the patient make certain lesions more likely at different stages of life. For example, anovulation is an underlying etiology for abnormal bleeding at both ends of the reproductive spectrum.

Endometrial biopsies may provide abundant or scant tissue, based on the lesion, the age and hormonal status of the patient, and sometimes the skill of the operator. Clinicians should be aware that what appears as a great deal of tissue may be mostly blood clot. A clinical history is extremely helpful for the pathologist, as there are many processes that, while benign, do not match up with what is in histology books. Pertinent history includes age, last menstrual period, any recent pregnancy, any prior pertinent surgery such as curettage, myomectomy, or ablation, endometrial instrumentation or IUD use, and any hormonal therapy that may impact on the endometrium. In the absence of an appropriate history, for example of exogenous hormones, a longer and less clear report may result (see Tables 6.1 and 6.2).

6.2 Infections and Inflammations of the Endometrium

6.2.1 Acute Endometritis

Acute endometritis is not a common finding. It was more commonly seen in the era of illegal septic abortions. Histologically, a neutrophilic infiltrate is seen within glands, forming microabscesses and involving and "chewing on" the

© Springer International Publishing Switzerland 2015

D.S. Heller, *OB-GYN Pathology for the Clinician*,

DOI 10.1007/978-3-319-15422-0_6

Table 6.1 Importance of providing clinical history with an endometrial biopsy

Report 1 without history
– Endometrium showing decidualized stroma and small inactive glands. This finding may represent exogenous progestin effect. Clinical correlation suggested
Report 1 with history
– Benign endometrium with features consistent with progestin effect
Report 2 without history
– Irregularly developed endometrium with proliferative areas and secretory areas. There is focal glandular crowding
Report 2 with history
– Irregularly developed benign endometrium consistent with history of hormone replacement therapy

Table 6.2 Key points about endometrial pathology

– An abundant biopsy may represent estrogen effect, hyperplasia, neoplasia, or benign endometrium stimulated by hormones (late proliferative, secretory)
– A scant biopsy may represent atrophy, prolonged bleeding, Asherman's syndrome, drug effect (i.e., GnRH agonists, progestins), cervical stenosis, or operator inexperience
– Partially treated (by progestins) atypical endometrial hyperplasia may show glandular crowding but atypia can no longer be assessed

glandular epithelium (Fig. 6.1). This needs to be distinguished from the normal physiologic neutrophils associated with breakdown of endometrium with menses, or decidua after a gestation, where inflammation does not signify infection. In menstrual breakdown, there is not the formation of microabscesses, and the neutrophils are not specifically involving glandular epithelium.

6.2.2 Chronic Endometritis

Chronic endometritis may be caused by identifiable organisms such as actinomyces or tuberculosis; however, an etiology is usually not apparent. Chronic endometritis may be associated with IUD use, history of instrumentation, submucous leiomyomata, or retained placenta, but often it is unclear what the underlying etiology is. It is debated in the literature whether the histologic finding of chronic endometritis corresponds to abnormal uterine bleeding, or is just an incidental finding. Histologically, chronic endometritis is diagnosed when plasma cells are seen in the endometrium (Fig. 6.2a). A hypercellular or spindled stroma (Fig. 6.2b)

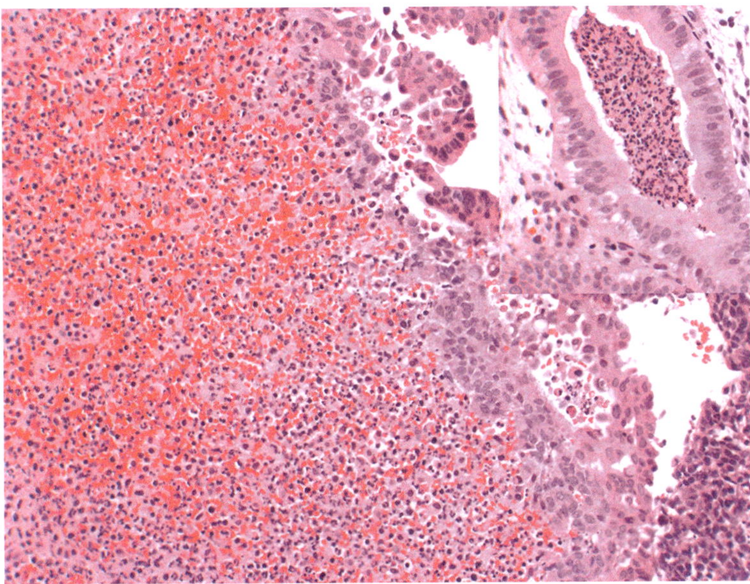

Fig. 6.1 Acute endometritis, with a neutrophilic infiltrate replacing stroma. This purulent exudate can also be seen involving glands (*inset*)

suggests that plasma cells should be sought. Other types of inflammatory cells (lymphocytes, neutrophils) are present physiologically during the menstrual cycle and do not indicate chronic endometritis.

6.3 Exogenous Hormones

Exogenous hormones exert varying influences on the endometrium. Age and hormonal milieu of the patient as well as the type of drug and duration of use influence the findings, so it is important to provide a clinical history, so that appropriate correlation can be made [1]. It should be remembered that endogenous hormones also may affect the endometrium, such as an estrogen-producing granulosa cell tumor, and these neoplasms should also be considered in clinically appropriate situations.

6.3.1 Oral Contraceptives and Progestins

Histologic manifestations of oral contraceptives on the endometrium relate to the progestin-dominant effects. Early on in administration, the stroma appears spindled,

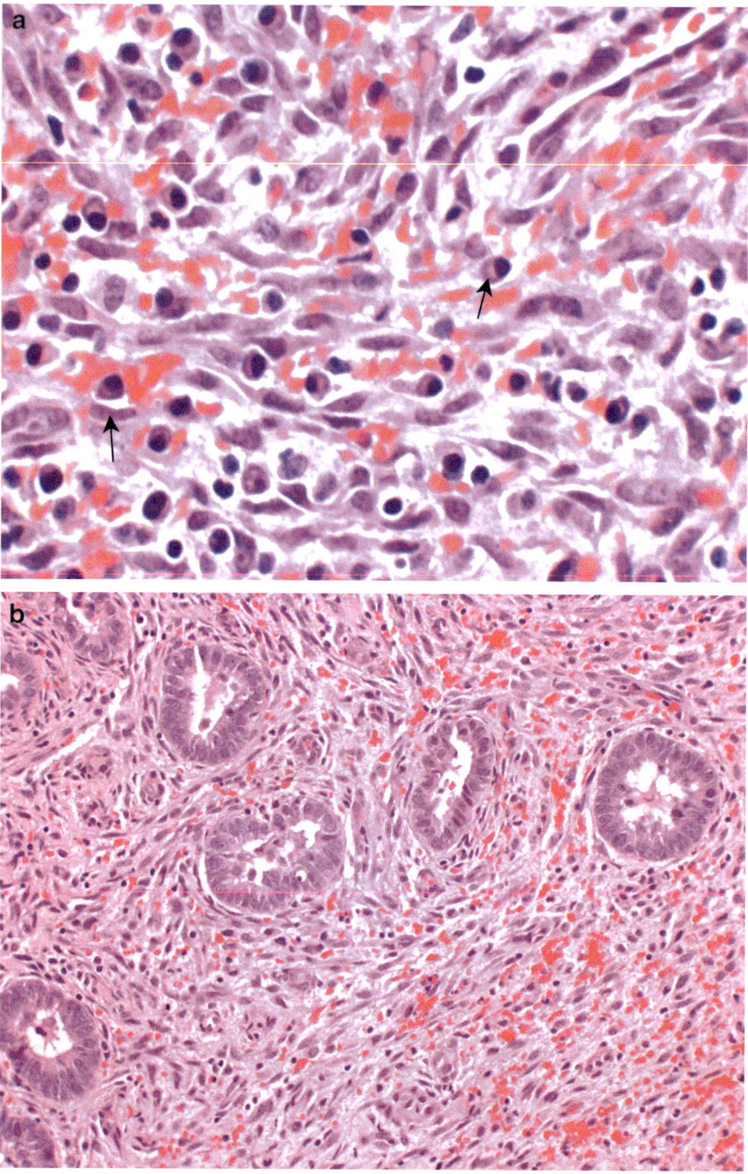

Fig. 6.2 Chronic endometritis is assessed by identifying plasma cells in the stroma (**a**, *arrows*). A spindled cell (**b**) or hypercellular stroma is a clue that plasma cells should be sought

and the glands become small and inactive (Fig. 6.3a). Over time, the stroma becomes decidualized. It is this combination of decidualized stroma and tiny inactive glands that confirms exogenous progestin exposure. Progestins used therapeutically for abnormal bleeding usually show stromal decidualization directly, without a spindle cell stromal phase (Fig. 6.3b).

6.3.2   Hormone Replacement Therapy

Hormone replacement comes in many combinations, so there is no one finding. In general, the effects tend to be a mix of estrogenic and progestational, hence a mix of proliferative and secretory changes may be seen. This "confused" endometrium does not appear neoplastic, but doesn't fit textbook categorization. A history provided to the pathologist will lead to a shorter more comprehensible diagnosis (see Table 6.1).

6.3.3   Ovulation Induction

Ovulation induction can lead to unusual patterns. Clomiphene-affected endometrium can show an exaggerated day 17 pattern with prominent subnuclear vacuoles. Administration of follicle-stimulating hormone/luteinizing hormone may lead to gland-stromal dating dissociation, with the glands showing day 17–18 features and stroma showing day 22–23 features.

6.3.4   GnRH agonists

Gonadotropin-releasing hormone agonists may lead to atrophic endometrium.

6.3.5   Tamoxifen

A variety of hyperplastic and neoplastic lesions have occasionally been associated with tamoxifen. Most often, tamoxifen exerts a weak estrogenic effect on the post-menopausal endometrium. Endometrial polyps are also not uncommon.

6.4   Benign Lesions of the Endometrium

6.4.1   Organic (Structural) Lesions

6.4.1.1 Endometrial Polyps

Endometrial polyps are common. They are polypoid lesions composed of irregular, and sometimes, dilated endometrial epithelial-lined glands in a stroma more fibrotic than native endometrium and containing prominent stalk vessels.

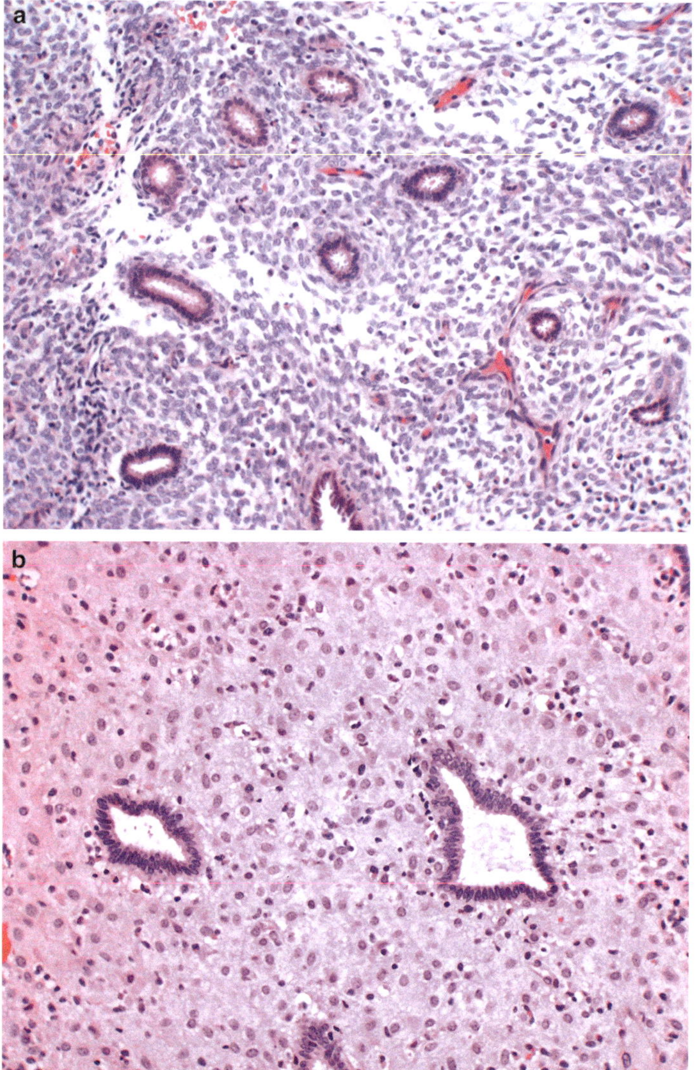

Fig. 6.3 Oral contraceptive pills affect the endometrium by leading to small inactive glands. Initially the stroma is spindled (**a**). Later, the stroma is decidualized (**b**) and appears similar to progestational therapy

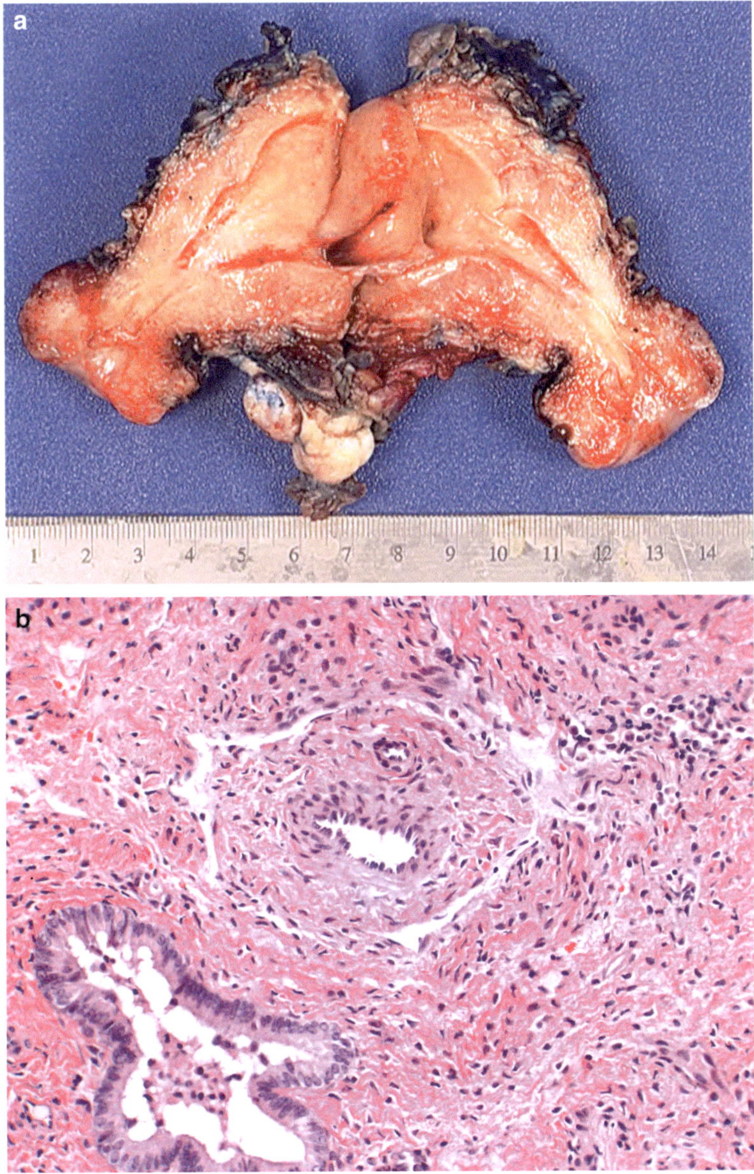

Fig. 6.4 Endometrial polyp distorting the cavity (**a**). The irregular glands are in a fibrotic stroma with thick stalk vessels (**b**)

If intact, a surface lining of endometrial-type epithelium may be seen. If fragmented, as can occur during removal by curettage, not all of the features may be discernable, leading the pathologist to make a diagnosis of a possible polyp, rather than a definitive one (Fig. 6.4a, b).

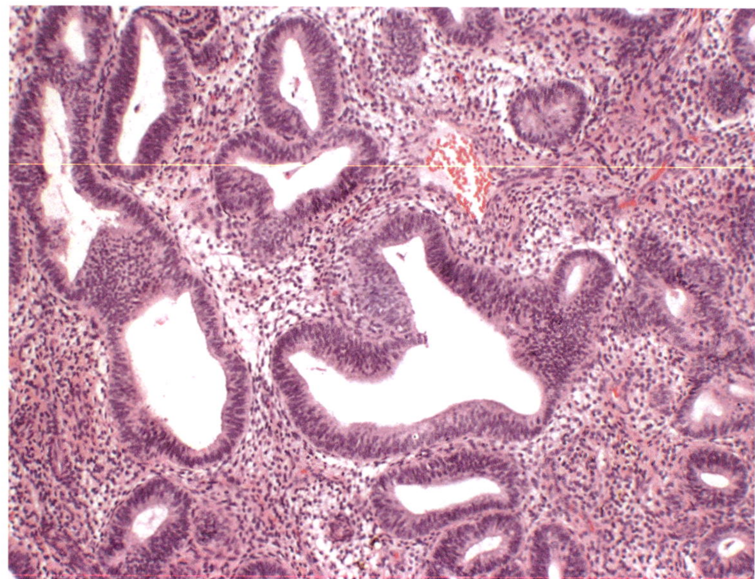

Fig. 6.5 Disordered proliferation shows occasional dilated glands, but no increase in gland to stromal ratio

6.4.1.2 Endometrium Overlying Submucous Leiomyomas

The endometrium overlying leiomyomas may become attenuated and even ulcerated, with resultant pressure atrophy. Chronic endometritis is sometimes associated.

6.4.2 Dysfunctional Uterine Bleeding

After organic (structural) abnormalities have been ruled out, the most common underlying etiology leading to an endometrial biopsy is probably dysfunctional uterine bleeding, which is essentially due to hormonal imbalance. In most cases, this is anovulatory. There is unopposed estrogen, which may not be of sufficient duration or effect to see hyperplasia or neoplasia. The most common associated histologic finding is disordered proliferation (Fig. 6.5), which shows a basically proliferative pattern with occasional dilated or crowded glands insufficient to warrant a diagnosis of hyperplasia.

6.4.3 Endometrial Hyperplasia

Endometrial hyperplasia is currently classified by two systems. The World Health Organization classification uses Simple, Complex, and Atypical (complex hyperplasia with atypia) hyperplasia (Figs. 6.6a, b, 6.7, and 6.8a, b). Simple and complex

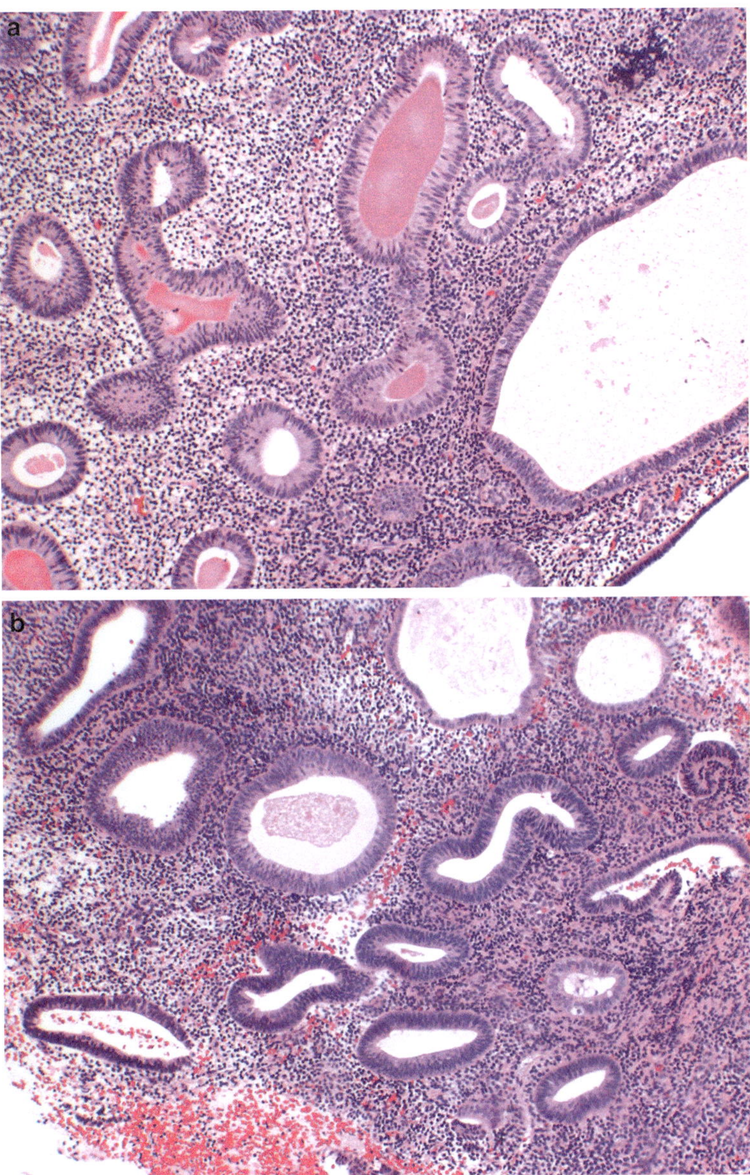

Fig. 6.6 Simple hyperplasia shows a mild increase in gland to stromal ratio (**a**), with dilated glands (**b**)

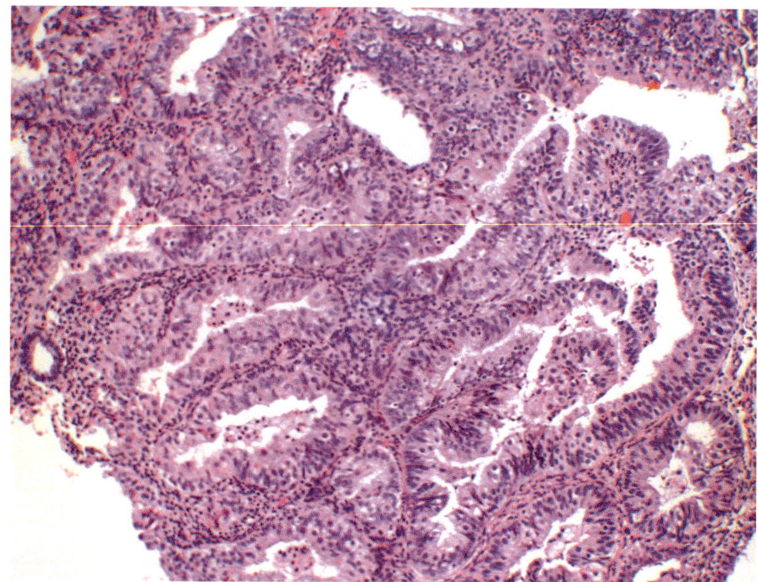

Fig. 6.7 Complex hyperplasia shows increased glandular crowding compared to simple hyperplasia, but stroma is still present

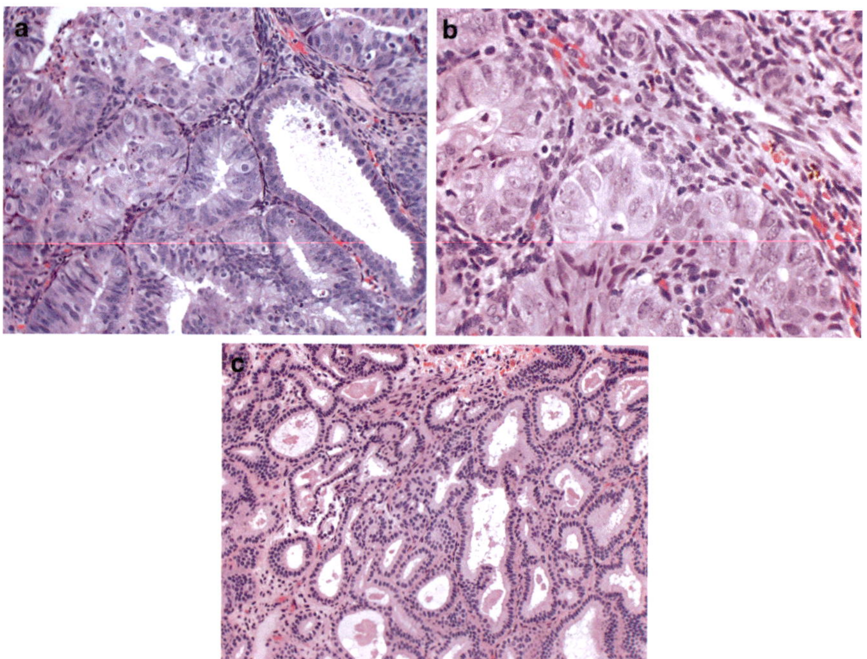

Fig. 6.8 Atypical hyperplasia (complex hyperplasia with atypia) shows crowded glands with nuclear atypia as well as tubal metaplasia seen on the left (**a**). A non-atypical gland is seen on the right. On higher power, nuclear atypia with rounded nuclei and prominent nucleoli are seen (**b**). Treated atypical hyperplasia (**c**) shows incomplete resolution in this case, with glandular crowding. The progestins make assessment of nuclear atypia no longer possible

refer to the degree of glandular crowding, with simple hyperplasia showing mild crowding and mildly increased gland to stroma ratio. Glands may be cystic and show outpouchings resembling "rabbit ears." Complex hyperplasia shows more glandular crowding, with a significantly increased gland to stroma ratio, but still some stroma between. Atypical hyperplasia refers to nuclear atypia, where the nuclei of the glandular epithelial cells, instead of their usual oval shape, become rounded, with margination of chromatin and prominent nucleoli. While there is such a thing as simple atypical hyperplasia, it is so uncommon that it often gets dropped from the usage of the terminology. This terminology was created to distinguish the only lesion significantly associated with either an unsampled adjacent carcinoma or risk of developing carcinoma in the future, which is atypical hyperplasia [2, 3].

It has been found that discrimination between grades of hyperplasia may not always be reproducible, and a second terminology is also in use in some laboratories. Based originally on morphometric measurements, as well as molecular alterations, but converted to applicable histopathologic criteria that assess amount of relative stroma to glands, the EIN system (endometrial intraepithelial neoplasia) separates hyperplasia (no significant cancer risk) from EIN, with risk. Like the first system, there are some who favor its use more than others [4, 5]. Interested readers can review http://www.endometrium.org/ for examples of this methodology.

6.4.4   Treated Hyperplasia

A diagnosis of atypical hyperplasia may lead to hysterectomy, if the patient is finished with reproduction; however, uterine sparing therapy may be undertaken. Thus, some atypical hyperplasias, as well as the lesser degrees of hyperplasia, may be treated by progestins. As part of follow-up of hormonally treated hyperplasias, repeat biopsies may be taken after progestational therapy and may show a wide pattern of partially treated responses (Fig. 6.8c). Again, providing a clinical history is important in these cases and will lead to a diagnosis indicating a partially resolved hyperplasia, rather than a long descriptive paragraph for an endometrium that fits no textbook description. A variety of partial response patterns may be seen. The stroma may become decidualized as is usual with progestins, but degrees of glandular crowding may persist. If the hyperplasia was associated with squamous metaplasia with morules (see below), the squamous morules take a longer time to regress than the glandular changes. If the original diagnosis was atypical hyperplasia, the atypia tends to disappear histologically with progestins, so that while glandular crowding may persist, nuclear atypia may not be identifiable.

6.4.5   Endometrial Metaplasias

There are a number of metaplasias that can be seen in the endometrium. Metaplasia is the change from one benign cell type to another. The endometrial metaplasias are often associated with unopposed estrogen and seen in association with endometrial

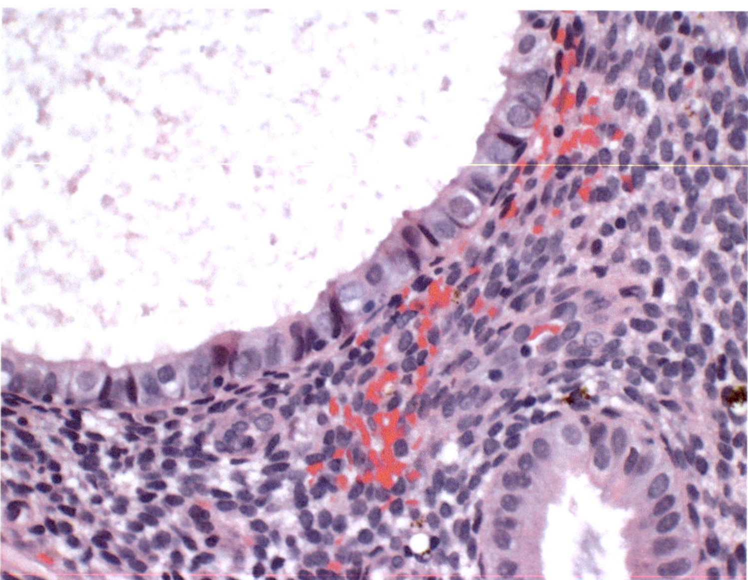

Fig. 6.9 Tubal metaplasia showing the epithelial types seen in fallopian tube. Cilia are present on some of the columnar cells

hyperplasia, but may be seen without hyperplasia as well. They may not be reported in pathology reports, as there is no therapy needed for metaplasia in the absence of other pathology however may signify need for follow-up, particularly in an older patient. Among the more commonly seen metaplasias are tubal metaplasia (Fig. 6.9) and squamous metaplasia, which may be mature squamous epithelium, or immature balls of squamous epithelium known as morules (Fig. 6.10). Squamous differentiation may also be seen in usual endometrioid endometrial adenocarcinoma (see section on endometrial carcinoma).

6.5   Malignant Lesions of Endometrium

6.5.1   Endometrial Adenocarcinoma

Endometrial adenocarcinoma occurs by two distinct molecular mechanisms. Usual, type I endometrial adenocarcinoma is associated with PTEN mutations and unopposed estrogen. Patients tend to be slightly younger than type II patients and more obese. Staging is currently a clinicopathologic one, and prognosis is based among other things on differentiation of the tumor and depth of invasion, both of which can sometimes be asked for during an intraoperative consultation at hysterectomy (frozen section) (Fig. 6.11a–d). Differentiation is easier to assess on a preoperative

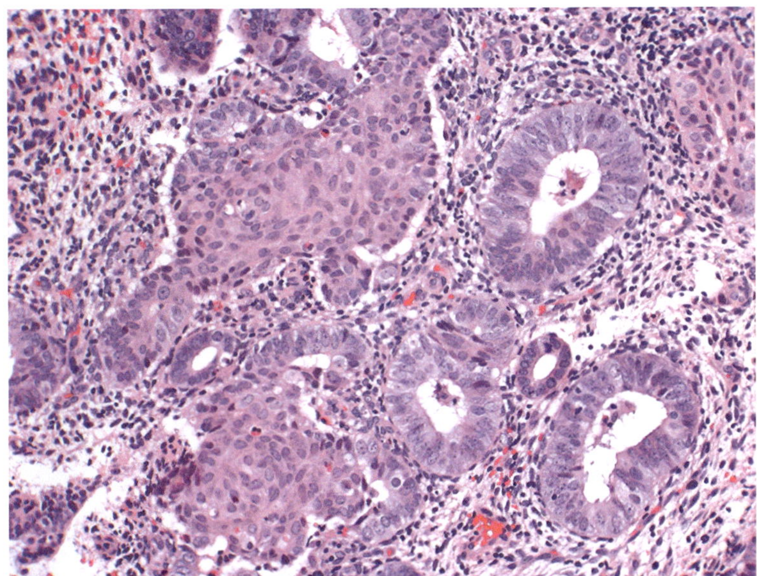

Fig. 6.10 Simple hyperplasia with squamous metaplasia. The squamous metaplasia seen in the center makes assessing degree of glandular crowding difficult

biopsy or curettage, but may potentially lead to under- or overgrading of the tumor, as differentiation is predominantly based on the percent of the tumor that is solid rather than glandular. This differs from most other malignancies, where cytologic features carry greater weight in grading. However, marked nuclear atypia permits upgrading 1° from the architecture in usual endometrioid adenocarcinoma. Both grading and staging are performed using the FIGO criteria. Grade 1 tumors are no more than 5 % solid, grade 2 are 6–50 %, and grade 3 are over 50 % solid. Extensive squamous differentiation can make this assessment difficult; however, squamous differentiation does not count in grading these lesions. A variant of usual endometrioid (type I) adenocarcinoma is a villoglandular pattern, mimicking a tubular adenoma of the colon (Fig. 6.11e). This should not be mistaken for a serous carcinoma of the endometrium, which shows a great deal more cytologic atypia.

The second group of molecular mechanisms for endometrial carcinoma is less common. Type 2 lesions are seen in slightly older, thinner women and are not related to unopposed estrogen. Most of these lesions are uterine serous carcinomas, which show p53 mutations (Fig. 6.12). Uterine serous carcinoma spreads similarly to the ovarian counterpart, over peritoneal surfaces, as opposed to the spread patterns of usual endometrioid carcinoma. Another lesion under this category, clear cell adenocarcinoma (Fig. 6.13a, b), is a much less common, aggressive lesion. Both uterine serous and clear cell adenocarcinomas are considered grade 3.

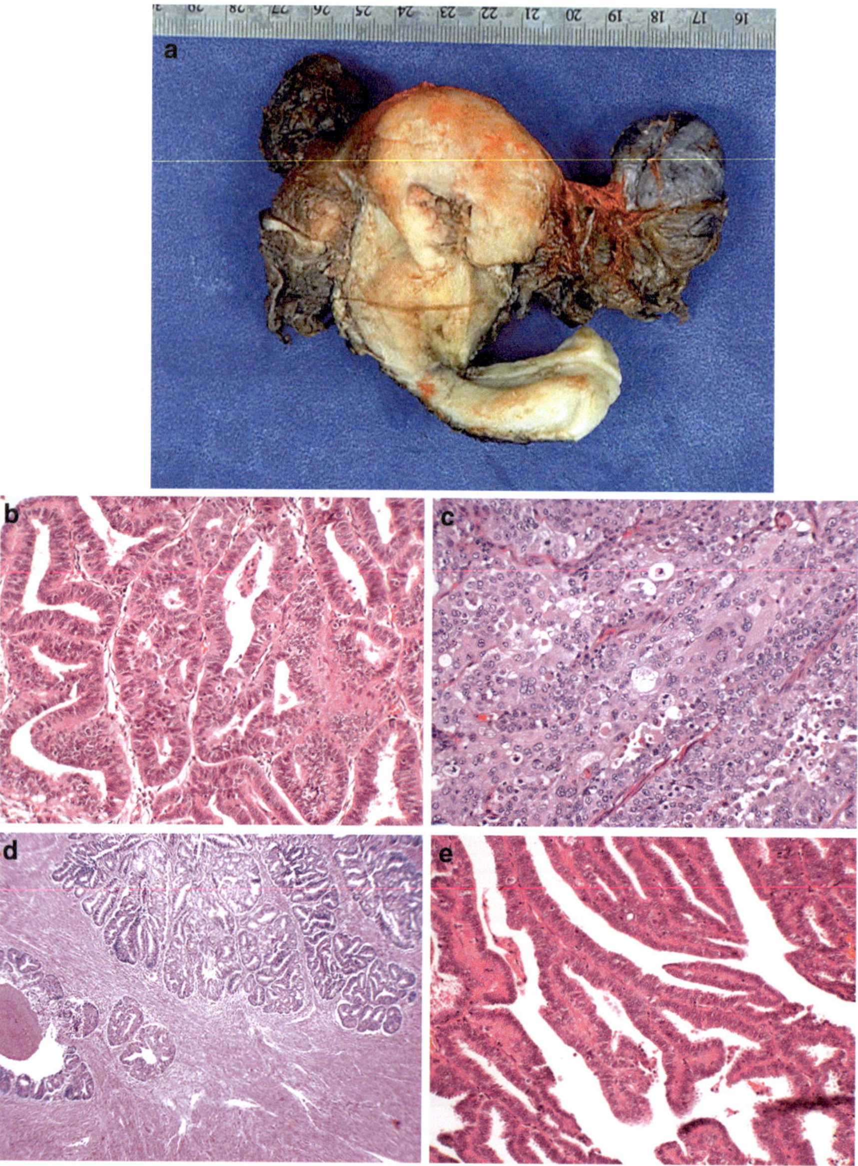

Fig. 6.11 Endometrial carcinoma. Grossly the lesion is involving the entire endometrium in this case (**a**). Well-differentiated adenocarcinoma is predominantly composed of back to back glands (**b**), while a poorly differentiated tumor is over 50 % solid (**c**). Moderately differentiation falls in between. Tumor is assessed for percentage of myometrial invasion (**d**) by measuring from the endometrial–myometrial junction to the deepest tumor depth, and assessing its percentage of myometrial thickness. The villoglandular pattern of endometrioid shows delicate fibrovascular cores (**e**) and should not be mistaken for uterine serous carcinoma

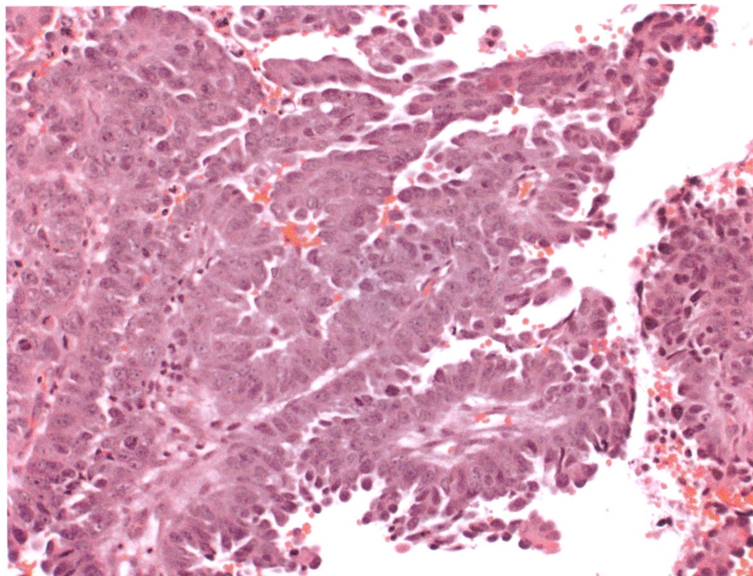

Fig. 6.12 Uterine serous carcinoma, with broad fibrovascular cores lined by markedly atypical epithelium with prominent nucleoli

6.5.2   Malignant Mixed Mesodermal (Müllerian) Tumor (MMMT) (Carcinosarcoma)

Carcinosarcomas are considered metaplastic carcinomas with sarcomatous differentiation. These aggressive lesions are grossly polypoid (Fig. 6.14a). Histologically, the carcinomatous component may be usual endometrioid adenocarcinoma, but serous and squamous areas may be seen. Sarcomatous differentiation may be homologous, with differentiation native to the uterus, such as stromal sarcoma, leiomyosarcoma, or undifferentiated sarcoma, or heterologous, not native to the uterus, such as chondrosarcoma or rhabdomyosarcoma (Fig. 6.14b, c). This is not thought to alter prognosis.

6.5.3   Adenosarcoma

Adenosarcomas are rare polypoid lesions composed of benign endometrial type glands cuffed by a sarcomatous stroma. They are less aggressive than carcinosarcoma.

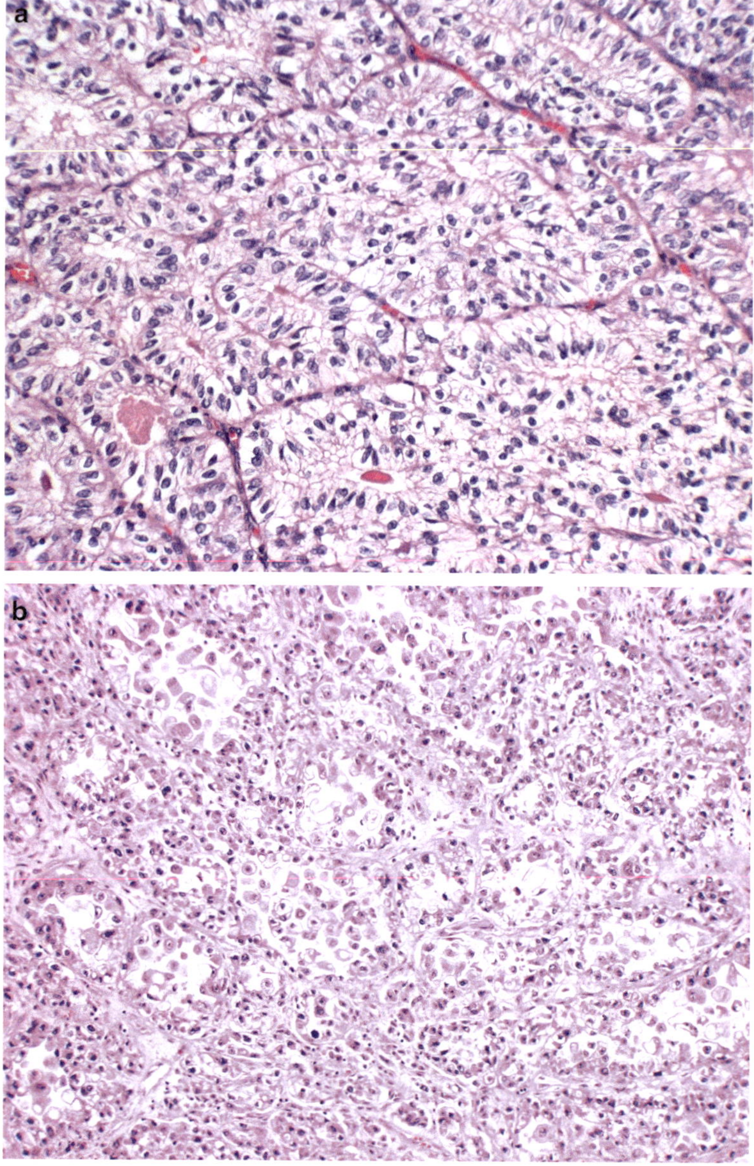

Fig. 6.13 Clear cell adenocarcinoma may appear as sheets of clear cells (**a**), or may show a tubulopapillary pattern (**b**)

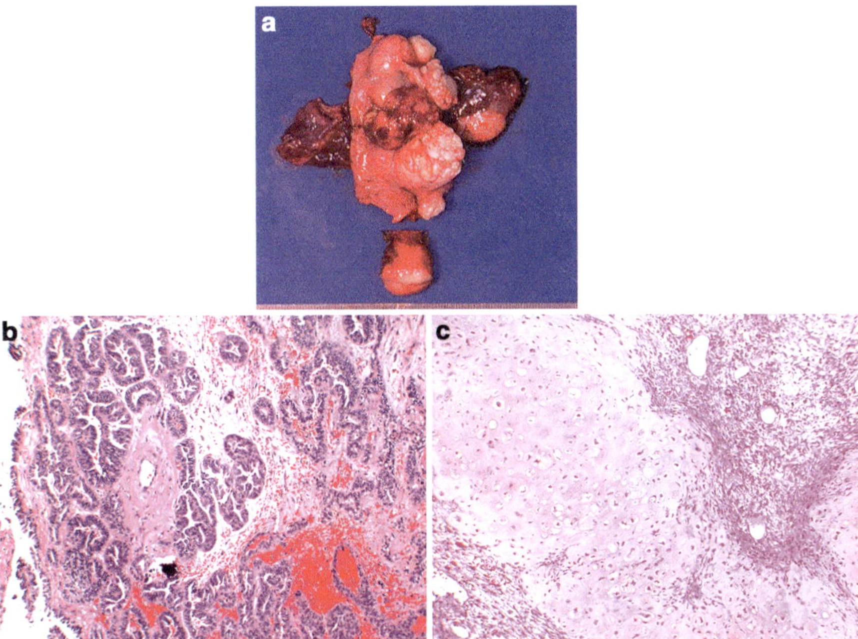

Fig. 6.14 Carcinosarcoma (MMMT) is often a polypoid lesion (**a**), composed of carcinomatous (**b**) and sarcomatous elements. A heterologous chondrosarcoma is shown (**c**)

References

1. Heller DS. Handbook of endometrial pathology. London: JP Medical Ltd; 2012.
2. Kurman RJ, Kaminski PF, Norris HJ. The behavior of endometrial hyperplasia: a long-term study of "untreated" hyperplasia in 170 patients. Cancer. 1985;56:403–12.
3. Clark TJ, Neelakantan D, Gupta JK. The management of endometrial hyperplasia: an evaluation of current practice. Eur J Obstet Gynecol Reprod Biol. 2006;125:259–64.
4. Owings RA, Quick CM. Endometrial intraepithelial neoplasia. Arch Pathol Lab Med. 2014;138:484–91.
5. Kane SE, Hecht JL. Endometrial intraepithelial neoplasia terminology in practice: 4-year experience at a single institution. Int J Gynecol Pathol. 2012;31:160–5.

Diseases of the Myometrium

7

7.1 Lesims of the Myometrium

Specimens received by pathology laboratories for myometrial pathology sometimes pose unique challenges (Table 7.1). Diseases of the myometrium are discussed in this chapter.

7.2 Congenital Anomalies of the Uterus

The uterus is formed by fusion of the two Müllerian ducts and resorption of the resultant intervening septum. Anomalies are uncommon, but may include agenesis, dysgenesis, or varying types of duplication. Agenesis or dysgenesis may present as lack of onset of menses in adolescence. Lesions that are associated with obstruction to menstrual egress may present at menarche with symptoms of pain and an expanding mass, such as in duplication with a blind uterine horn. Lesions with menstrual egress may not show symptoms or may present with issues relating to fertility.

7.3 Benign Lesions of the Myometrium

7.3.1 Adenomyosis

Adenomyosis is an extremely common finding in hysterectomy specimens. While the old name "endometriosis interna" referred to the nests of endometrial glands and stroma within the myometrium, which are required for histologic confirmation, the mechanism is thought to be totally different in adenomyosis than endometriosis. Adenomyosis is thought to connect with the surface endometrium [1], essentially representing diverticular outpouchings. Grossly, adenomyosis may markedly enlarge the uterus (Fig. 7.1a), although this enlargement is lacking in circumscription as seen in leiomyomata. On cut surface, small punctate bleeding sites are

© Springer International Publishing Switzerland 2015
D.S. Heller, *OB-GYN Pathology for the Clinician*,
DOI 10.1007/978-3-319-15422-0_7

Table 7.1 Key points about myometrial pathology

The distinction between an endometrial stromal nodule and a low-grade endometrial stromal sarcoma can rarely be made on a biopsy or curettage specimen and often necessitates hysterectomy
Adenomyosis involved by adenocarcinoma should be reported, but does not factor into the measurement of tumor depth of invasion
Confirmation of leiomyosarcoma requires consideration of additional factors besides mitotic count, including hemorrhage, lack of circumscription, atypia, and tumor cell necrosis. This may require many sections
It may not be feasible to distinguish leiomyoma from leiomyosarcoma on frozen section

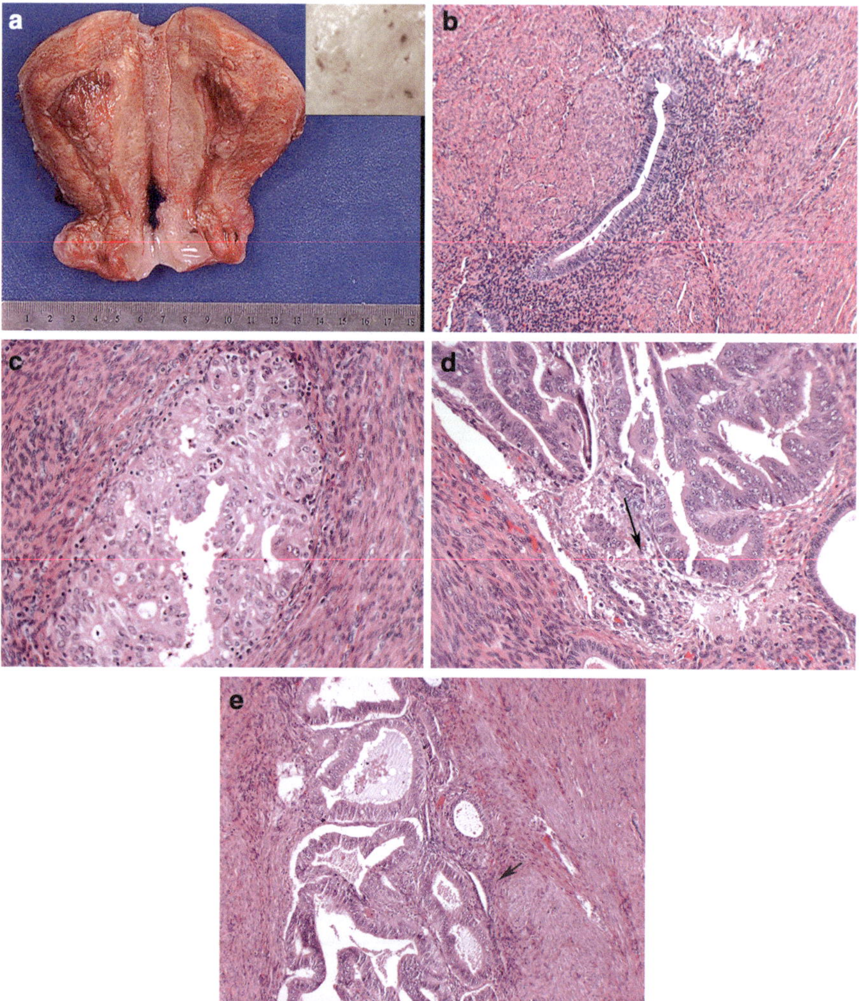

Fig. 7.1 Uterus diffusely enlarged by adenomyosis (**a**). Punctate areas may show hemorrhage (*inset*). Histologically the lesion is composed of endometrial glands and stroma within the myometrium (**b**). Endometrial carcinoma can involve adenomyosis, with features including rounded nests away from invading carcinoma (**c**), stroma seen amid the glands (**d**, *arrow*), and (**e**) benign glands (*arrow*) admixed with malignant serving as diagnostic clues

sometimes apparent in adenomyosis. Histology shows endometrial glands and stroma within the myometrium ((Fig. 7.1b). Occasionally, adenomyosis forms partially circumscribed nodules, "adenomyomas," which may be clinically interpreted as leiomyomas, but which lack the well-defined pseudocapsule of leiomyomas, leading at times to increased operative blood loss when "myomectomy" is attempted and cleavage planes are less well-defined.

A potential pitfall for pathologists is distinguishing myometrial invasion of an endometrial adenocarcinoma from carcinomatous transformation of an adenomyotic focus, thought to be a field effect (Fig. 7.1c–e). Identification of stroma around the crowded atypical glands or residual benign glands is helpful, but immunohistochemistry may show overlapping features between carcinoma in adenomyosis and true myometrial invasion, limiting utility [2]. The depth of invasion of an endometrial carcinoma is measured to the deepest true invasion, not from tumor in adenomyotic foci, although these foci should be reported separately. It has been suggested that adenocarcinomatous transformation of adenomyotic foci is a risk factor for associated myometrial invasion [3].

7.3.2   Leiomyoma

Symptomatic leiomyomata are among the most common reasons for performance of a hysterectomy. Upon receipt of a hysterectomy for uterine fibroids, the specimen is weighted and the location of the fibroids described (submucous, intramural, subserosal) (Fig. 7.2a). The location may explain some of the symptomatology, with submucous fibroids more likely to cause abnormal uterine bleeding, and anterior subserosal or intramural large fibroids more likely to cause urinary symptoms, etc. Leiomyomas are well circumscribed, with a pseudocapsule. This is not a true capsule with a delineating membrane, but a compression of surrounding myometrium. This pseudocapsule (Fig. 7.2b) is what creates the surgical planes that permit ease of myomectomy. Histologically, leiomyomas usually resemble the adjacent uterine smooth muscle, with elongated cells with oval cigar-shaped nuclei (see Fig. 2.27). Leiomyomas have a tendency to outgrow their blood supply. They are estrogen-sensitive, and hence may grow rapidly in pregnancy and tend to regress in menopause. Degenerative changes of varying types may be seen. Some of these may raise both clinical and histopathological concern for leiomyosarcoma (see below). Benign degenerative changes that are commonly seen histologically and not likely to raise concern for the pathologist include hyalinization, with areas of acellular pink material and calcification.

7.3.3   Symplastic Leiomyoma

An uncommon but potentially concerning variant of leiomyoma is symplastic leiomyoma. This variant is benign, and of no additional clinical significance, but may raise concern of malignancy for the pathologist due to the pronounced cytologic atypia (Fig. 7.3). However, symplastic leiomyoma lacks the other diagnostic hallmarks of leiomyosarcoma (see below).

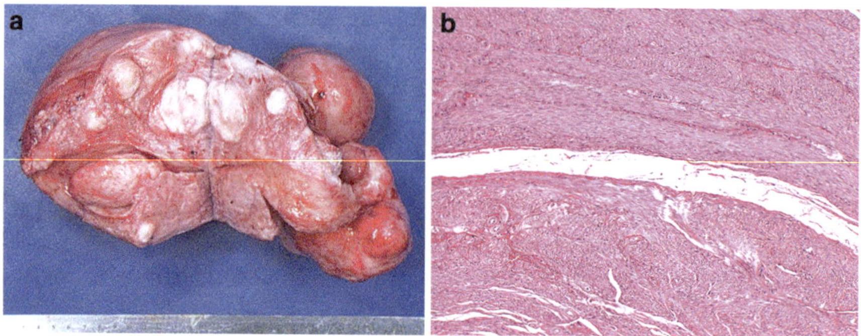

Fig. 7.2 Submucous and intramural well-circumscribed leiomyomas (**a**). Histologically (**b**) the pseudocapsule is composed of compressed myometrium (*top* of image), which is delineated from the leiomyoma (*bottom* of image)

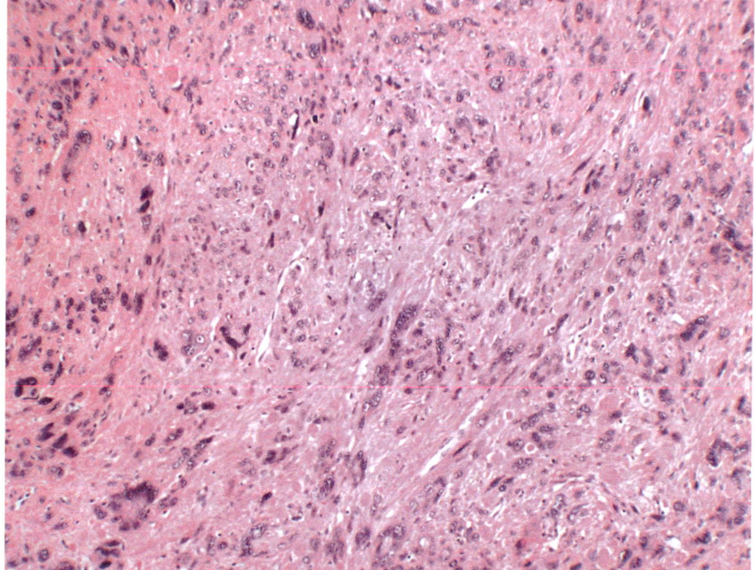

Fig. 7.3 Symplastic leiomyoma showing diffuse atypia but no mitotic activity

7.3.4   Extrauterine Leiomyomas

A variety of lesions histologically identical to benign leiomyomas but in unusual places can rarely be seen. These include parasitic leiomyomas, benign metastasizing leiomyomas, diffuse peritoneal leiomyomatosis, and intravenous leiomyomatosis.

Parasitic leiomyomas are leiomyomas that have lost their uterine blood supply and reestablished blood flow from a peritoneal surface, hence becoming "parasitic."

They may occur spontaneously, but reports of cases associated with surgical procedures such as the uterine morcellator have appeared [4]. Benign metastasizing leiomyoma is composed of multiple benign smooth muscle nodules, most often in the lungs, although a variety of other locations have occurred. The condition may be interpreted clinically as metastatic disease. Diffuse peritoneal leiomyomatosis consists of multiple peritoneal implants, grossly mimicking peritoneal carcinomatosis [5]. Intravenous leiomyomatosis is a rare condition with cords of histologically benign smooth muscle identical to a leiomyoma getting into the venous system. Although a benign lesion, intravenous leiomyomatosis can get into the inferior vena cava and reach the right heart, causing death [5].

7.3.5 Stromal Nodule

Stromal nodules are composed of cells that resemble the stroma of proliferative endometrium. This is an uncommon benign lesion. The issue that may arise is that histologically these lesions look identical to low-grade endometrial stromal sarcoma (see below), but are distinguished by circumscription and lack of invasion. This makes the distinction between the two lesions unfeasible on most curettage specimens where the periphery can't be assessed, and a hysterectomy may be the only way to make the distinction. As this lesion may occur during reproductive age, this can pose a significant problem.

7.4 Malignant Neoplasms of the Myometrium

7.4.1 Leiomyosarcoma

Both clinicians and pathologists worry about missing a diagnosis of leiomyosarcoma. Leiomyosarcomas are uncommon lesions, with malignant degeneration of leiomyomas extremely rare. Clinically, rapid growth of a smooth muscle neoplasm may raise concern. Grossly, the first factor to raise concern for the pathologist may be a "fish flesh" appearance of sarcomas, instead of the usual firm white whorled nodule, but this may simply represent edema and degeneration. Gross hemorrhage and lack of circumscription are important gross clues (Fig. 7.4). Histologically, there are several things to look for (Fig. 7.5a–e). Mitotic activity (mitoses per ten high power fields), atypia and atypical mitoses, tumor cell necrosis with apoptosis, and hemorrhage are all significant factors. In different permutations, these features will designate a lesion as benign, malignant, or of uncertain malignant potential [6]. There is not one single diagnostic criterion, but among the most significant is tumor cell necrosis (Fig. 7.5a), with apoptotic debris, which differs from the non-apoptotic hyalinization seen in benign degeneration.

Because of the complexity of establishing a diagnosis of leiomyosarcoma on histology, a frozen section diagnosis may not be possible. Frozen section slides are

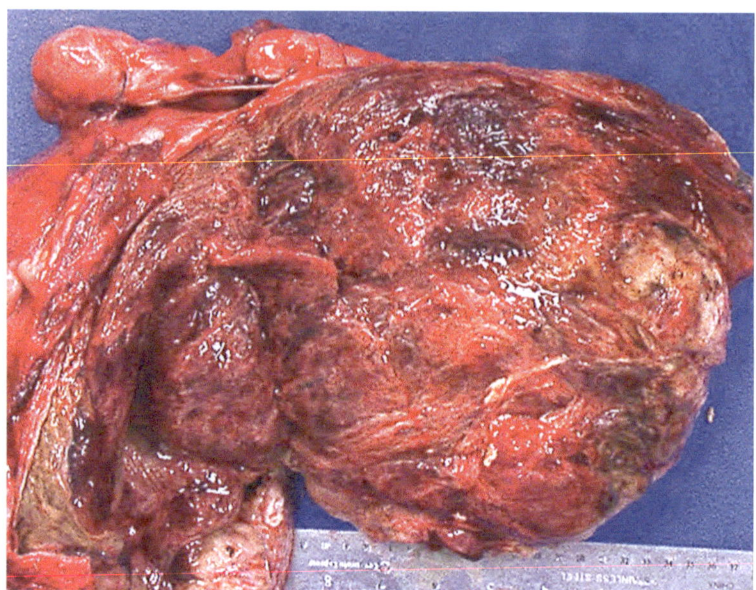

Fig. 7.4 Leiomyosarcoma. The lesion is hemorrhagic and poorly circumscribed

not of as high quality as a permanent section after fixation, and mitoses may not be readily discernable. In addition, extensive sampling of a lesion may be required to assess all the diagnostic features. Clinicians should be cognizant that a deferral may be provided in frozen section consultations on such a case.

7.4.2   Endometrial Stromal Sarcoma

Low-grade endometrial stromal sarcoma is an indolent low-grade malignancy. This unusual lesion has a propensity to extend into lymphvascular spaces of the uterus and adnexa in a worm-like pattern (Fig. 7.6). Histologically, the lesion resembles the stroma of benign proliferative endometrium (Fig. 7.7a, b). Low-grade stromal sarcoma shares a common translocation with stromal nodule, JAZF1–SUZ12. The more unusual high-grade endometrial stromal sarcomas are distinguished by greater atypia with retention of resemblance to endometrial stroma, and a different translocation, YWHAE–FAM22. Their behavior is more aggressive than low-grade stromal sarcomas, but less aggressive than undifferentiated sarcomas, which have a variety of chromosomal aberrations [7], and simply resemble an undifferentiated spindle cell sarcoma, similar to the sarcomatous portion seen in some carcinosarcomas. Sometimes the distinction between an endometrial stromal lesion and a smooth

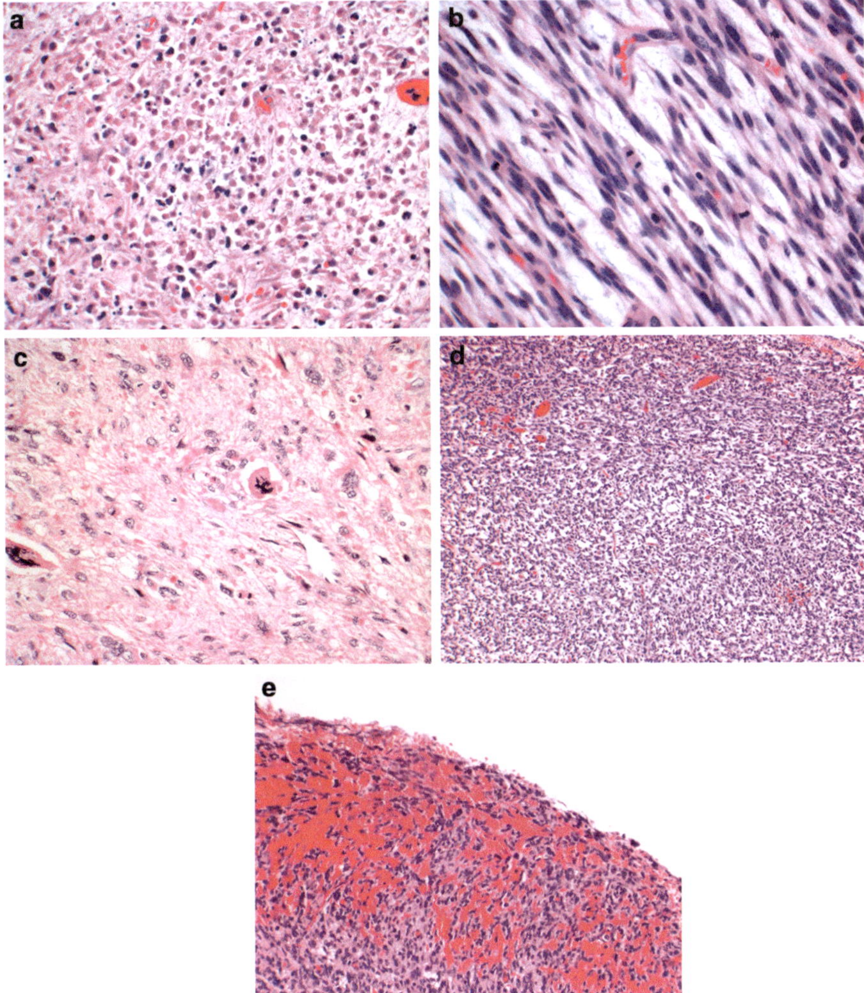

Fig. 7.5 Leiomyosarcoma. Diagnostic features to consider include tumor cell necrosis (**a**), mitotic activity (**b**), and atypical mitoses (**c**). Other features to consider include hypercellularity (**d**) and hemorrhage (**e**)

muscle lesion can be difficult. Histology may be similar, and there may be variants of morphology with overlapping differentiation. A broad panel of immunohisto-chemical stains can be helpful in such cases. Both endometrial stromal lesions and smooth muscle lesions can stain for CD10, but desmin and h-caldesmon positivity favor smooth muscle [7].

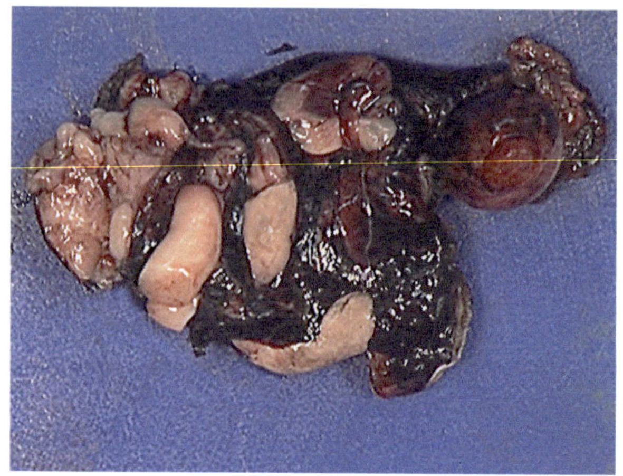

Fig. 7.6 Low-grade endometrial stromal sarcoma protruding as worm-like plugs in the lymphvascular space of this adnexum

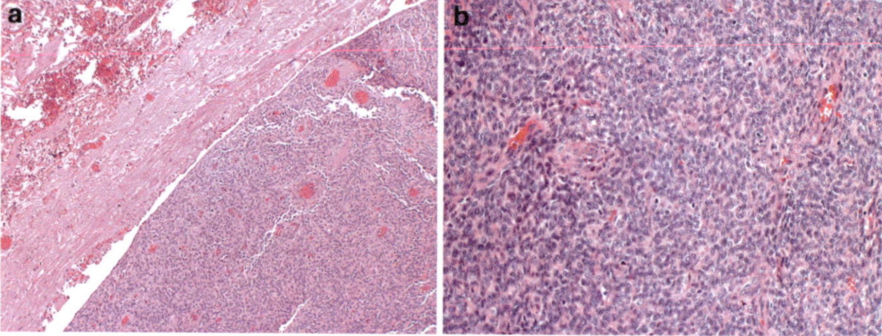

Fig. 7.7 Low-grade endometrial stromal sarcoma. The lesion involves lymphvascular spaces (**a**). Histologically, it resembles the stroma of proliferative endometrium, with thick-walled vessels (**b**)

References

1. Reeves MF, Goldstein RB, Jones KD. Communication of adenomyosis with the endometrial cavity: visualization with saline contrast sonohysterography. Ultrasound Obstet Gynecol. 2010;36:115–9.
2. Srodon M, Klein WM, Kurman RJ. CD10 immunostaining does not distinguish endometrial carcinoma invading myometrium from carcinoma involving adenomyosis. Am J Surg Pathol. 2003;27:786–9.
3. Ismiil ND, Rasty G, Ghorab Z, Nofech-Mozes S, Bernardini M, Thomas G, Ackerman I, Covens A, Khalifa MA. Adenomyosis is associated with myometrial invasion by FIGO 1 endometrial adenocarcinoma. Int J Gynecol Pathol. 2007;26:278–83.
4. Leren V, Langebrekke A, Qvigstad E. Parasitic leiomyomas after laparoscopic surgery with morcellation. Acta Obstet Gynecol Scand. 2012;91:1233–6.

5. Mahmoud MS, Desai K, Nezhat FR. Leiomyomas beyond the uterus; benign metastasizing leiomyomatosis with paraaortic metastasizing endometriosis and intravenous leiomyomatosis: a case series and review of the literature. Arch Gynecol Obstet. 2015;291(1):223–30.
6. Bell SW, Kempson RL, Hendrickson MR. Problematic uterine smooth muscle neoplasms: a clinicopathologic study of 213 cases. Am J Surg Pathol. 1994;18:535–58.
7. Conklin CM, Longacre TA. Endometrial stromal tumors: the new WHO classification. Adv Anat Pathol. 2014;21:383–93.

Diseases of the Fallopian Tube

8

8.1 Diseases of the Fallopian Tubes

The Fallopian tube can pose some unique challenges for evaluation by pathologists, and there are newer developments in our understanding of the origin of some of the epithelial malignancies of the ovaries now felt to derive from Fallopian tube fimbria (Table 8.1). This chapter addresses these and other diseases of the Fallopian tubes.

8.2 Congenital Anomalies of the Fallopian Tubes

The Fallopian tubes derive from the upper non-fused portions of the Müllerian ducts. Isolated anomalies are rare, but partial or total atresia has been reported [1]. Atresias are more likely to occur in association with uterine anomalies, such as a unicornuate uterus, than in isolation.

8.3 Infectious and Inflammatory Lesions of Fallopian Tubes

8.3.1 Acute Salpingitis

Acute salpingitis may be secondary to a variety of organisms, including gonorrhea, chlamydia, and occasionally actinomyces (Fig. 8.1), the latter usually in association with IUD usage. Grossly, if the fimbria become adherent, the tube becomes dilated with purulent material, forming a pyosalpinx. Histologically, purulent material, composed of neutrophils and necrotic debris, is seen within the mucosa and the tubal lumen (Fig. 8.2).

© Springer International Publishing Switzerland 2015
D.S. Heller, *OB-GYN Pathology for the Clinician*,
DOI 10.1007/978-3-319-15422-0_8

Table 8.1 Key points about Fallopian tube pathology

Acid fast bacilli are not reliably identified on acid fast histochemical stains, due to the rarity of organisms. Patients with granulomatous salpingitis may benefit from other diagnostic modalities to rule out tuberculosis
Implantation site should be sought in cases of tubal abortion with only hematosalpinx seen, to confirm ectopic pregnancy
For atypical epithelial proliferations in the fallopian tube, a positive p53 indicates a p53 signature and requires increased Ki-67 proliferation index in addition, to diagnose a serous tubal intraepithelial carcinoma (STIC), the putative precursor lesion of high grade ovarian and peritoneal serous carcinoma

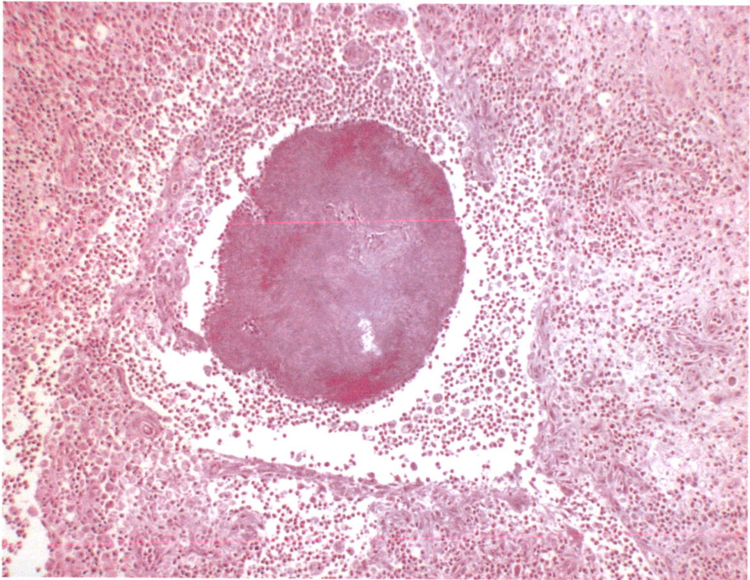

Fig. 8.1 Actinomyces. A typical radiating colony of organisms is seen. Grossly, these colonies are sometimes *yellow* in appearance, leading to the name "sulphur granules"

8.3.2 Chronic Salpingitis

Patterns of chronic salpingitis depend on how the Fallopian tube heals after an episode of acute salpingitis. The fimbria may remain open or may be sealed shut by adhesions. If the tube remains patent, there may be no changes at all, or there may be chronic salpingitis, characterized by a chronic inflammatory infiltrate composed of lymphocytes, plasma cells, and/or histiocytes. The folds of the tube may agglutinate, and although no inflammation is seen, there are numerous blind pouches created, termed follicular salpingitis (Fig. 8.3). This is thought to increase the risk of tubal ectopic pregnancies, as the fertilized ovum can get trapped in one of these areas. If the fimbria are sealed, and pyosalpinx resolves, what is left is flattened epithelium in a tube filled with nonpurulent fluid, a hydrosalpinx (Fig. 8.4).

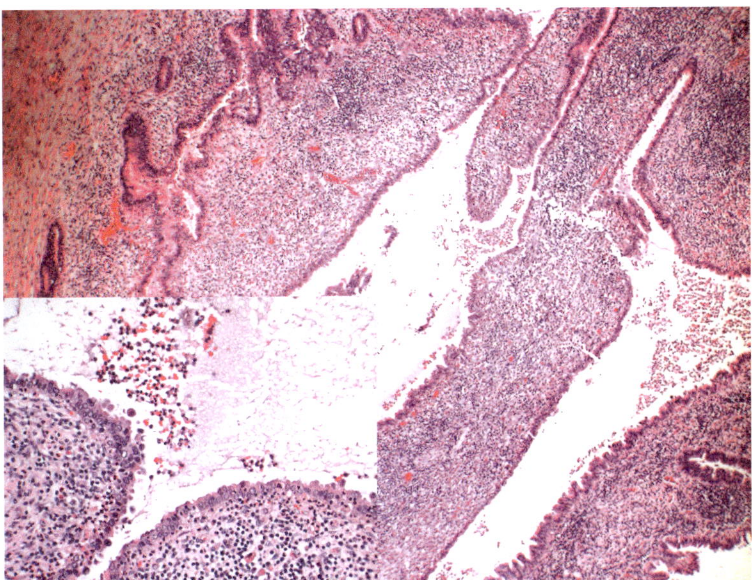

Fig. 8.2 Pyosalpinx. The tube is dilated by purulent exudate (pus). Histologically, the purulent material involves both the tubal epithelial folds and the lumen. The inset shows the purulent material, composed of neutrophils and necrotic debris

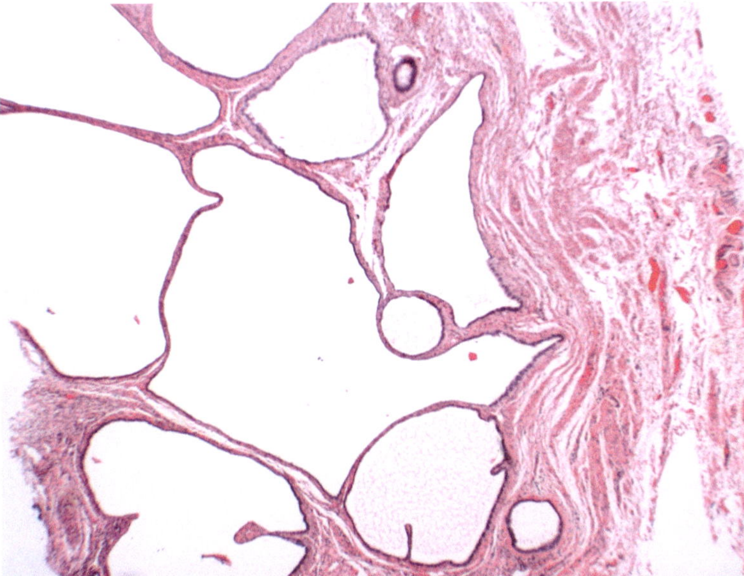

Fig. 8.3 Follicular salpingitis. Numerous blind spaces are seen due to agglutination of the folds of tubal epithelium

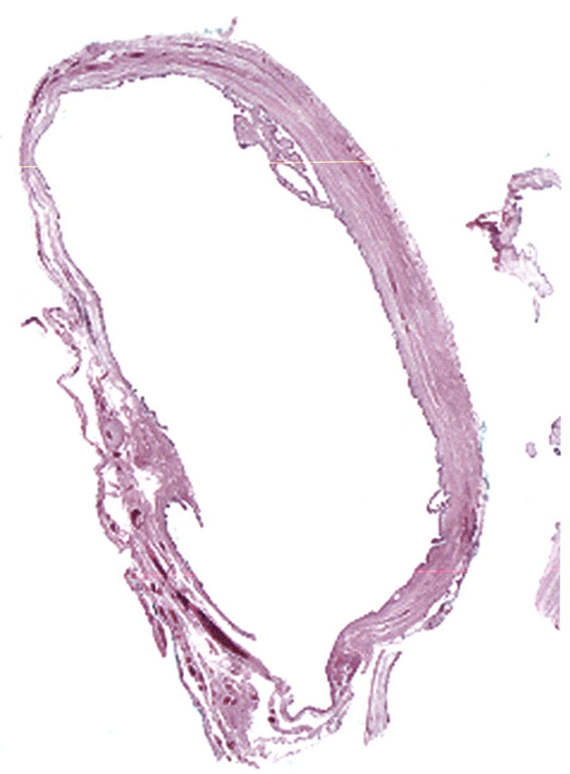

Fig. 8.4 Hydrosalpinx. The epithelium is flattened and the folds are lost, leaving behind a dilated sac of fluid

8.3.3   TB Salpingitis

Although rare in developed countries, tuberculous salpingitis is a common cause of infertility in endemic areas, where it may spread to the genital tract through hematogenous or lymphatic spread, or rarely through sexual contact [2]. It has also been reported in association with immunosuppression [3]. Clinically, the tube has been described as sometimes having a beaded appearance [2]. Histopathologically, the hallmark of tuberculosis is granulomatous inflammation (Fig. 8.5), usually with central necrosis called caseation, due to the gross cheesy appearance. However, even in the absence of central necrosis, stains for fungi and acid fast bacilli should be performed on cases of granulomatous salpingitis. Clinicians need to be aware that the stain for acid fast bacilli is very insensitive for confirmation of tuberculosis, due to the rarity of identifiable microorganisms, differing from some other strains of mycobacterium. If suspected clinically, other modalities, such as culture and PCR, should be considered.

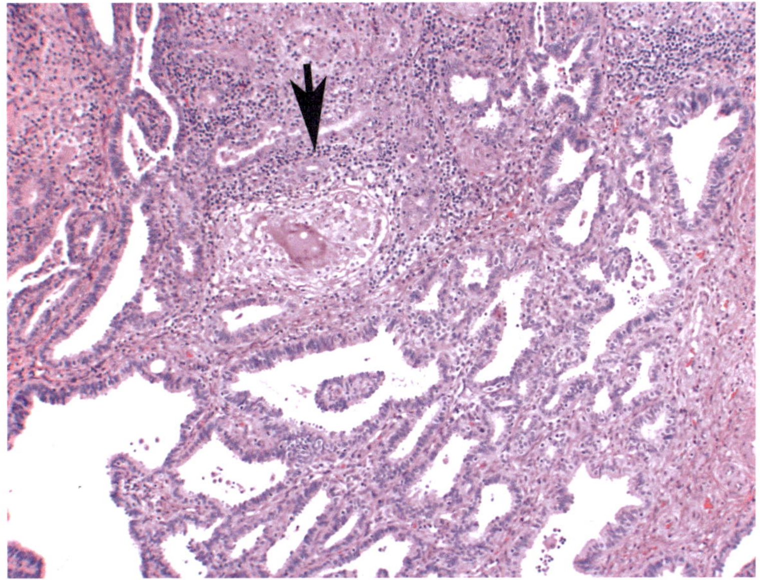

Fig. 8.5 Granulomatous salpingitis. This tube shows chronic salpingitis with fused epithelial folds. A granuloma (*arrow*) composed of epithelioid histiocytes surrounding a multinucleated giant cell is seen. No necrosis was present in this case

8.3.4 Salpingitis Isthmica Nodosa

Salpingitis isthmica nodosa is a lesion of unclear etiology, but with an association with infertility and ectopic pregnancy [4, 5]. Grossly there is nodular thickening of the proximal tube, and imaging studies have demonstrated that these are diverticular outpouchings from the lumen [4, 5]. Histologically, glandular spaces lined by tubal epithelium are seen out in the tubal muscular wall, away from the lumen. Sometimes there is distinct muscular cuffing around these glandular spaces (Fig. 8.6).

8.4 Benign Lesions of the Fallopian Tubes

8.4.1 Fallopian Tube Prolapse

The Fallopian tube, most often the fimbria, may prolapse into the vaginal vault after hysterectomy, particularly if the cuff remains open over a period of time. Grossly prolapsed Fallopian tube appears as granulation tissue at the vaginal vault. Histologically, swollen inflamed tubal mucosa may be appreciated.

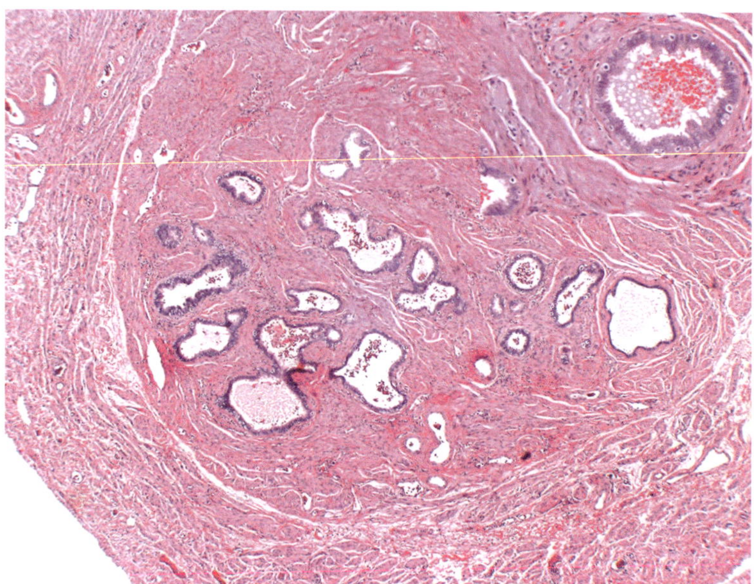

Fig. 8.6 Salpingitis isthmica nodosa. The lesion is composed of glandular spaces within the muscular wall of the tube. The epithelium is tubal or flattened, and muscular cuffing may be seen around glands (*inset upper right*)

8.4.2 Tubal Ectopic Pregnancy

Tubal ectopic pregnancies are common specimens in the pathology laboratory. The term "ectopic" means "wrong place" and doesn't necessarily indicate a Fallopian tube location. However, since most ectopic pregnancies do occur in the Fallopian tube, the term "ectopic" is generally taken to be synonymous with Fallopian tubal pregnancy. The pathology laboratory may receive a dilated tube, or a ruptured specimen. Rarely is the pregnancy advanced enough to see an actual fetus, unless the pregnancy is cornual, where it can develop further before rupture. Histologically, immature chorionic villi (Fig. 8.7a), and rarely fetal tissue, can be seen within the tube. As there is no decidua in the tube, this is technically a form of acreta, and implantation site trophoblasts can be seen in the tubal wall (Fig. 8.7b). These should be sought in cases of tubal abortion, where the products of conception have passed into the peritoneal cavity via rupture site or fimbriated end. This invasiveness is why a tubal ectopic pregnancy can persist after treatment by salpingostomy rather than salpingectomy. Villi seen with tubal ectopics are usually first trimester (Fig. 8.7c), and although they may have exuberant trophoblast proliferation, it is generally polar, pointing towards the implantation site, rather than the circumferential, and hence unlikely to represent hydatidiform mole, a potential pitfall. Adjacent Fallopian tube may show evidence of chronic salpingitis or salpingitis isthmica nodosa.

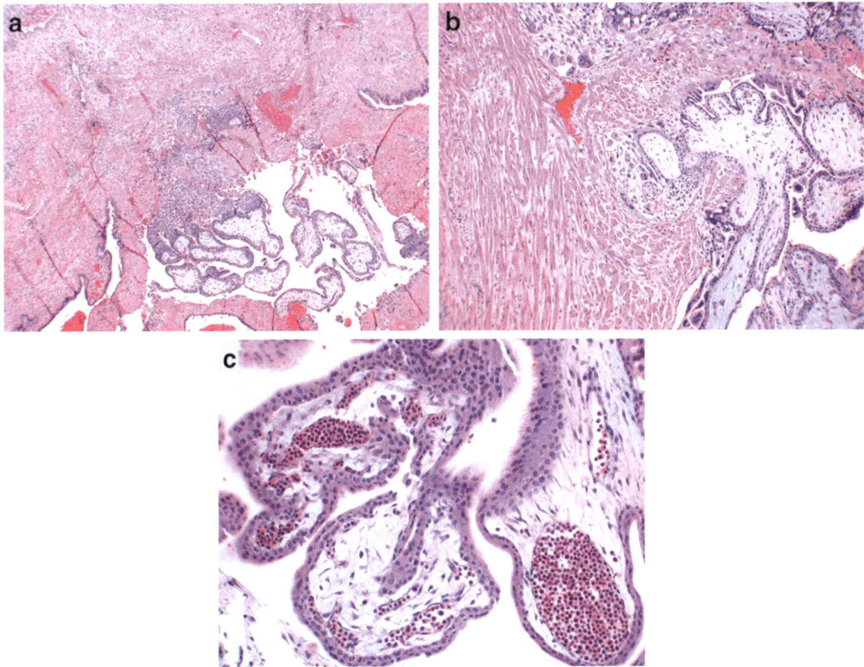

Fig. 8.7 Tubal ectopic pregnancy. The tubal lumen contains blood and immature chorionic villi (**a**), with trophoblast cells invading into the muscular wall of the tube (**b**). Histologically, most ectopics show first trimester villi such as these (**c**), with a two cell layer of trophoblast, inner cyto-trophoblast, and outer syncytiotrophoblast. In this case there are many nucleated red blood cells in fetal villous capillaries, consistent with a first trimester gestation

8.4.3   Paratubal Cyst

Paratubal cysts are extremely common. The origin is unclear, but may be mesothelial, or from Müllerian or Wolffian remnants. Most cases are incidental, where they appear as small thin-walled cystic structures (Fig. 8.8a). Histologically they are lined by flat or tubal-type epithelium (Fig. 8.8b). However, occasionally paratubal cysts may become large, presenting as a mass, may hemorrhage, torse, or develop neoplasia. "Borderline"/low malignant potential neoplasms have been reported to develop in paratubal cysts [6], as well as extremely rare carcinomas are possible.

8.4.4   Endometriosis

The Fallopian tube is a common site for endometriosis, which requires endometrial glandular epithelium and stroma to histopathologically confirm the diagnosis (Fig. 8.9).

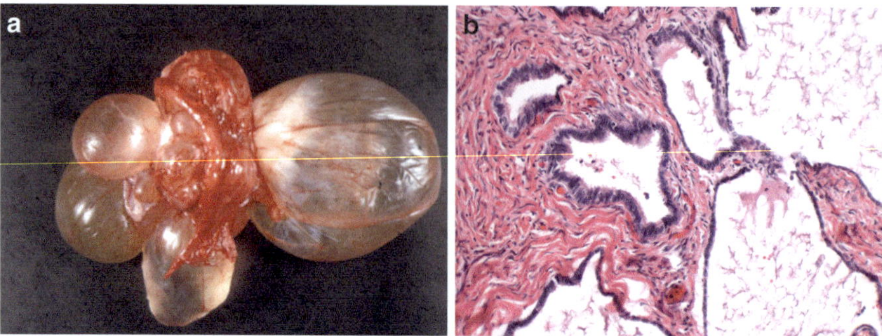

Fig. 8.8 Paratubal cyst. These common lesions show thin-walled cysts (**a**) lined by flattened or tubal type epithelium (**b**) (Fig. 8.8a, Reprinted with permission, originally published in Timor-Tritsch, IE, Kurjak A, Ultrasound and the Fallopian Tube. Parthenon, 1996, Chapter 2, Figure 20, p. 19)

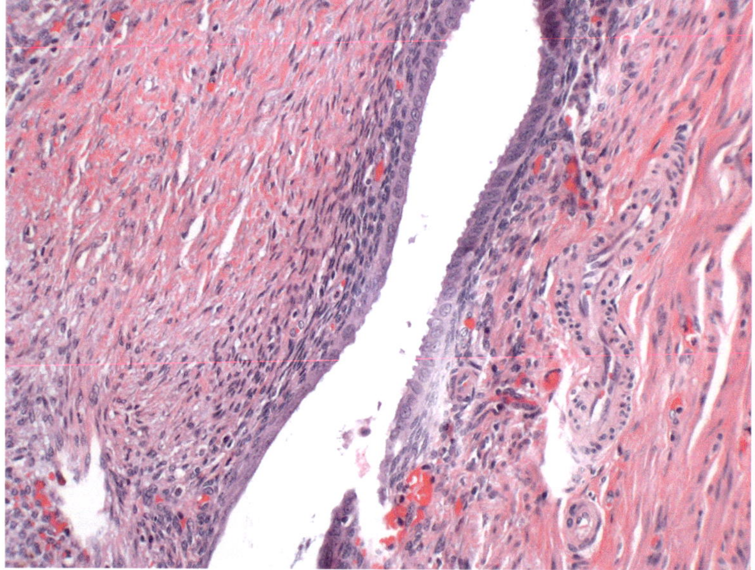

Fig. 8.9 Endometriosis. Endometrial glandular epithelium and stroma involving peritubal tissue. Smooth muscle is seen to the right

8.4.5   Adenomatoid Tumor

Adenomatoid tumors are benign tumors of mesothelial origin. They may be incidental findings in the Fallopian tube or uterus. Histologically they are composed of numerous small spaces lined by a flattened mesothelium that can stain for mesothelial markers such as calretinin (Fig. 8.10).

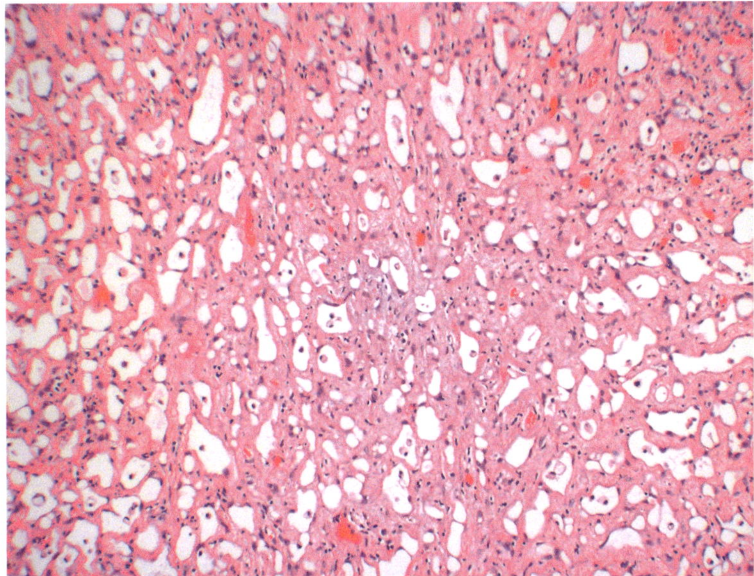

Fig. 8.10 Adenomatoid tumor showing numerous spaces lined by flat mesothelium

8.4.6 Adrenal Rest

Occasional incidental adrenal cortical rests may be found in Fallopian tube (Fig. 8.11).

8.5 Malignant Neoplasms of the Fallopian Tube

8.5.1 Serous Tubal Intraepithelial Carcinoma

Recent evidence suggests that high grade ovarian and peritoneal serous carcinomas may derive from lesions of the fimbria. Some of the histopathologic findings that have contributed to this newer theory of carcinogenesis have been detected in the detailed pathological evaluation that is performed in the tubes and ovaries of patients who undergo prophylactic excision of tubes and ovaries for BRCA mutations, where there may be detection of early lesions. Early tubal neoplasia shows focal piling up of epithelium with some degree of atypia, possible mitoses, and papillary formations or stratification. There is mutation of p53. Immunostaining for p53 and Ki-67, a proliferation marker, should be performed. If p53 immunohistochemistry is positive, indicating aberrant p53, but Ki-67 proliferation isn't increased, the lesion is said to show the p53 signature, which is not thought to have clinical significance [7]. If Ki-67 index is also increased, the lesion is diagnosed as serous tubal intraepithelial carcinoma (STIC), the putative precursor lesion of high-grade serous carcinomas of ovary and peritoneum [7] (Fig. 8.12a, b).

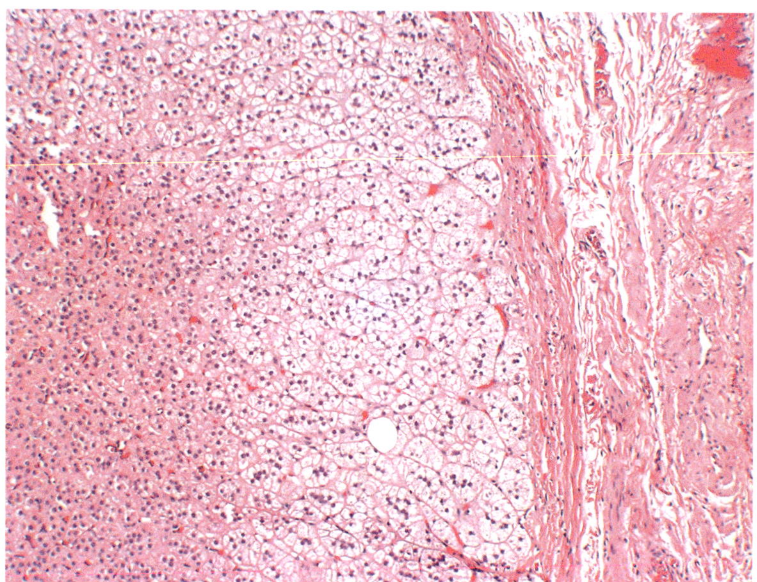

Fig. 8.11 Adrenal cortical rest seen in peritubal tissue

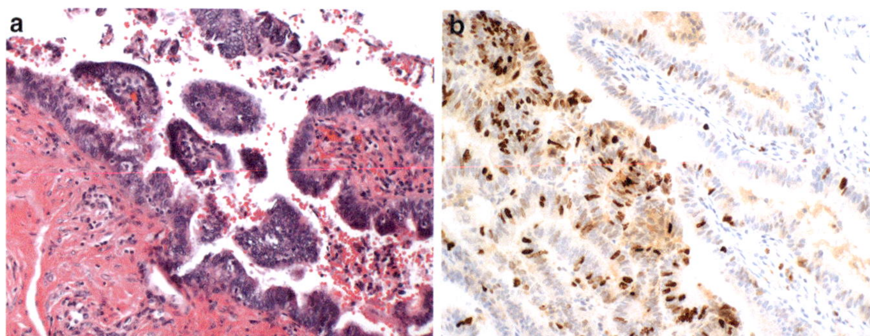

Fig. 8.12 STIC, showing epithelial stratification and papillary fronds (**a**). Ki-67 proliferation was increased (**b**) on the *left*, compared to the normal epithelium on the *right*. P53 (not shown) immunostain was positive as well

8.5.2 Primary Fallopian Tube Carcinoma

Like other Müllerian-derived tissues, Fallopian tube carcinoma may show a variety of histologies; however, most such lesions are either papillary serous or undifferentiated carcinomas (Fig. 8.13). Recently, FIGO staging has been updated, to reflect the emerging molecular concepts of carcinogenesis [8].

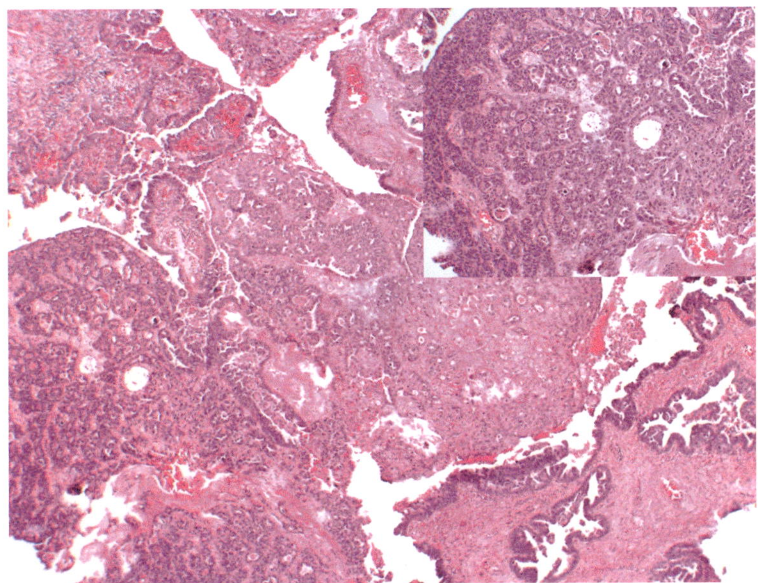

Fig. 8.13 Fallopian tube carcinoma infiltrating mucosa, and showing glandular architecture (*inset upper right*)

References

1. Vallerie AM, Breech LL. Update in Müllerian anomalies: diagnosis, management, and outcomes. Curr Opin Obstet Gynecol. 2010;22:381–7.
2. Bhanothu V, Theophilus JP, Reddy PK, Rozati R. Occurrence of female genital tuberculosis among infertile women: a study from a tertiary maternal health care research centre in South India. Eur J Clin Microbiol Infect Dis. 2014;33(11):1937–49.
3. Ilmer M, Bergauer F, Friese K, Mylonas I. Genital tuberculosis as the cause of tuboovarian abscess in an immunosuppressed patient. Infect Dis Obstet Gynecol. 2009;2009:745060. doi:10.1155/2009/745060. Epub 2010 Mar 8.
4. Yaranal PJ, Hegde V. Salpingitis isthmica nodosa: a case report. J Clin Diagn Res. 2013;7: 2581–2.
5. Jenkins CS, Williams SR, Schmidt GE. Salpingitis isthmica nodosa: a review of the literature, discussion of clinical significance, and consideration of patient management. Fertil Steril. 1993;60:599–607.
6. Kiseli M, Caglar GS, Cengiz SD, Karadag D, Yılmaz MB. Clinical diagnosis and complications of paratubal cysts: review of the literature and report of uncommon presentations. Arch Gynecol Obstet. 2012;285:1563–9.
7. Rutgers JK, Lawrence WD. A small organ takes center stage: selected topics in Fallopian tube pathology. Int J Gynecol Pathol. 2014;33:385–92.
8. Mutch DG, Prat J. 2014 FIGO staging for ovarian, Fallopian tube and peritoneal cancer. Gynecol Oncol. 2014;133:401–4.

9.1 Diseases of the Ovaries

The ovary is made up of several tissue types, so it is not surprising that the range of ovarian tumors is so broad. The ovarian surface is lined by the Müllerian epithelium, which is of the same derivation as the mesothelium lining the peritoneal cavity. While older literature theorized an origin of epithelial tumors from this epithelium, current literature suggests different pathogenetic pathways (see below). The germ cells of the ovaries give rise to germ cell tumors. The specialized stroma surrounding the germ cells, the granulosa and theca cells, can give rise to sex cord stromal tumors. In addition, due to blood supply, a large number of neoplasms, both genital and nongenital, can metastasize to ovaries. There are a variety of challenges for pathologic evaluation of ovarian masses (Table 9.1).

9.2 Non-neoplastic Masses

Ovarian masses may be non-neoplastic in nature. Functional cysts are common and often resolve on their own.

9.2.1 Follicle Cyst

The most common functional cyst is a follicle cyst (Fig. 9.1). Follicle cysts are lined by the same cells as normal follicles, with an inner granulosa cell layer, and a visible outer theca interna. The theca externa blends with the ovarian stroma and is not easily detectable on routine stains.

© Springer International Publishing Switzerland 2015
D.S. Heller, *OB-GYN Pathology for the Clinician*,
DOI 10.1007/978-3-319-15422-0_9

Table 9.1 Key points about ovarian pathology

Endometrioma requires evidence of endometrial glandular epithelium and stroma, not just hemorrhage, to confirm the diagnosis histopathologically
Frozen section diagnosis may be limited in cases requiring extensive sampling for a final diagnosis, particularly large multiloculated mucinous neoplasms
Hyperplastic ovarian masses are usually bilateral
Metastatic lesions to ovaries are usually bilateral
Pseudomyxoma peritoneii is thought to arise from appendiceal mucinous neoplasms, which may coexist with mucinous tumor in the ovary

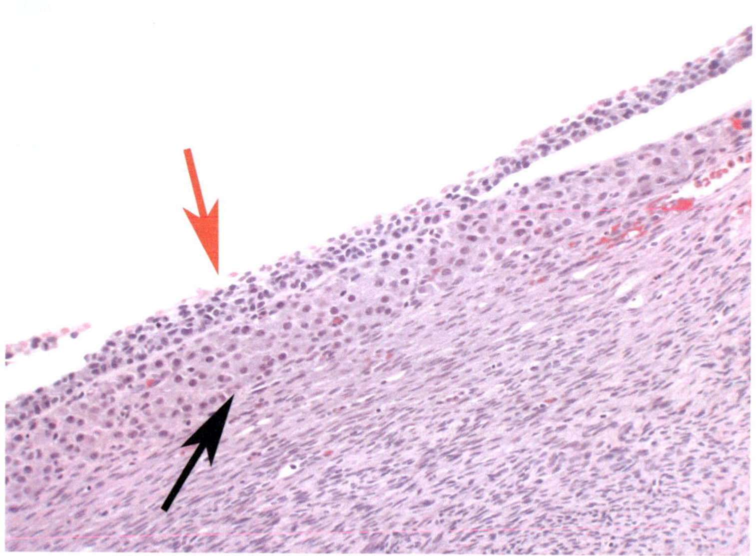

Fig. 9.1 Follicle cyst lined by inner granulosa (*red arrow*) layer, and outer theca interna (*black arrow*)

9.2.2 Corpus Luteum Cyst

Corpus luteum cysts (Fig. 9.2) are lined by luteinized granulosa and theca interna cells, in the characteristic cerebriform pattern of folding. Corpus luteal cysts are hemorrhagic in the center. Very rarely, rupture of one of these cysts can cause peritoneal hemorrhage of a degree that may mimic a ruptured tubal ectopic pregnancy.

9.2.3 Polycystic Ovary

Polycystic ovaries contain numerous cystic follicles that have not gone on to ovulation, under a dense capsule. Occasionally patients with polycystic ovarian disease do ovulate, so the finding of a corpus luteum or a corpus albicans or two does not rule out the diagnosis, which is a clinical one. Polycystic ovaries may also show cortical stromal hyperplasia and stromal hyperthecosis (see next section).

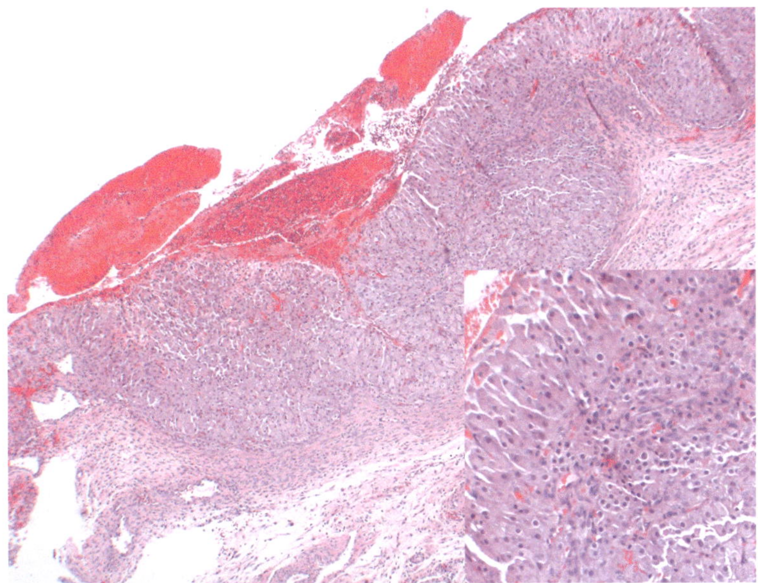

Fig. 9.2 Hemorrhagic corpus luteum showing cerebriform configuration. At higher power, the larger luteinized granulosa, and smaller luteinized theca cells may be seen (*inset*)

9.2.4 Cortical Stromal Hyperplasia and Stromal Hyperthecosis

Cortical stromal hyperplasia and stromal hyperthecosis are seen in two clinical instances, polycystic ovarian disease and in menopause. As these findings are hyperplastic, not neoplastic, they are generally bilateral. Cortical stromal hyperplasia is characterized by increased amounts of nodular cortical stroma. Grossly, this may be very yellow in appearance, rarely raising concern for the clinician of a masculinizing sex cord stromal tumor. Histologically cortical stromal hyperplasia appears as dense blue nodular ovarian stroma with its characteristic spindle cells. It is often associated with stromal hyperthecosis, a subtle finding of nests of luteinized stromal cells (Fig. 9.3a, b), which may be hormonally active, secreting androstenedione. This androgenic compound may be masculinizing, and if the patient is obese, androstenedione may aromatize to estrone in peripheral adipose. This has the potential then of leading to hyperstimulation of the endometrium due to unopposed estrogen.

9.2.5 Theca Lutein Cysts

Theca lutein cysts are seen in two main clinical scenarios. Ovarian hyperstimulation syndrome after ovulation induction is a clinical diagnosis, and often associated with major fluid imbalance and symptomatology. Although these ovaries are rarely surgical specimens, what is seen are numerous non-ovulated follicle cysts. A similar histopathologic picture is seen with hyperreactio luteinalis, usually presenting in the third trimester, as opposed to the earlier presentation of hyperstimulation syndrome,

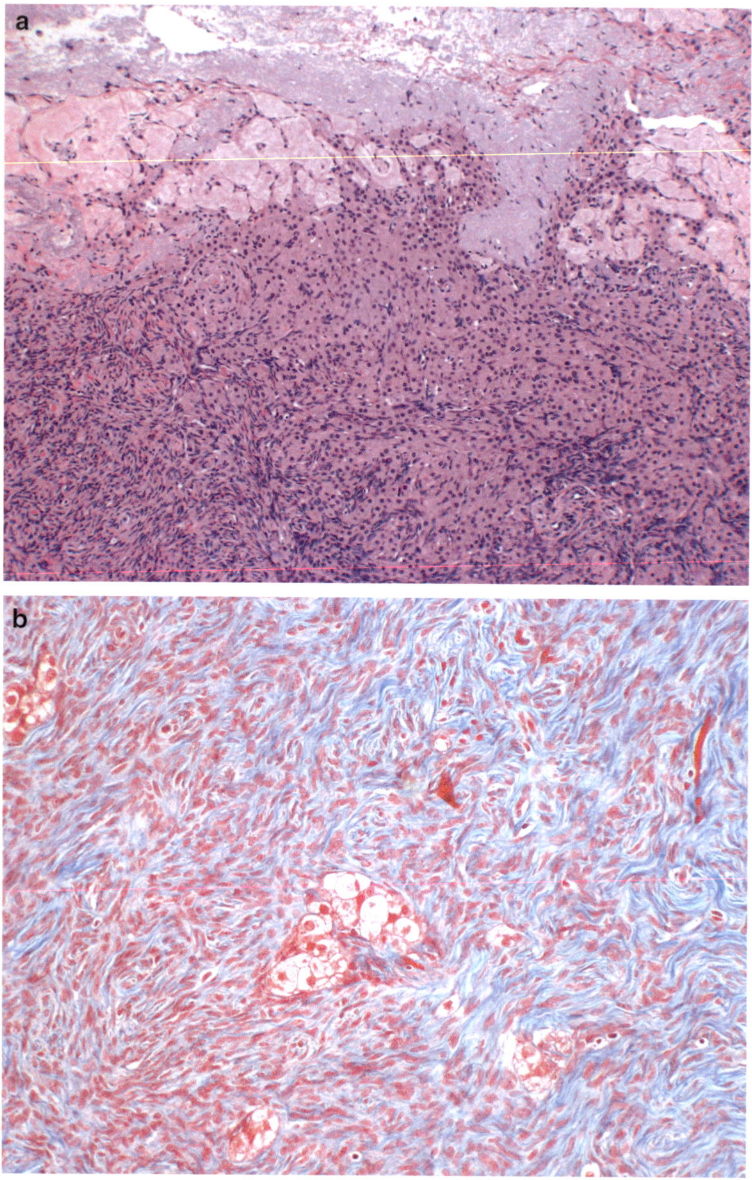

Fig. 9.3 Stromal hyperthecosis. Luteinized stromal cells may be seen adjacent to the pale corpora albicantia (**a**). Trichrome stain makes these nests more prominent, here seen in the center (**b**)

and seen in association with high levels of beta-hCG, which can occur with molar disease and multiple gestations. Lack of clearance of beta-hCG is thought to be the mechanism of hyperreactio seen with chronic renal disease [1]. Hyperreactio is usually less associated with fluid imbalance, and again, unlikely to provide a specimen for pathology review unless the diagnosis is unsuspected clinically. Both conditions, being hyperplastic rather than neoplastic, are generally bilateral and regress after the hormonal stimulus is removed.

9.2.6 Endometrioma

Endometriosis can form an enlarging ovarian cyst, an endometrioma. The cyst enlarges due to cyclic bleeding. The blood has no egress, so thickens and darkens and becomes "chocolate" fluid. This fluid may compress and destroy the histologically diagnostic lining, so that a diagnosis of endometrioma may only be inferred. To confirm histologically, as in sites elsewhere, endometriosis must show endometrial glandular type epithelium and stroma, not merely evidence of a cyst with old bleeding lined by hemosiderin-laden macrophages.

9.2.7 Ovarian Pregnancy

Not all ectopic pregnancies are tubal, and rarely, an ovarian pregnancy occurs, usually within the corpus luteum (Fig. 9.4). The incidence is quite low, but appears to be greater with assisted reproductive technology [2]. It is possible that a tubal abortion leads to implantation in a rupture site of a corpus luteum. There are specific

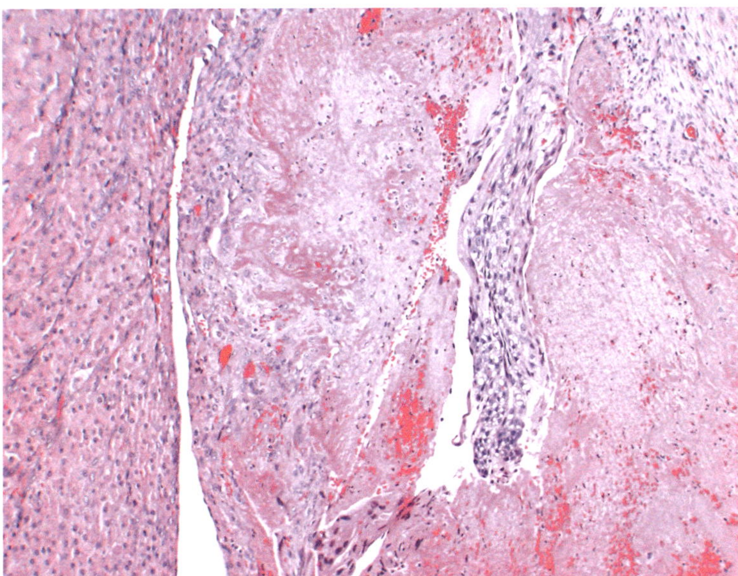

Fig. 9.4 Ovarian pregnancy showing implantation site trophoblasts (*right*) adjacent to the corpus luteum (*left*)

criteria for the diagnosis of an ovarian pregnancy. Spiegelberg's criteria, first described in 1878 [3], include that the ipsilateral fallopian tube is intact, the gestational sac must be in the position of the ovary, and this must be attached to the uterus by the uteroovarian ligament, and finally that there must be ovarian tissue in the wall of the gestational sac.

9.3　Epithelial Neoplasms

Epithelial ovarian neoplasms were initially thought to derive from the lining of the ovary, the Müllerian epithelium (mesothelium), possibly from invaginations associated with prior ovulation, so-called inclusion cysts. As our understanding of molecular genetic mechanisms has progressed, newer theories have been put forward for epithelial ovarian malignancies, particularly of serous type [4]. This newer evidence suggests that ovarian carcinogenesis falls into two main types, a type I which is low grade and more indolent, and associated with different mutations than the type II aggressive lesions. Papillary serous cystadenocarcinoma, the usual high grade type, is associated with p53 mutations and is now thought to derive from the fimbriated end of the fallopian tube. In tubes removed prophylactically in BRCA individuals, areas of histologic proliferation are sometimes seen. If they show aberrant p53 expression on immunohistochemistry, they are said to show the p53 signature. If, in addition, they show increased proliferation as evidenced by Ki-67 immunostaining, they are designated as serous tubal intraepithelial carcinoma (STIC), thought to be the precursor of high-grade ovarian and peritoneal serous carcinomas. Endometrioid and clear cell carcinomas have been associated with and may derive from endometriosis. Mucinous and Brenner tumor derivations are less clear. A good review of current thinking has been published [4]. The subsequent discussion pertains to the histopathological features of these neoplasms.

9.3.1　Serous Cystadenoma

Serous cystadenomas are often unilocular, but may be multilocular. Some are paper thin and can be transilluminated. Grossly, the outer surface is smooth, and the lining is smooth. Histologically, the cyst is lined either by fallopian tubal type epithelium, or the epithelium may have become flattened (Fig. 9.5a–c). A variant neoplasm, papillary serous cystadenofibroma (Fig. 9.5d), has papillary excrescences inside the cystic cavities, but they are lined by benign serous epithelium. It is also possible to have cystadenofibromas lined by other types of Müllerian epithelium.

Although not definitively diagnostic, a clue that papillary structures represent a papillary serous cystadenofibroma rather than a low malignant potential tumor is the finding of increased firmness to the touch of cystadenofibroma papillae, due to the stromal predominance of these structures, as well as the finding that they may only occupy a portion of the cyst.

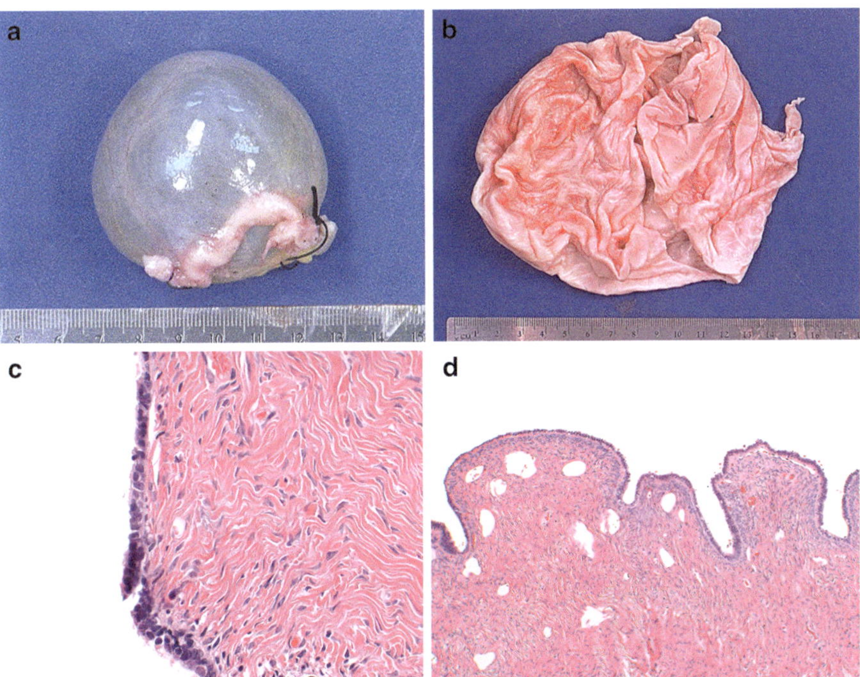

Fig. 9.5 Serous cystadenoma. The lesion is smooth externally (**a**), and internally (**b**). The lining (**c**) resembles fallopian tube epithelium. A variant papillary serous cystadenofibroma shows dense fibrous papillae lined by the same benign serous epithelium (**d**)

9.3.2 Serous Tumor of Low Malignant Potential ("Borderline")

Serous neoplasms of low malignant potential (also called "borderline," "atypical proliferative serous tumor") show papillary excrescences inside the cysts that comprise the lesion. These are comprised of fibrovascular cores lined by mildly atypical epithelium, which may show stratification and mitoses. The outer surface of the mass may contain these papillary excrescences as well, or may be smooth. The hallmark of this lesion is the lack of stromal invasion, distinguishing it from an invasive papillary serous carcinoma (Fig. 9.6). Serous tumors of low malignant potential may extend beyond the ovary and are staged the same way as frank malignancies, although they are prognostically better. As such they may have omental implants, which are separated into noninvasive implants (subdivided into epithelial and desmoplastic noninvasive implants), which hug the lobules of omental adipose, and invasive implants, which are thought to be worse prognostically, and invade into the actual adipose. A variant pattern of borderline tumor, the micropapillary pattern, which shows increased generations of thin epithelial fronds, is thought to be the noninvasive variant of low-grade serous carcinoma. If confined to the ovary, the micropapillary variant has similar prognosis to the usual pattern of low malignant

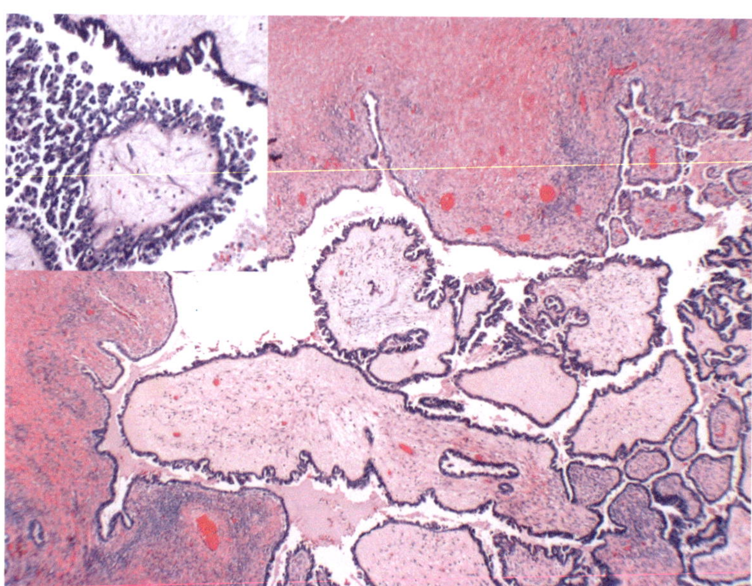

Fig. 9.6 Serous tumor of low malignant potential. The papillae are lined by somewhat more atypical epithelium than in the benign lesion, but there is no stromal invasion. The micropapillary variant (*inset*) shows increased thin branching

potential tumor, but is thought by some authors to be worse than usual borderline tumor when extending beyond the ovary. Nomenclature and prognostication in the area of borderline tumors and tumors in transition between them and frankly invasive carcinoma are still in flux [5].

9.3.3 Papillary Serous Cystadenocarcinoma

Papillary serous cystadenocarcinomas are usually bilateral and may be grossly a mix of cystic and solid. Papillary areas may be seen on the surface of the ovaries and on cut surface. Low-grade serous carcinomas show more uniform cellularity histologically. The more usual high-grade tumors are generally either papillary or solid in configuration. Papillary high-grade tumors are comprised of fibrovascular cores lined by markedly atypical epithelium, or by solid sheets with similar cells, often with prominent nucleoli. Serous tumors may frequently show psammoma bodies, concentric calcifications thought to be degenerative, but these are not diagnostic (Fig. 9.7a–d).

9.3.4 Mucinous Neoplasms

Mucinous ovarian neoplasms are among the more challenging to evaluate histopathologically. These neoplasms are more frequently unilateral. Regardless of

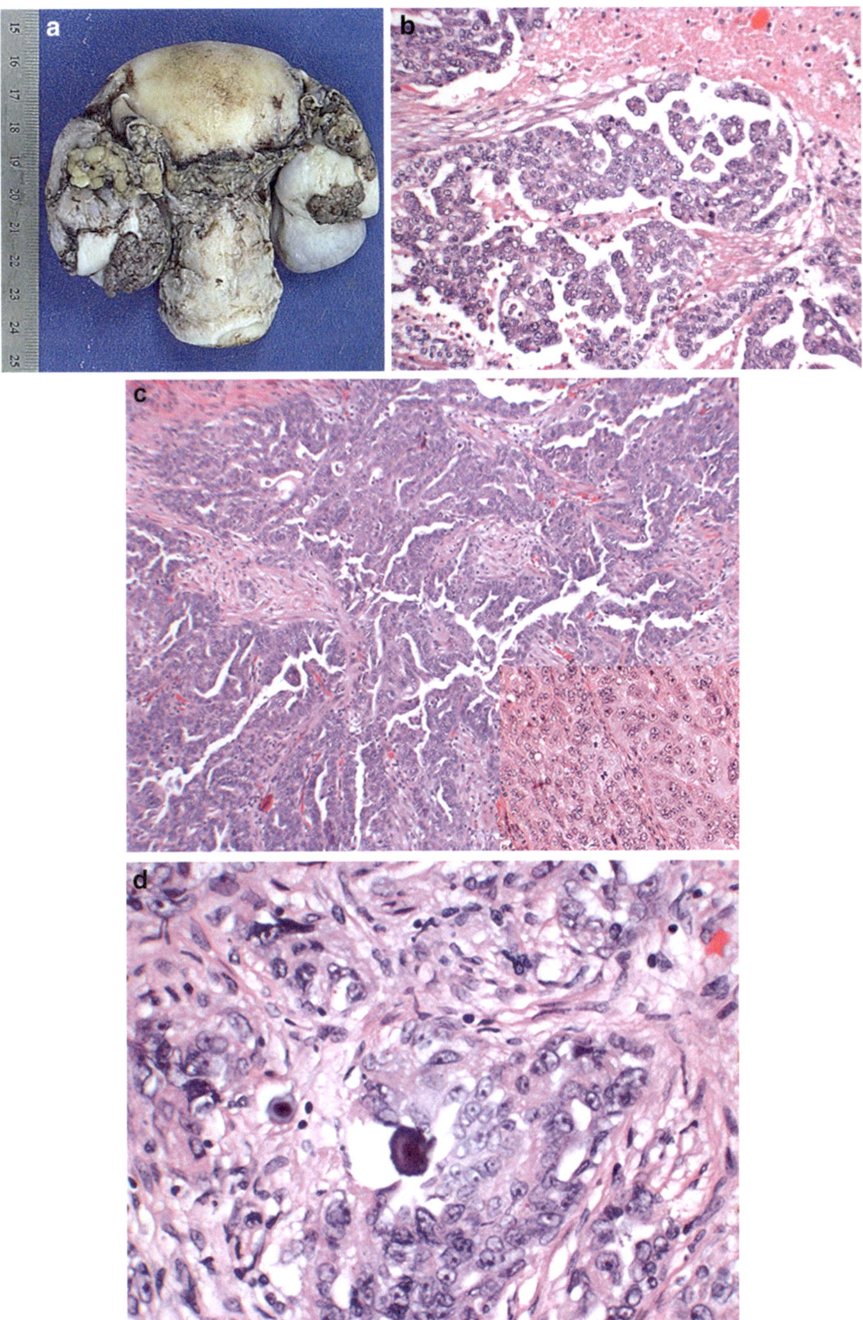

Fig. 9.7 Papillary serous cystadenocarcinoma of the ovary is usually bilateral (**a**). Low-grade carcinoma shows less atypia and more uniformity (**b**). High-grade papillary cystadenocarcinoma (**c**) shows increasingly atypical epithelium lining the fibrovascular cores, or the tumor may be solid (*inset*). A characteristic but not diagnostic finding is psammoma bodies (**d**), laminated calcifications. Note prominent nucleoli

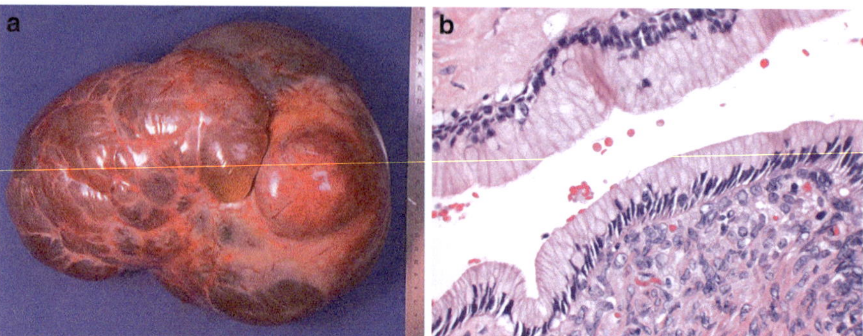

Fig. 9.8 Mucinous cystadenoma. Mucinous neoplasms, even benign, are often large and multi-loculated (**a**). Benign mucinous cystadenoma is lined by a single layer of mucinous columnar epithelium resembling endocervix (**b**)

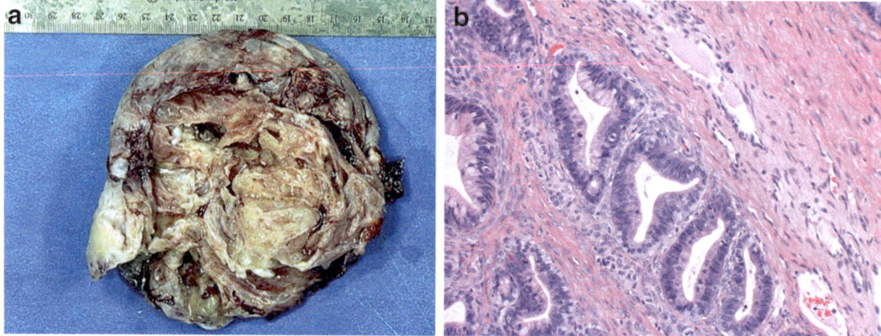

Fig. 9.9 Mucinous neoplasm of low malignant potential. Low malignant potential and malignant mucinous neoplasms may appear grossly similar to the benign ones, or may look more ominous grossly as seen here (**a**). In low malignant potential tumors (**b**), histology shows loss of mucin and increase in atypia and mitotic activity in the epithelium but no stromal invasion

where they fall on the spectrum of benign to low malignant potential to malignant, they may be similar in gross appearance, often very large and multiloculated (Fig. 9.8a). As such, it requires extensive sectioning, at least one section per centimeter of tumor, to appropriately evaluate these neoplasms. This is why a deferral may be received by the gynecologic surgeon at the time of frozen section, where it is not feasible to process more than a couple of sections.

9.3.5 Mucinous Cystadenoma

Mucinous cystadenomas may be unilocular or multilocular. They are lined by a single layer of mucinous columnar epithelium resembling endocervix (Fig. 9.8b).

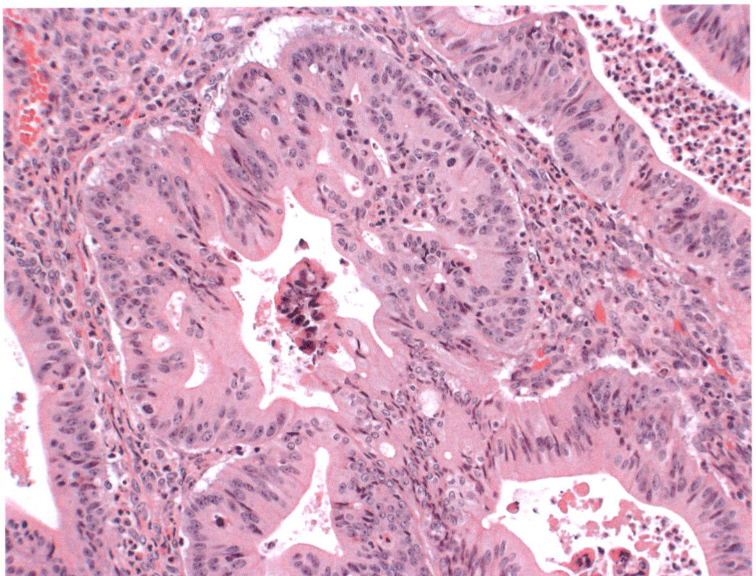

Fig. 9.10 Malignant mucinous cystadenocarcinoma showing cribriforming consistent with stromal invasion

9.3.6 Mucinous Tumor of Low Malignant Potential ("Borderline")

Mucinous neoplasms of low malignant potential and malignant mucinous tumors cannot usually be distinguished grossly. They tend to appear more solid than the benign lesions, but this is actually due to more complex multiloculation in many cases (Fig. 9.9a). Mucinous neoplasms of low malignant potential show epithelial atypia, stratification, and mitotic activity with loss of intracellular mucin, but there is no stromal invasion (Fig. 9.9b).

9.3.7 Mucinous Cystadenocarcinoma

Mucinous cystadenocarcinoma differs from mucinous borderline tumors by the presence of frank invasion (Fig. 9.10). Bilaterality is less common than in papillary serous cystadenocarcinoma. Unlike serous tumors which invade by papillary or solid outgrowths into the stroma, mucinous neoplasms are already loculated, so sections appear to have neoplastic cells sitting within stroma in borderline tumors as well, making the evaluation of true invasion challenging at times. The hallmark of invasive carcinoma, then, is a stromal reaction, either desmoplastic (fibrotic) or inflammatory around the tumor. Cribriforming of the epithelium may also qualify as stromal invasion. It may take many sections to confirm this diagnosis, which is why

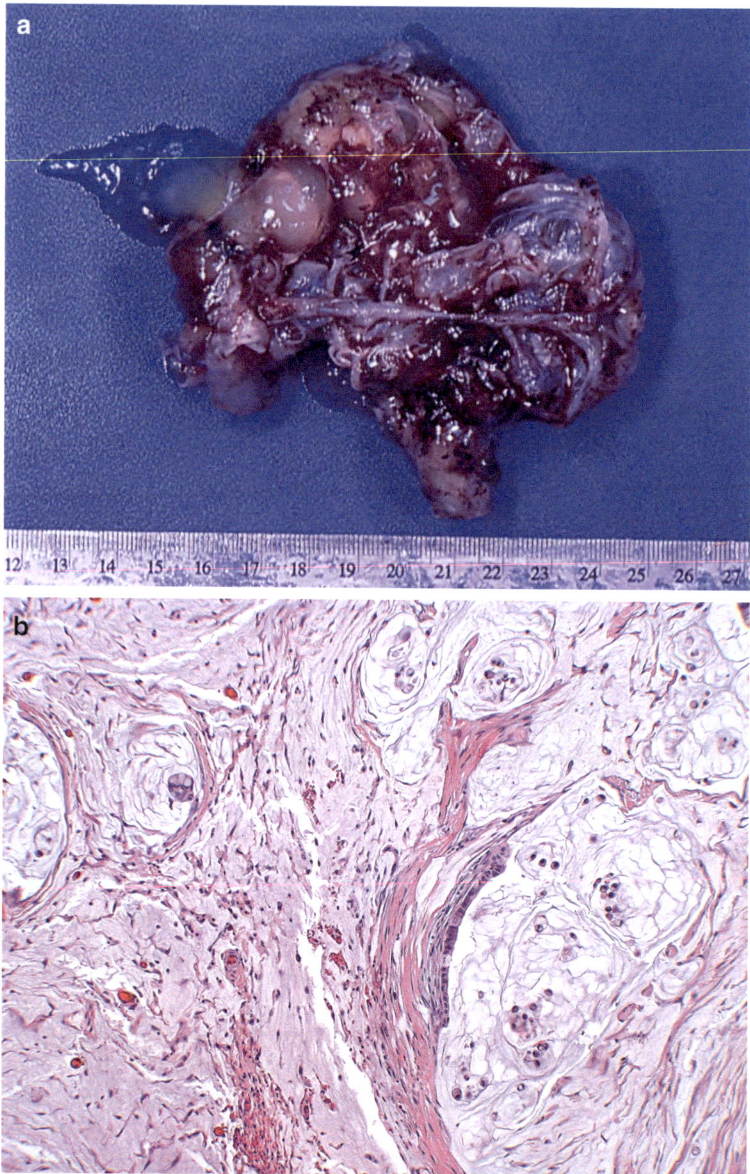

Fig. 9.11 Pseudomyxoma peritonei. This lesion, usually of appendiceal origin, but often associated with ovarian involvement, is comprised of loculated mucinous ascites (**a**). Histologically, there is abundant mucin with minimal amounts of epithelium, often low grade, as in this case of diffuse peritoneal adenomucinosis (**b**)

frozen section diagnosis can be unreliable. In addition, metastatic tumors to ovary that may resemble primary mucinous cystadenocarcinoma of ovary, such as metastatic colonic adenocarcinoma, sometimes need to be considered as well and require immunohistochemical stains to establish the origin, not possible at frozen section.

9.3.8   Pseudomyxoma Peritonei

Pseudomyxoma peritoneii is mucinous ascites (Fig. 9.11). It was once thought to be due to implants of ovarian mucinous neoplasms, most often of low malignant potential. Pseudomyxoma is now thought to originate in an appendiceal mucinous neoplasm in most cases. There is sufficient coexistence of mucinous appendiceal neoplasms with an ovarian mucinous neoplasm that the appendix should be evaluated at surgery in all ovarian mucinous cases, with liberal excision. It is possible in such cases that the ovarian neoplasm spreads from the appendix. Pseudomyxoma is a problem because it reoccurs and can obstruct bowel, necessitating repeat procedures. It cannot be easily drained, because it is loculated. It consists of predominantly mucus, with a minimal amount of mucinous epithelium floating in the pools. Most pseudomyxoma has low grade epithelium, which has been termed diffuse peritoneal adenomucinosis (DPAM), distinguished from epithelium with more atypia, termed peritoneal mucinous carcinomatosis (PMCA), which is thought to be more aggressive [6].

9.3.9   Endometrioid Adenocarcinoma

Endometrioid adenocarcinoma of the ovary has been described as grossly appearing like necrotic brain tissue. It may be unilateral or bilateral. Histologically, the tumor is similar in appearance to the uterine counterpart (Fig. 9.12), with back to back crowded glands, often with squamous metaplasia. Current thinking is that these tumors may arise from endometriosis [4].

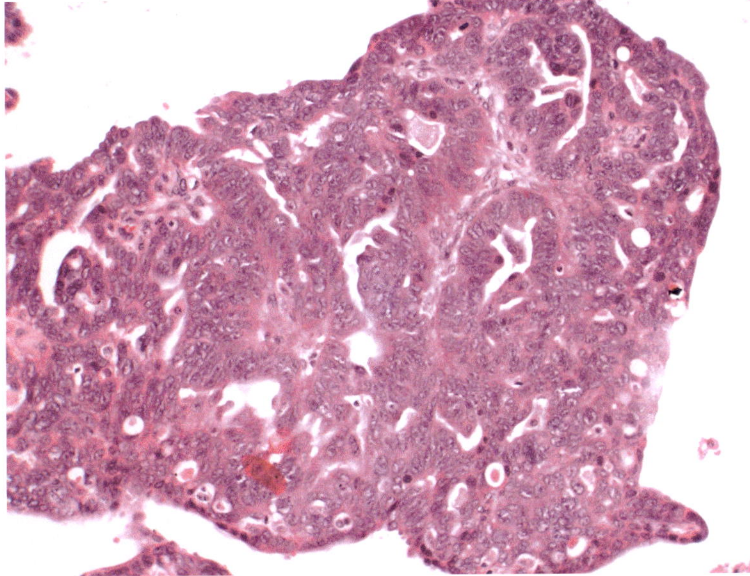

Fig. 9.12 Endometrioid carcinoma. Histologically, the lesion is similar in appearance to the endometrial counterpart

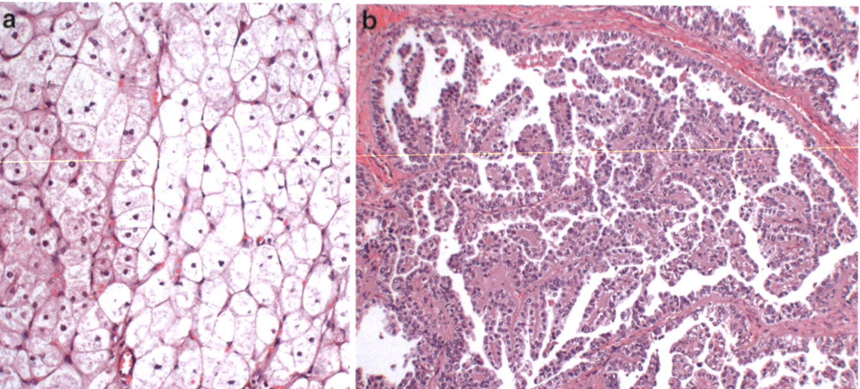

Fig. 9.13 Clear cell adenocarcinoma. This lesion may appear as clear cells in solid sheets (**a**), or may present as the tubulopapillary pattern (**b**)

9.3.10 Clear Cell Adenocarcinoma

Clear cell adenocarcinoma of the ovary may also arise from endometriosis [4]. Histologically, it is similar to clear cell adenocarcinomas elsewhere and may have a clear cell pattern or a tubulopapillary pattern. These lesions tend to be unilateral (Fig. 9.13a, b).

9.3.11 Brenner Tumor

Grossly, Brenner tumors resemble fibromas. Histologically (Fig. 9.14), these usually benign lesions are composed of nests of transitional type epithelium in a fibromatous stroma. The nests have cells with grooved ("coffee-bean") nuclei. The nests are usually solid, but may be cystic as well. The distinction between a malignant Brenner tumor and a transitional cell carcinoma is the identification of benign Brenner tumor adjacent to and transitioning into the malignant component in malignant Brenner tumor, whereas transitional cell carcinoma only shows the malignant component, which resembles transitional cell carcinoma seen in genitourinary locations.

9.3.12 Undifferentiated Carcinomas

Some epithelial neoplasms defy categorization due to lack of differentiation and are classified as undifferentiated carcinoma.

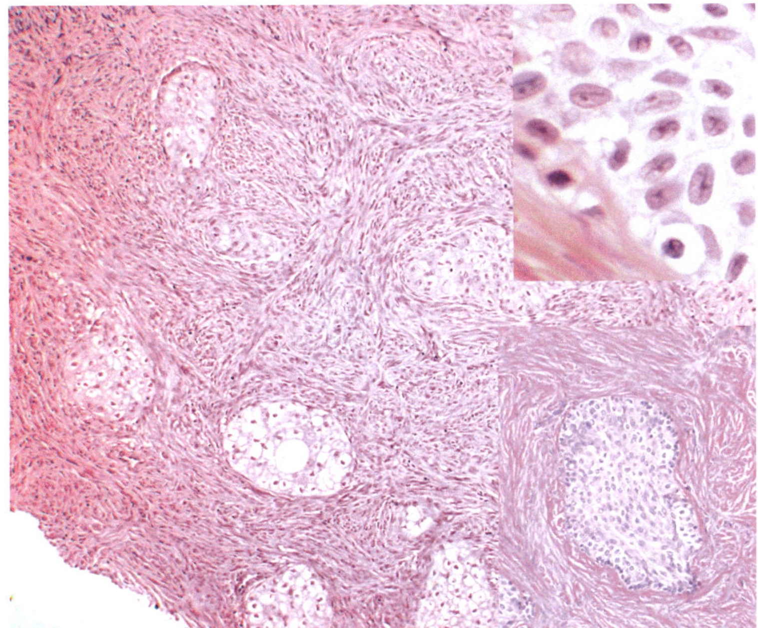

Fig. 9.14 Brenner tumor. Nests of solid (*lower inset*) and occasionally cystic transitional cells with grooved nuclei (*upper inset*) in a fibromatous background

9.3.13 Small Cell Carcinoma, Hypercalcemic Type

This rare aggressive tumor is associated with hypercalcemia. It has a wide variety of histologic appearances, including sheets of cells, with pseudofollicular spaces. This lesion needs to be distinguished from the rare small cell neuroendocrine carcinoma of the ovary.

9.3.14 Malignant Mixed Mesodermal (Müllerian) Tumor (Carcinosarcoma)

While more common in the uterus, carcinosarcomas can arise as ovarian primary tumors.

9.4 Germ Cell Tumors

Benign cystic teratomas are benign neoplasms derived from the germ cells of the ovary. The other lesions discussed are malignant. Germ cell neoplasms tend to present at a younger age than the epithelial neoplasms.

9.4.1 Benign Cystic Teratoma

Benign cystic teratomas ("dermoid") are among the more common adnexal neoplasms, often seen in younger women. They are heavy for their size, and hence have a tendency to undergo torsion. If they rupture, they can provoke a florid chemical peritonitis, due to the sebaceous contents. Although the cystic contents are liquid-based at body temperature, they solidify when at room temperature, so appear as solid greasy contents in the Pathology Laboratory, admixed with hair, and occasionally teeth (Fig. 9.15a). If these contents are removed, the neoplasm is noted to be

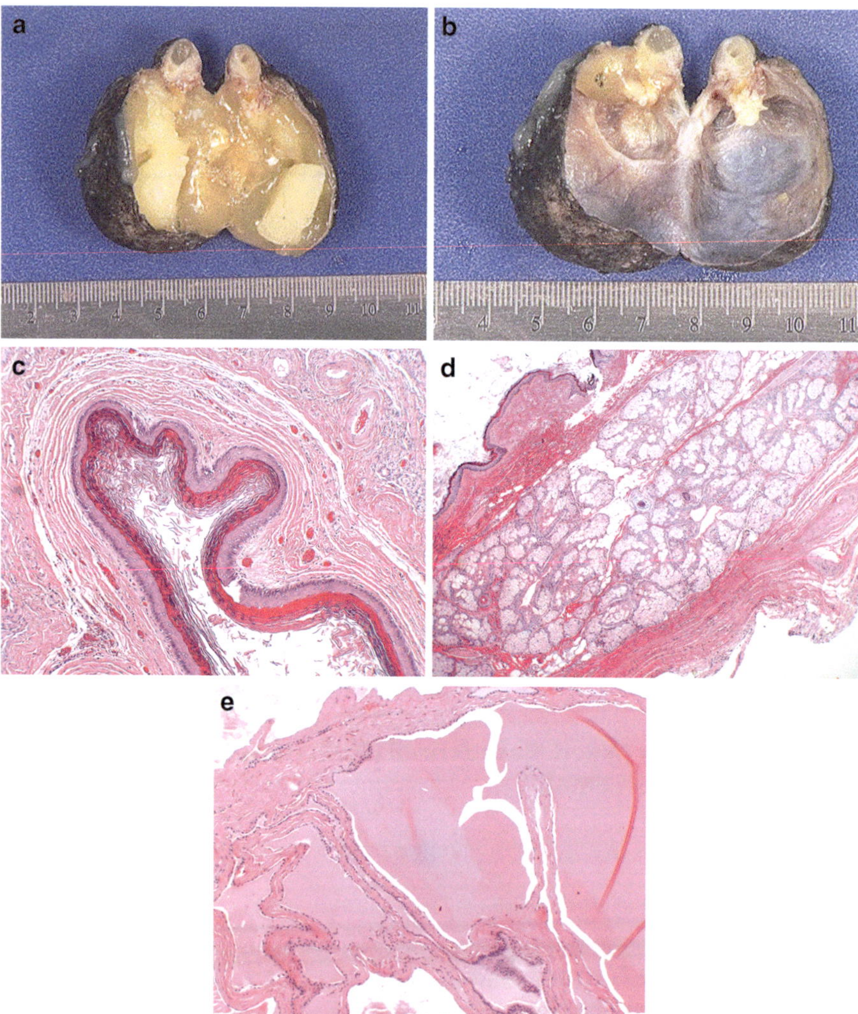

Fig. 9.15 Benign cystic teratoma. At room temperature in the laboratory, the contents appear as solid greasy material with hair (**a**). Once evacuated, the lesion is predominantly cystic with a solid Rokitansky protuberance (**b**). Histologically the ectodermal components predominate, with squamous epithelium shedding keratinaceous debris (**c**), and abundant sebaceous glands (**d**). Struma ovarii (**e**) showing recognizable thyroid tissue at the lowermost aspect of the tumor

predominantly cystic, usually with a single solid protuberance, the Rokintansky's protuberance (Fig. 9.15b). This solid area is what gives rise to the tissues from the three germ cell layers, with the ectodermal component predominating over the endoderm and mesoderm. Thus, it is not surprising that in the rare dermoid that undergoes malignant transformation, the most common malignancy is squamous cell carcinoma. This is a completely different entity than immature teratoma (see below), which is malignant from the start. Histologically, all manner of mature tissues may be seen in dermoids, most commonly squamous epithelium and sebaceous glands (Fig. 9.15c, d), but other mature tissues, including brain, respiratory epithelium, and cartilage, are common. A variant of benign cystic teratoma is the struma ovarii. The definitions for struma ovarii vary, but all have a major component of thyroid tissue. Some define struma ovarii as mainly thyroid, some as entirely thyroid, and some as grossly identifiable thyroid (Fig. 9.15e). Potential functionality and/or malignant behavior of the thyroid tissue cannot be predicted based on histologic appearance.

9.4.2 Malignant Germ Cell Tumors

Except for benign cystic teratomas with variants, germ cell tumors fall into the malignant category. Malignant germ cell tumors occur predominantly in younger patients, often adolescent. Although they may be of pure type, mixed germ cell tumors are common and must be looked for. Features of the more common lesions are described.

9.4.3 Immature Teratoma

Immature teratomas tend to be larger than the benign counterpart and more solid (Fig. 9.16a). There is no distinct gross appearance to this or any of the germ cell tumors, but the appearance is worrisome for malignancy. Immature teratomas can be comprised of a mix of mature and immature histologic elements, and so must be

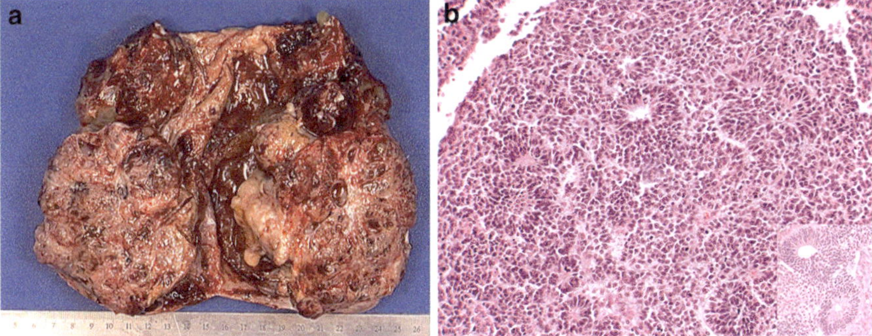

Fig. 9.16 Immature teratoma. Grossly (**a**) there isn't a distinct appearance, but it is clearly worrisome for malignancy. The hallmark is the presence of immature neural tubules (**b** and *inset*)

adequately sampled to look for the immature portions that define the lesion, as well as for a mixed germ cell component, particularly yolk sac tumor, which may be more aggressive. The hallmark tissue that defines immature teratoma is the presence of immature neuroepithelium, usually in the form of neural tubules, and the lesion is graded by how many low power fields of this tissue are present on the worst slide (Fig. 9.16b).

9.4.4 Dysgerminoma

Dysgerminoma is histologically identical to the analogous male seminoma, comprised of large germ cells separated by fibrous stroma containing variable amounts of lymphocytes (Fig. 9.17).

9.4.5 Yolk Sac Tumor

Yolk sac tumor (endodermal sinus tumor) may be pure or often comprises part of a mixed germ cell tumor. The hallmark findings are globules composed of alpha-fetoprotein, which can be stained for via immunohistochemistry, and the presence of Schiller–Duval bodies (Fig. 9.18) a distinct formation of a vessel surrounded by tumor residing in a space surrounded a by more tumors.

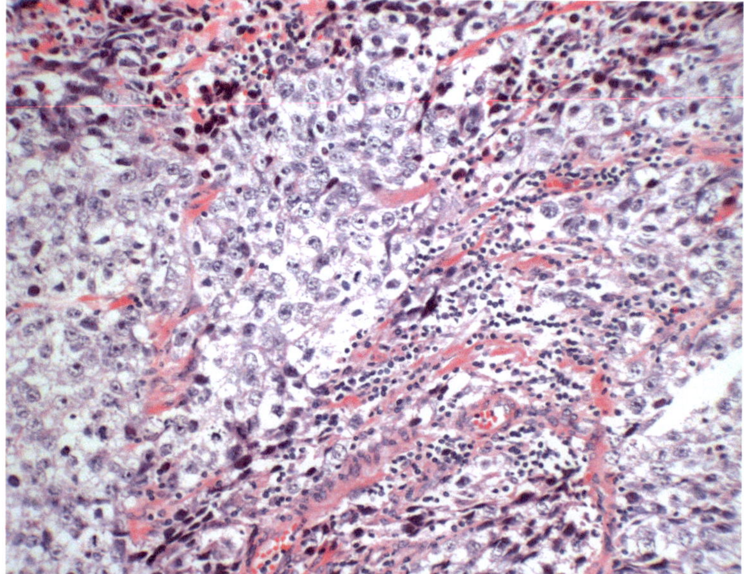

Fig. 9.17 Dysgerminoma. A good mnemonic is "dysgerminoma with the lymphocytic stroma" for the lymphocyte-containing fibroconnective tissue between the nests of germ cells

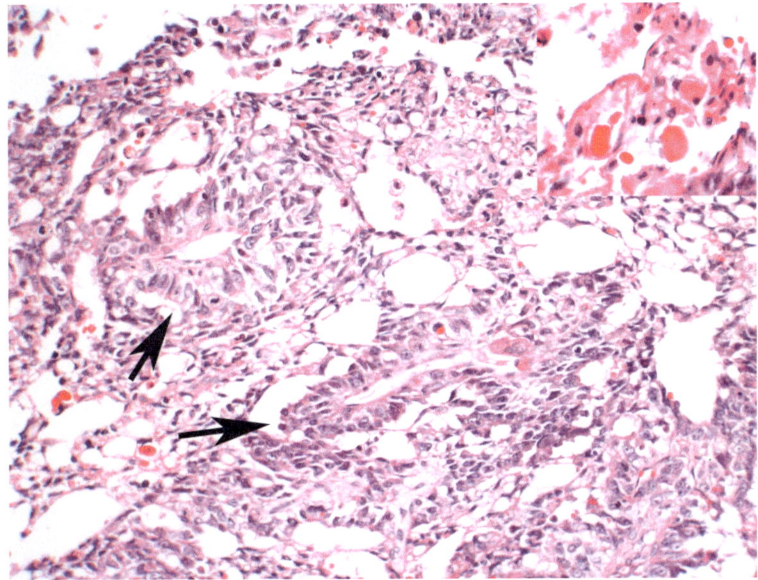

Fig. 9.18 Yolk sac tumor. The hallmark is the presence of Schiller–Duval bodies (*arrows*), a vessel surrounded by tumor in a space surrounded by tumor. *Pink* globules that stain for AFP are sometimes seen (*inset*)

9.4.6   Other Germ Cell Tumors

Other germ cell elements may be seen, usually in mixed germ cell tumors, including choriocarcinoma, embryonal carcinoma, and rarely polyembryoma, with embryoid bodies that resemble an early embryo. These are rarely pure ovarian lesions.

9.5   Sex Cord-Stromal Tumors

Although not distinguishing between the tumor types, a positive stain for inhibin helps characterize an ovarian tumor as falling into the sex cord-stromal category.

9.5.1   Granulosa Cell Tumor

Granulosa cell tumors are low-grade indolent malignancies. They may be functional, and unopposed estrogen can stimulate the endometrium, leading to hyperplasia or neoplasia. Grossly, granulosa cell tumors are often cystic and solid and may be very hemorrhagic (Fig. 9.19a). There are a wide variety of histologic appearances, but the most recognizable is the microfollicular pattern with Call–Exner bodies, which are degenerative spaces, not glands (Fig. 9.19b). The cells of granulosa cell tumors, except for a juvenile variant, have grooved nuclei ("coffee bean" nuclei).

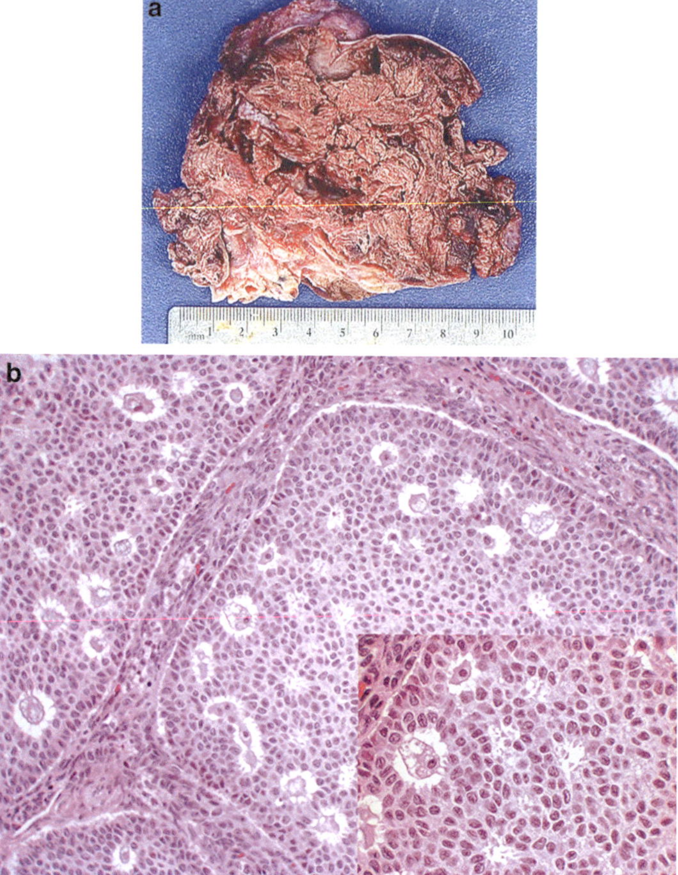

Fig. 9.19 Granulosa cell tumor. The lesions are cystic, solid, and hemorrhagic (**a**). Histologically, the most recognizable pattern is the microfollicular pattern (**b**). The degenerative Call–Exner bodies are lined by cells with grooved nuclei (*inset*)

9.5.2 Fibrothecoma

In pathology, there are lumpers and splitters in the classification of lesions. The splitters separate lesions into fibromas for white lesions that grossly resemble leiomyomas, and thecomas for more yellow lesions with more likelihood of endocrine activity (Fig. 9.20a, b). The lumpers call all these lesions together fibrothecomas. Grossly, they are solid well-circumscribed lesions. Histologically, they are composed of benign appearing spindle cells, which may appear more vacuolated in thecomatous regions (Fig. 9.20c). The lesions may occasionally produce estrogen. These lesions are almost always benign, and usually unilateral.

9.5.3 Sertoli–Leydig Cell Tumor

Sertoli–Leydig cell tumors are less common than granulosa cell tumors and fibrothecomas. They can be functional and may be masculinizing. If well-differentiated, they

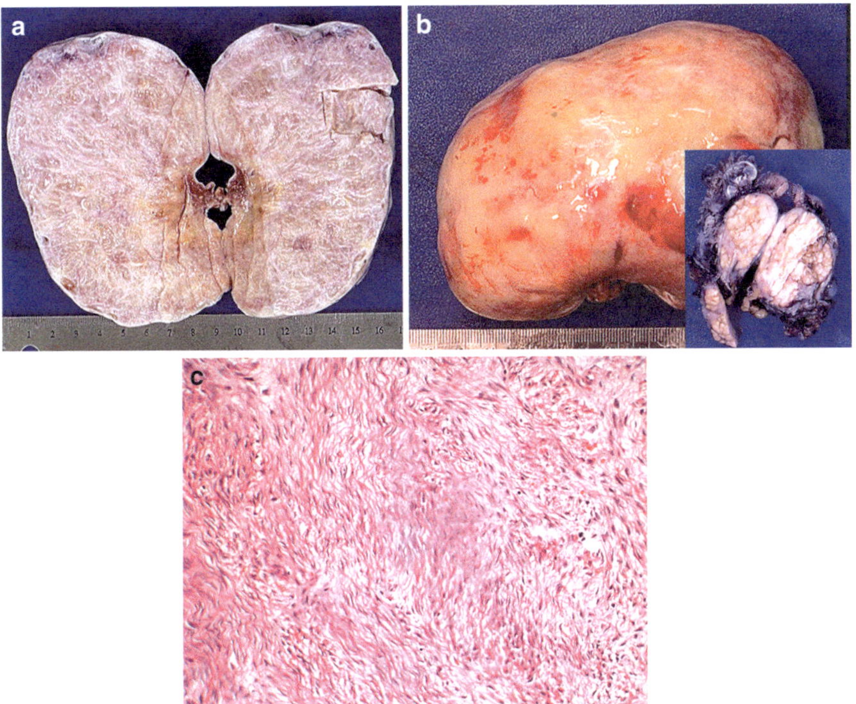

Fig. 9.20 Fibrothecoma. Fibroma, appearing similar grossly to a leiomyoma (**a**). Thecoma is more *yellow*, here seen externally and on cut surface (**b**). Many pathologists call both lesions fibrothecoma. Histologically, they are composed of bland spindle cells. Unlike the cigar shape nuclei of leiomyomata, these are pointed at the ends (**c**)

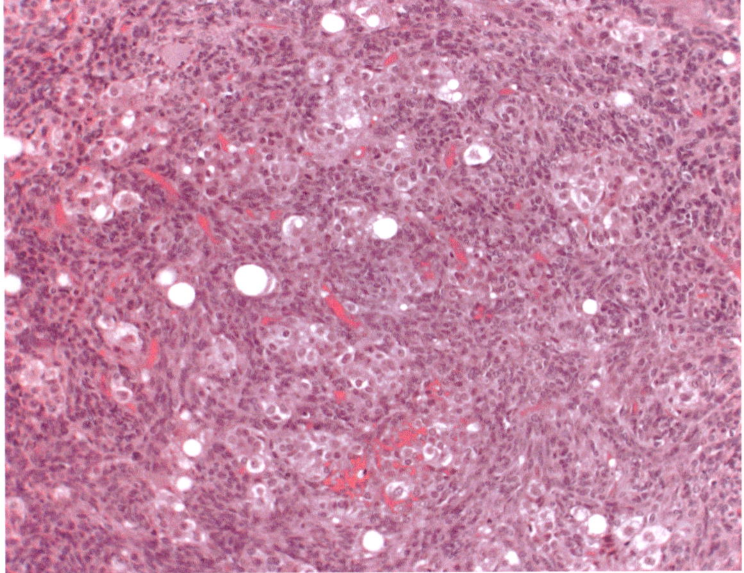

Fig. 9.21 Sertoli–Leydig cell tumor. Although this moderately differentiated lesion is not making tubules, the biphasic nature can be seen

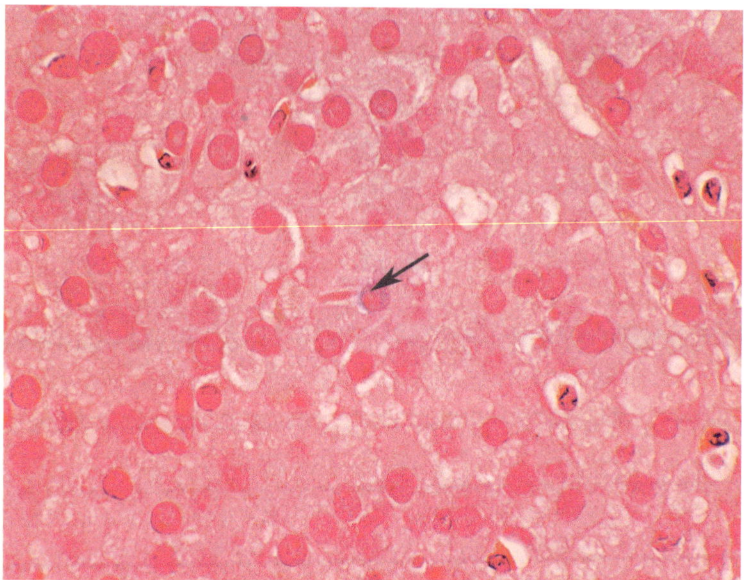

Fig. 9.22 Leydig cell tumor, composed of sheets of eosinophilic cells, showing Reinke crystalloids (*arrow*)

resemble the Sertoli and Leydig cells of the testis in both cytology and architecture, with well-formed Sertoli tubules with interspersed Leydig cells between the tubules, but the less well-differentiated ones may show sheets of cells, with the biphasic nature more subtle (Fig. 9.21).

9.5.4   Steroid Cell Tumor

These lesions have been called a variety of other terms, including lipid tumor, lipoid tumor, and Leydig cell tumor. They can be functional and may be masculinizing. Grossly, they have a characteristic brown-gold to yellow cut surface and are composed of sheets of cells with abundant eosinophilic cytoplasm, resembling corpus luteum cells. Currently they are classified as stromal luteoma, for small benign lesions surrounded by ovarian tissue, or as hilar or nonhilar steroid cell tumors for larger tumors, which may have malignant potential. The term Leydig cell tumor is reserved for those steroid cell tumors that have identifiable Reinke crystalloids in the cytoplasm of the cells (Fig. 9.22).

9.6   Metastatic Tumors

9.6.1   Krukenberg Tumor

A wide variety of malignant neoplasms, both genital and nongenital, can metastasize to ovaries, most likely due to the rich vascular supply. A hallmark of metastatic lesions is their frequent bilaterality, which assists in the evaluation of these lesions. A unique

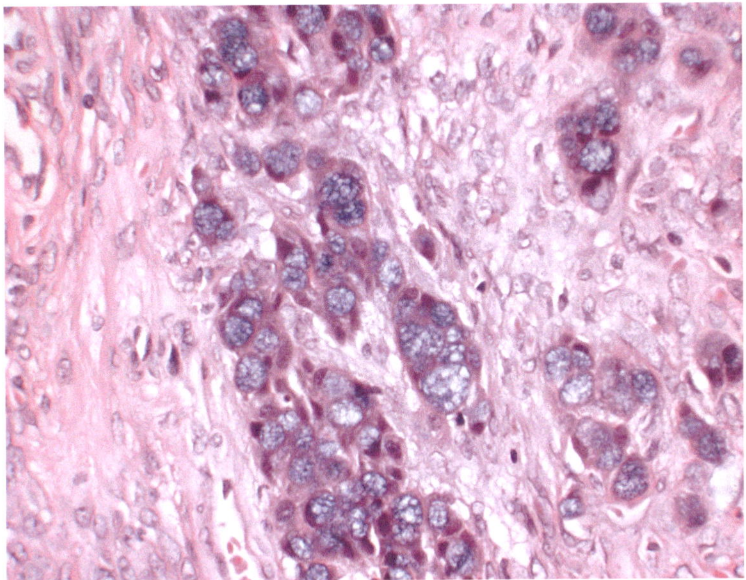

Fig. 9.23 Krukenberg tumor. Histologically, metastatic signet-ring cell adenocarcinoma, with mucin pushing the nuclei to one side ("signet ring cells"), is seen

neoplasm in this category is the Krukenberg tumor. This term is used specifically for metastatic signet ring cell carcinoma to the ovaries (Fig. 9.23). As in other metastatic lesions, it is generally bilateral, and the ovaries, while markedly enlarged, tend to keep their usual shape. Signet ring cell carcinomas are most commonly metastatic from the stomach, then breast and colon. Metastases from stomach, breast or colonic primaries that are not signet ring cell carcinomas are not termed Krukenberg tumors.

9.7 Miscellaneous Tumors

9.7.1 Sex Cord Tumor with Annular Tubules

These rare neoplasms are seen most often in association with Peutz-Jeghers syndrome. They can occasionally exhibit malignant behavior and may be hormonally active. They have a distinct appearance of tubules containing abundant eosinophilic basement membrane material.

9.7.2 Gonadoblastoma

Gonadoblastomas occur in association with intersex conditions where there is testicular tissue. They are considered in situ germ cell neoplasms that can overgrow into malignant germ cell tumors, most commonly dysgerminoma. They are comprised of nests of mixed sex cord stromal and germ cells (sertoli-like cells and germ

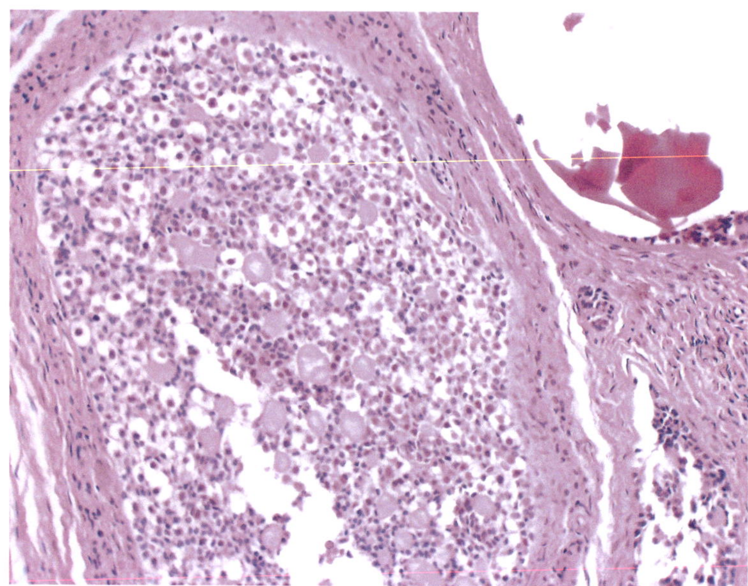

Fig. 9.24 Gondoblastoma showing a calcification (*upper right*) adjacent to a nest containing larger pale germ cells, smaller sex cord stromal cells, and eosinophilic basement membrane material. The most common invasive malignancy associated with this in situ malignancy is dysgerminoma, due to overgrowth of the germ cells breaking out of the nests

cells) with basement membrane material and frequent calcification separated by nonspecific stroma which may contain Leydig-like cells (Fig. 9.24).

9.7.3 Gynandroblastoma

These exceptionally rare sex cord stromal tumors contain both male (Sertoli) and female (granulosa) cells.

References

1. Cavoretto P, Giorgione V, Sigismondi C, Mangili G, Serafini A, Dallagiovanna C, et al. Hyperreactio luteinalis: timely diagnosis minimizes the risk of oophorectomy and alerts clinicians to the associated risk of placental insufficiency. Eur J Obstet Gynecol Reprod Biol. 2014;176:10–6.
2. Plotti F, DiGiovanni A, Oliva C, Battaglia F, Plotti G. Bilateral ovarian pregnancy after intrauterine insemination and controlled ovarian stimulation. Fertil Steril. 2008;90:e3–5.
3. Spiegelberg O. Casuistry in ovarian pregnancy. Arch Gynecol. 1878;13:73–9.
4. Kurman RJ, Shih I-M. The origin and pathogenesis of epithelial ovarian cancer—a proposed unifying theory. Am J Surg Pathol. 2010;34:433–43.
5. Bell DA. Low-grade serous tumors of ovary. Int J Gynecol Pathol. 2014;33:348–56.
6. Ronnett BM, Zahn CM, Kurman RJ, Kass ME, Sugarbaker PH, Shmookler BM. Disseminated peritoneal adenomucinosis and peritoneal mucinous carcinomatosis. A clinicopathologic analysis of 109 cases with emphasis on distinguishing pathologic features, site of origin, prognosis, and relationship to "pseudomyxoma peritonei". Am J Surg Pathol. 1995;19:1390–408.

10.1 Lesions of the Broad Ligament

Lesions arising in the broad ligament are uncommon, and most commonly endometriotic implants, leiomyomata, and hernias occurring through broad ligament defects. Rare broad ligament pregnancies have occurred (Table 10.1).

10.1.1 Female Tumor of Probably Wolffian Origin (FATWO)

The most common site of origin of this rare neoplasm is the broad ligament, but they have also occurred in the ovary and retroperitoneum [1]. These lesions may be grossly cystic or solid and histologically have a variety of patterns, including solid, with characteristic sieve-like areas, and with a variety of cellular morphologic features (Fig. 10.1). The lesions stain for C-kit, which is helpful in establishing the diagnosis. Although most of these lesions behave in a benign manner, some have exhibited metastases, sometimes years later [1].

10.1.2 Rare Broad Ligament Neoplasms and Broad Ligament Neoplasms More Often Occurring in Other Pelvic Locations

Epithelial neoplasms may occur in the broad ligament, including benign serous cystadenoma, as well as low malignant potential ("borderline") serous neoplasms. Rare malignancies of various Müllerian epithelial types, sometimes in association with endometriosis, have been reported [1, 2]. A small number of cases of a papillary cystadenoma of mesonephric rather than Müllerian origin have been reported in association with von Hippel Lindau syndrome [3].

Rare germ cell neoplasms and mesenchymal tumors such as leiomyomata have also arisen in the broad ligament. Leiomyomas are the most common lesion of the

© Springer International Publishing Switzerland 2015
D.S. Heller, *OB-GYN Pathology for the Clinician*,
DOI 10.1007/978-3-319-15422-0_10

Table 10.1   Key points about broad ligament pathology

Most broad ligament lesions are leiomyomata or implants of endometriosis
A variety of epithelial lesions arising elsewhere in the upper female genital tract can arise in the broad ligament as well
Female Adnexal Tumor of Probable Wolffian Origin (FATWO) is a rare lesion that usually arises in the broad ligament

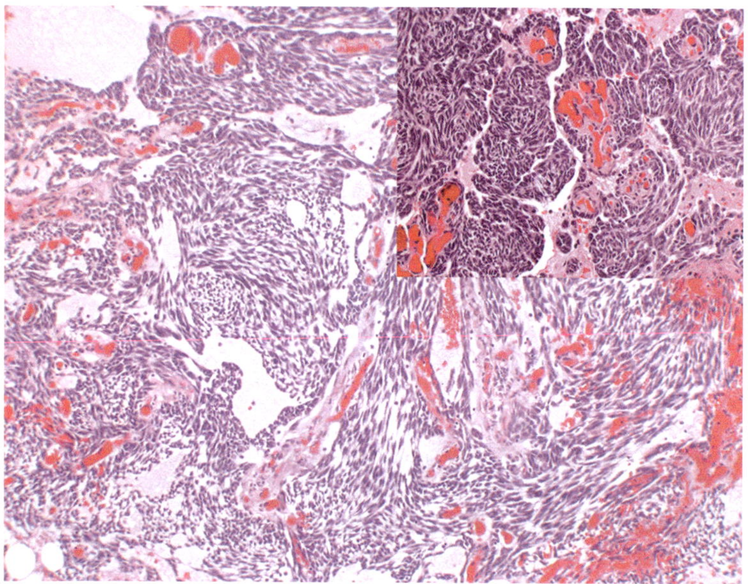

Fig. 10.1   Female adnexal tumor of probably Wolffian origin (FATWO) often shows a characteristic sieve-like pattern, but may appear more solid (*inset, upper right*)

broad ligament [3], and only rare leiomyosarcomas have been reported [4]. Adenomyomas have occurred as well [3].

10.2   Lesions of the Peritoneum

A variety of sometimes histologically challenging lesions can affect the peritoneum. An index of suspicion, and sometimes immunohistochemistry, can be helpful in difficult cases (Table 10.2).

10.3   Benign Lesions of the Peritoneum

10.3.1 Endometriosis

Endometriosis involving peritoneum is often a clinical diagnosis and may not yield material for histopathological evaluation. Endometriosis often elicits a dense

Table 10.2   Key points about peritoneal pathology

A variety of benign and malignant mesothelial proliferations may appear similar histologically and be difficult to distinguish. True invasion may be the only definitive histologic sign of malignancy
Distinguishing papillary serous cystadenocarcinoma from peritoneal malignant mesothelioma usually requires an immunohistochemical panel of several antibodies
Primary peritoneal high-grade serous carcinoma is thought to arise from serous tubal intraepithelial carcinoma and is diagnosed after tubal or ovarian primaries are ruled out
Pseudomyxoma peritonei is most likely of primary appendiceal origin

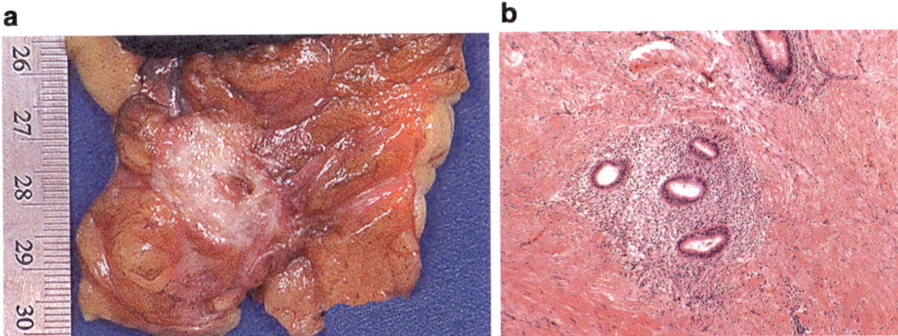

Fig. 10.2   Endometriosis. Endometriosis often provokes a dense fibrotic response around the hemorrhagic foci (**a**). Histologically, there are endometrial glands and stroma surrounded by dense fibroconnective tissue (**b**)

fibrotic response, particularly in omentum and abdominal wall (Fig. 10.2a). As in other sites, the histologic diagnosis requires endometrial glandular epithelium and stroma to confirm the diagnosis (Fig. 10.2b), which cannot be confirmed by hemosiderin-laden macrophages alone. A variety of Müllerian epithelial-derived malignancies (in particular clear cell adenocarcinoma and endometrioid adenocarcinoma) arising from pelvic soft tissues as well as ovary have arisen in association with endometriosis.

10.3.2 Endosalpingiosis

Endosalpingiosis is a common, clinically insignificant finding in peritoneum and pelvic and paraaortic lymph nodes and is comprised of small inclusions lined by a flattened or tubal-type epithelium (Fig. 10.3). Distinction from endometriosis is assisted by the lack of surrounding endometrial stroma in endosalpingiosis. Although endosalpingiosis may be an incidental finding in isolation, it is frequently associated with serous tumors of low malignant potential, and there may be some difficulties distinguishing endosalpingiosis from tumor implants histologically.

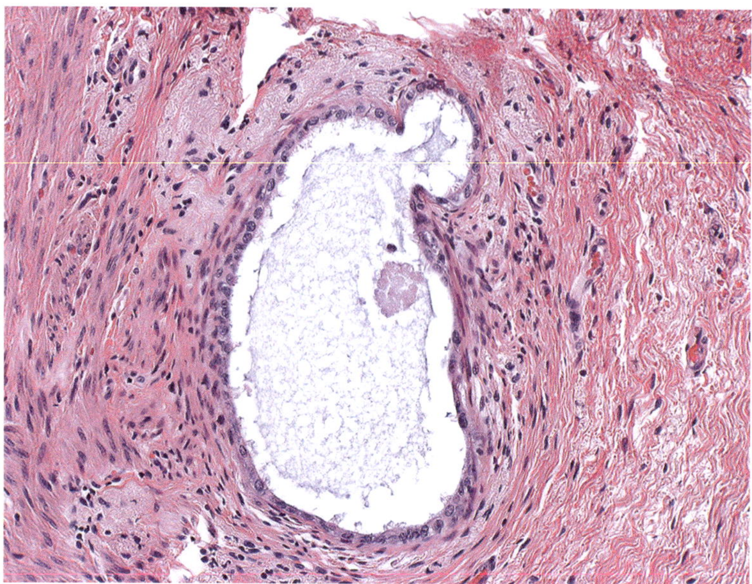

Fig. 10.3 Endosalpingiosis. There is a tubal epithelial type lining, and no cuff of endometrial stroma around the glandular space, distinguishing the lesion from endometriosis

10.3.3 Paraovarian/Paratubal Cyst

Paraovarian/paratubal cysts are usually benign thin-walled smooth serous lesions lined by a flat or tubal-type epithelium, although low malignant potential ("borderline") and malignant neoplasms have occurred. These lesions may undergo torsion or present as a pelvic mass, or be asymptomatic. A histologic hallmark is in the wall of the benign tubal or flattened epithelial-lined cyst, which is composed of neither ovarian tissue nor tubal smooth muscle (Fig. 10.4). Most of these lesions are of Müllerian origin, but mesonephric (Wolffian) cysts can rarely occur [5].

10.3.4 Ectopic Decidua (Decidualization, Deciduosis)

While usually an incidental histologic diagnosis involving peritoneal surfaces, Fallopian tube or cervix (Fig. 10.5a) of recently pregnant women, rarely ectopic decidua can form peritoneal nodules that mimic malignancy clinically and can even cause significant peritoneal hemorrhage, with rare fatalities reported [1, 6, 7]. Histologically, ectopic decidua appears much as decidua in the endometrium (Fig. 10.5b), with sheets of cells with abundant eosinophilic cytoplasm. Ectopic decidualization can also be seen in cases of endometriosis in women exposed to progestins, such as pregnancy or medication. Here glands as well as stroma may be seen.

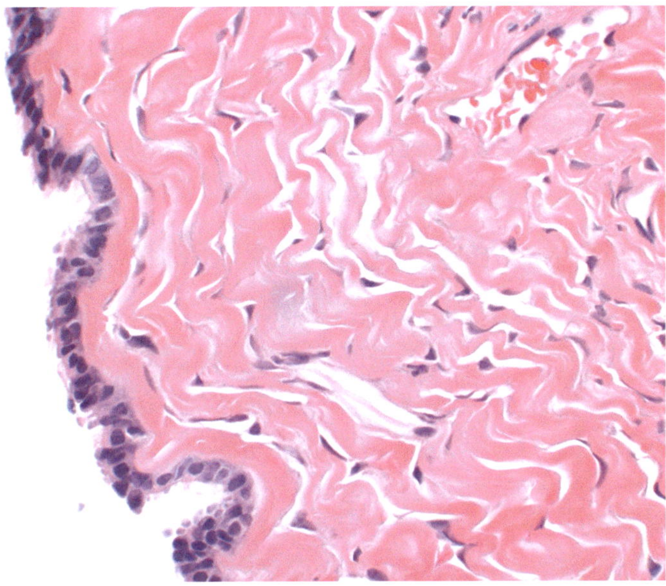

Fig. 10.4 Paraovarian cyst. The cyst can be lined by a flattened epithelium, or a tubal one, as shown here, reflecting the usual Müllerian origin. The wall lacks ovarian stroma as well as tubal smooth muscle, consistent with a cyst arising outside these two structures

10.3.5 Ectopic Pregnancy

While rare, ectopic pregnancy is not always tubal and can occur in the abdomen, on peritoneal surfaces as well as the previously mentioned broad ligament. It is possible that these abdominal implantations are secondary to a tubal pregnancy that has ruptured or aborted through the fimbria, and then established a secondary implantation site [8].

10.3.6 Mesothelial Hyperplasia

Mesothelial hyperplasia is a reactive process seen in association with a variety of benign, malignant, and inflammatory peritoneal processes. It is usually an incidental microscopic finding (Fig. 10.6), but if florid can raise concern for a malignant mesothelioma. Although distribution of the process and immunohistochemical markers may provide some assistance, at times only frank invasion can establish a histologic diagnosis of malignancy in mesothelial proliferations.

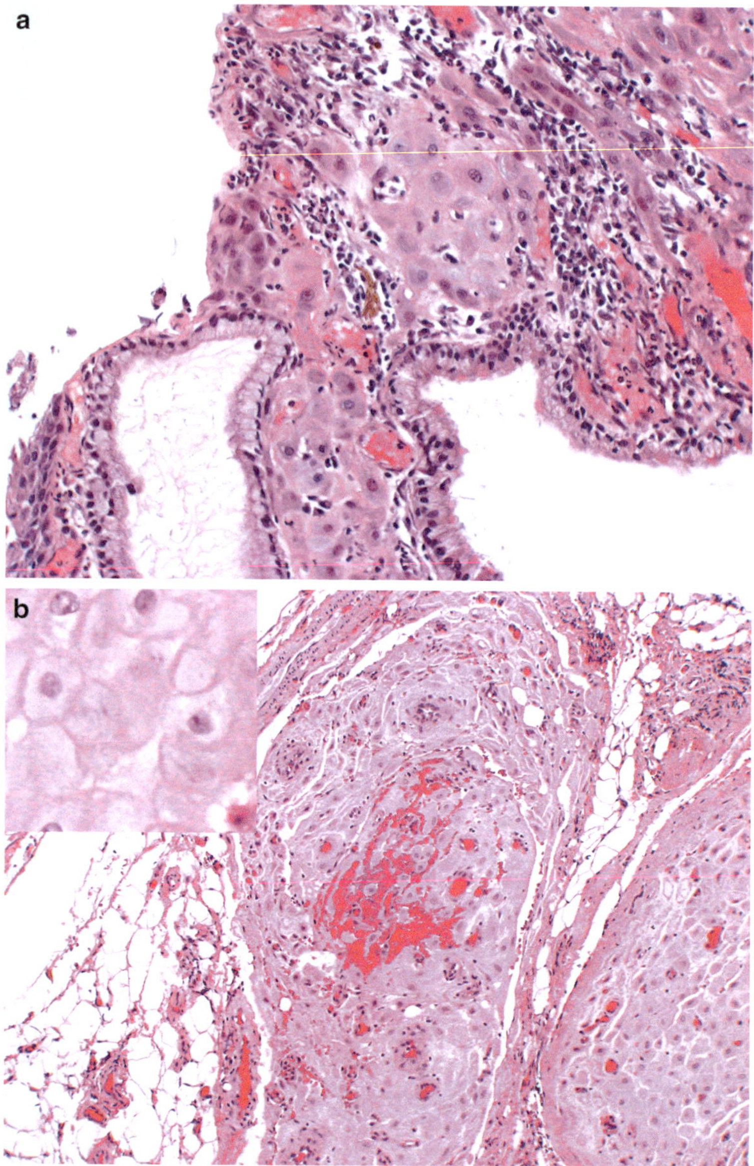

Fig. 10.5 Decidual change in the endocervix (**a**). Deciduosis of omentum (**b**). There is decidualization of the fibroadipose tissue, forming nodules, with some hemorrhage seen. The decidualized cells are large with abundant eosinophilic cytoplasm (*inset upper left*)

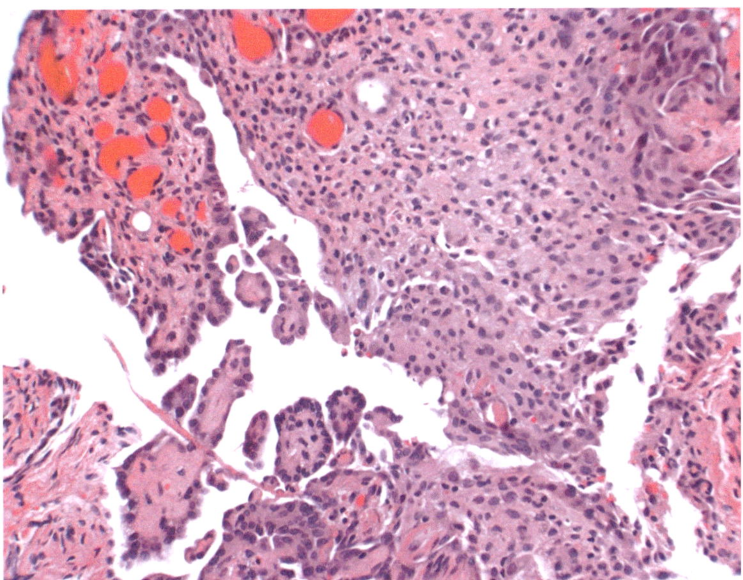

Fig. 10.6 Mesothelial hyperplasia. This usually incidental histologic finding can occasionally be florid enough to mimic malignant mesothelioma

10.3.7 Benign Multicystic Mesothelioma

This rare multiloculated lesion can present as a pelvic mass and may be associated with prior surgery or endometriosis. Whether the lesion is a true neoplasm or a reactive process is a matter of debate [9]; however, the lesion can recur after excision. Grossly, the lesion is composed of thin-walled multiloculated cysts, which may be thought to be peritoneal cysts associated with adhesions. Histologically, bland mesothelial cells line cystic spaces (Fig. 10.7). This lesion should be distinguished from the extremely rare well-differentiated papillary mesothelioma, a true neoplasm that is usually benign.

10.3.8 Diffuse Peritoneal Leiomyomatosis (Leiomyomatosis Peritonealis Disseminata)

Numerous peritoneal nodules of histologically benign smooth muscle may be seen in this rare condition, usually in association with pregnancy or hormonal administration [1], and often regressing when the stimuli are removed. The overwhelming majority of these cases behave in a benign manner.

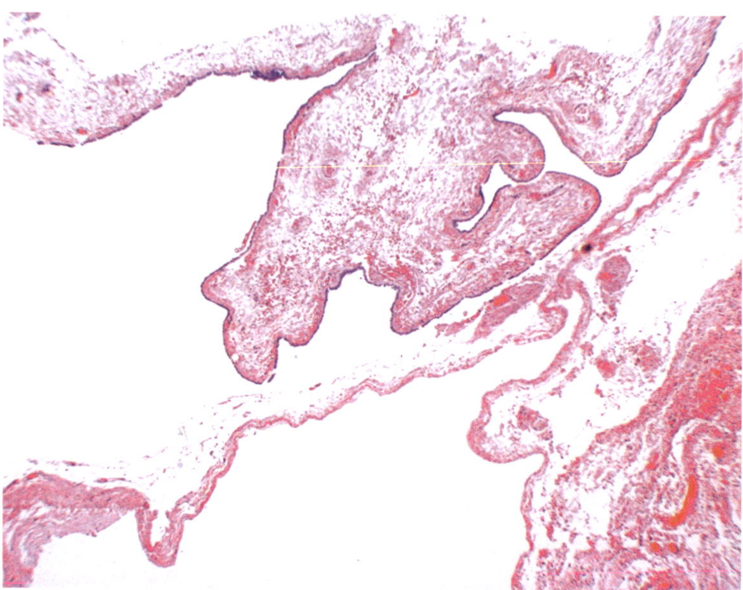

Fig. 10.7 Benign multicystic mesothelioma. Multiloculated cysts lined by a flattened mesothelium are seen

10.4   Malignant Neoplasms of the Peritoneum

10.4.1 Primary Peritoneal Serous Carcinoma

Primary peritoneal high-grade papillary serous cystadenocarcinoma presents similarly to the ovarian counterpart, and the tumor is histologically the same (Fig. 10.8a–c). The way to distinguish the lesion is that the ovaries are uninvolved, or only a small amount of ovarian surface is involved by tumor, and that the primary invasive carcinoma does not arise from the fallopian tubes. Primary peritoneal serous carcinomas are currently thought to arise from serous tubal intraepithelial carcinoma (STIC, see Chap. 8).

10.4.2 Malignant Mesothelioma

Peritoneal malignant mesothelioma is a rare neoplasm in women. Clinically, it can mimic ovarian carcinoma. Although there is an association with asbestos exposure in some patients [10], often no such exposure can be established. Histologically, the lesion may resemble papillary serous cystadenocarcinoma, although there is generally less cytologic atypia, with more uniformity of cells (Fig. 10.9a, b). Because of the histologic similarities, as well as some immunohistochemical overlap,

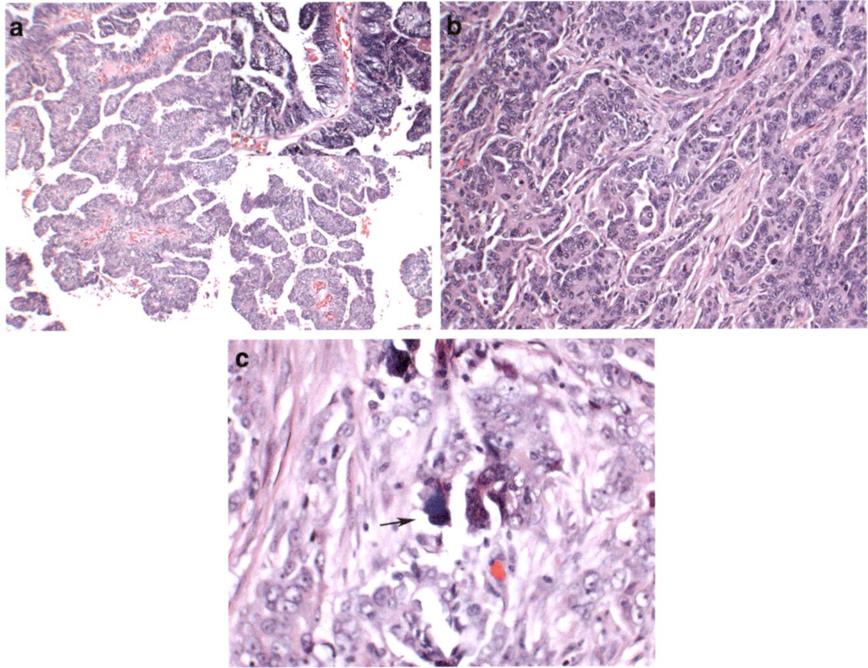

Fig. 10.8   Primary peritoneal serous carcinoma. The lesion is histologically identical to the ovarian counterpart and may be papillary (**a**), or more solid (**b**). Nuclear atypia is often pronounced (**a**, *inset upper right*). Psammoma bodies, thought to be degenerative calcifications showing a concentric configuration, while not diagnostic, are characteristic (**c**) (*arrow*)

pathologists often use a broad panel of immunohistochemical antibodies to help distinguish this lesion from the more common papillary serous cystadenocarcinoma [10, 11].

10.4.3 Pseudomyxoma Peritoneii

Pseudomyxoma peritoneii (mucinous ascites) is a difficult clinical problem, because it is recurrent, and complications unrelated to actual malignancy may cause morbidity and mortality. Unlike usual ascites, which is often not loculated, pseudomyxoma is usually loculated and hence not easily drained (Fig. 10.10a). The underlying etiology was originally thought to be a mucinous ovarian tumor, most often low malignant potential ("borderline") tumor of the ovary; however, most investigators currently consider a primary appendiceal mucinous neoplasm to be the origin [12]. The association of ovarian and appendiceal mucinous neoplasms is sufficiently frequent to warrant evaluating the appendix in patients with ovarian mucinous tumors. In cases of simultaneous tumor in both ovary and appendix, the ovarian neoplasm may well represent tumor metastatic from the appendix [13]. Histologically, what is

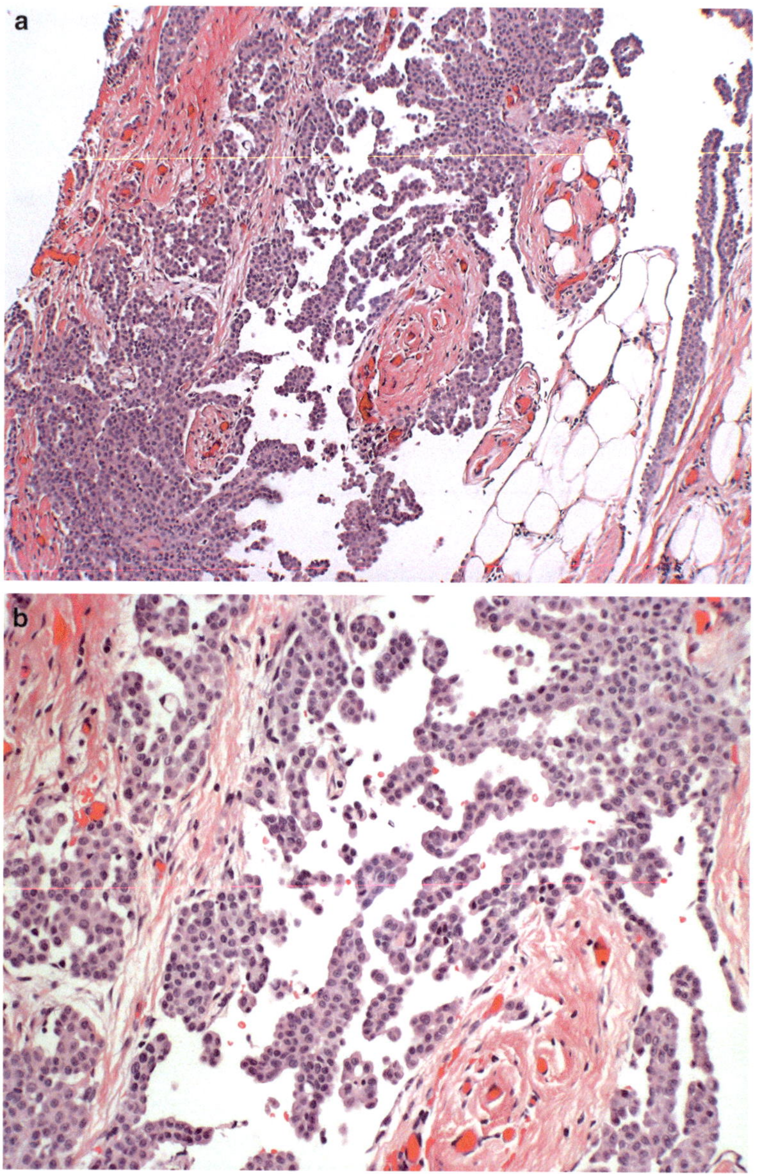

Fig. 10.9 Malignant mesothelioma. A papillary process is seen involving the omentum (**a**). While histologically similar to serous carcinoma, the cytologic atypia tends to be much less (**b**)

most often seen in pseudomyxoma are large pools of mucin with very small amounts of histologically bland or mildly atypical mucinous epithelium (diffuse peritoneal adenomucinosis, DPAM) (Fig. 10.10b, c), although frank mucinous carcinomatosis with more atypia and greater amounts of atypical epithelium can be seen in some cases, possibly with worse prognosis [14].

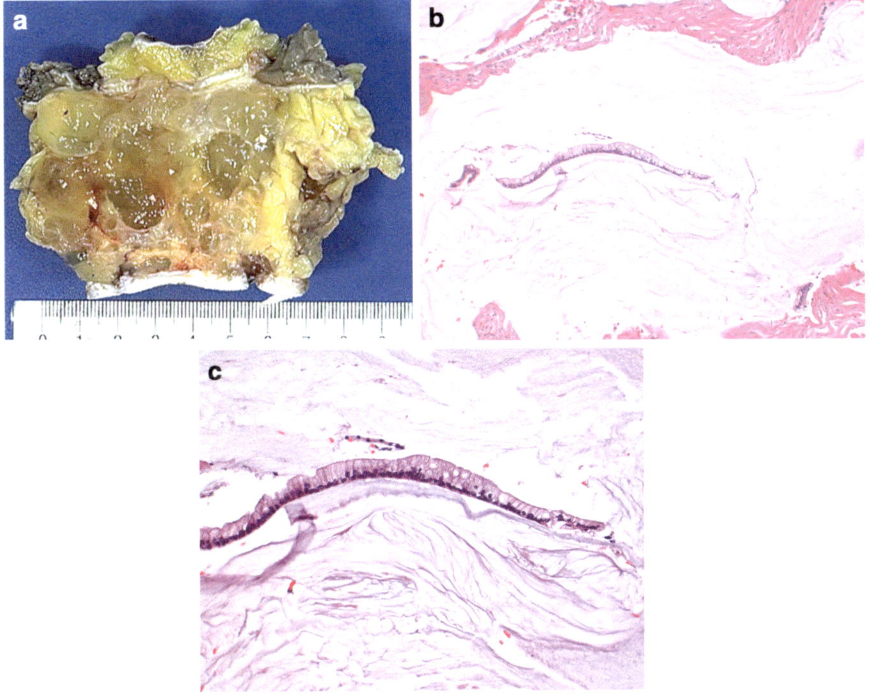

Fig. 10.10 Pseudomyxoma peritonei. The lesion is composed of loculated mucinous ascites (**a**). Histologically, what is usually seen is pools of mucin, with only rare fragments of low-grade mucinous epithelium (**b, c**)

References

1. Thor A, Young R, Clement PB. Pathology of the Fallopian tube, broad ligament, peritoneum, and pelvic soft tissues. Hum Pathol. 1991;22:856–67.
2. Handa Y, Kato M, Kaneuchi M, Saitoh Y, Yamashita K. High-grade broad ligament cancer of Müllerian origin: immunohistochemical analysis of a case and review of the literature. Int J Gynecol Cancer. 2007;17:705–34.
3. Young RH. Neoplasms of the fallopian tube and broad ligament: a selective survey including historical perspective and emphasizing recent developments. Pathology. 2007;39:112–24.
4. Kolusari A, Ugurluer G, Kosem M, Kurdoglu M, Yildizhan R, Adali E. Leiomyosarcoma of the broad ligament: a case report and review of the literature. Eur J Gynaecol Oncol. 2009;30(3):332–4.
5. Akkawi R, Valente AL, Badawy SZ. Large mesonephric cyst with acute adnexal torsion in a teenage girl. J Pediatr Adolesc Gynecol. 2012;25:e143–5.
6. Richter MA, Choudhry A, Barton JJ, Merrick RE. Bleeding ectopic decidua as a cause of intraabdominal hemorrhage. A case report. J Reprod Med. 1983;28:430–2.
7. O'Leary SM. Ectopic decidualization causing massive postpartum intraperitoneal hemorrhage. Obstet Gynecol. 2006;108:776–9.
8. Lee SW, Choi HJ, Lee YK, Yoon JH. Omental implantation secondary to ruptured tubal pregnancy with a negative urine pregnancy test: a case report. J Reprod Med. 2013; 58:89–92.

9. Witek TD, Marchese JW, Farrell TJ. A recurrence of benign multicystic peritoneal mesothelioma treated through laparoscopic excision: a case report and review of the literature. Surg Laparosc Endosc Percutan Tech. 2014;24:e70–3.
10. Nagata S, Tomoeda M, Kubo C, et al. Malignant mesothelioma of the peritoneum invading the liver and mimicking metastatic carcinoma: a case report. Pathol Res Pract. 2011;207(6):395–8.
11. Gao FF, Krasinskas AM, Chivukula M. Is PAX2 a reliable marker in differentiating diffuse malignant mesotheliomas of peritoneum from serous carcinomas of Müllerian origin? Appl Immunohistochem Mol Morphol. 2012;20:272–6.
12. Rouzbahman M, Chetty R. Mucinous tumours of appendix and ovary: an overview and evaluation of current practice. J Clin Pathol. 2014;67:193–7.
13. Carr NJ. Current concepts in pseudomyxoma peritonei. Ann Pathol. 2014;34:9–13.
14. Ronnett BM, Shmookler BM, Sugarbaker PH, et al. Pseudomyxoma peritonei: new concepts in diagnosis, origin, nomenclature, and relationship to mucinous borderline (low malignant potential) tumors of the ovary. Anat Pathol. 1997;2:197–226.

Pathology of the Female Genital Tract Related to Pregnancy

11

11.1 Lesims of the Female Genital Tract Related to Pregnancy

The hormonal milieu associated with pregnancy is the background for a unique group of genital tract lesions, many of which regress after the hormonal stimulus is removed. It is important to be familiar with these lesions to avoid overinterpretation of their clinical significance (Table 11.1).

11.2 Vulvo-Vaginal Lesions Associated with Pregnancy

11.2.1 Cellular Pseudosarcomatous Fibroepithelial Stromal Polyp of the Vulva and Vagina

Although fibroepithelial stromal polyps can affect a variety of locations, the genital tract lesions are most likely to be encountered in the vulva and vagina. During pregnancy, the stroma of these lesions may show increased cellularity (Fig. 11.1a), increased mitotic activity, atypical mitoses, and cytologic atypia (Fig. 11.1b). Awareness of this effect is important to avoid overdiagnosing these lesions as sarcomas. The lesion most likely to be confused with these hormonally stimulated polyps, sarcoma botryoides (embryonal rhabdomyosarcoma), occurs most often in children, rather than reproductive-aged women. True sarcoma botryoides stains for muscle markers, which are not present in fibroepithelial stromal polyps. Unlike the cambium layer of increased cellularity under the epithelium seen in sarcoma botryoides, cellular pseudosarcomatous fibroepithelial stromal polyps tend to be more cellular in the center [1].

© Springer International Publishing Switzerland 2015
D.S. Heller, *OB-GYN Pathology for the Clinician*,
DOI 10.1007/978-3-319-15422-0_11

Table 11.1 Key points about pregnancy-associated pathology

Vaginal fibroepithelial stromal polyps may look highly atypical in pregnancy, and these should not be mistaken for malignancy
Luteoma, hyperreactio luteinalis, and large solitary luteinized follicle cyst of pregnancy and puerperium are hyperplastic, not neoplastic processes
Uterine subinvolution shows histopathologic evidence of lack of involution of spiral arterioles of the implantation site
Arias-Stella reaction can be seen with pregnancy at any site, not just tubal ectopic pregnancy
If evaluating to confirm a spontaneous abortion, if villi aren't present, the implantation site with associated implantational trophoblasts should be sought

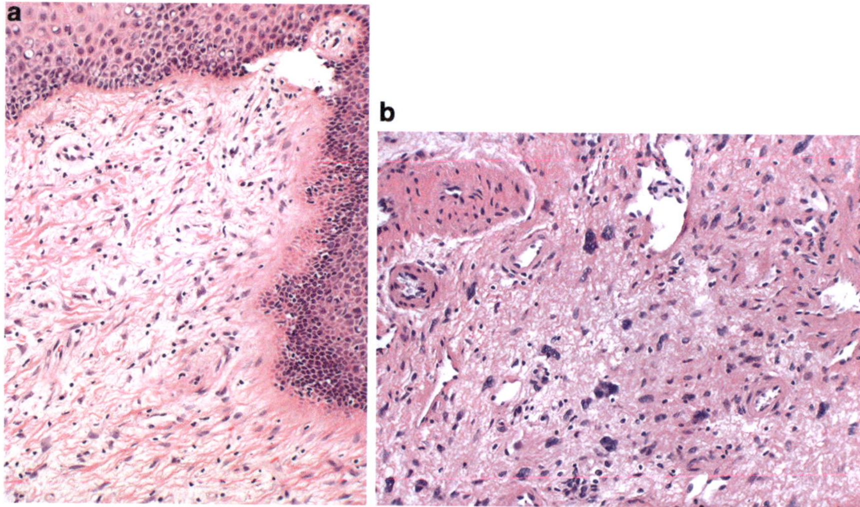

Fig. 11.1 Vaginal fibroepithelial stromal polyp. This polyp shows increased cellularity (**a**), with stellate cells extending to under the overlying epithelium. Additional findings that may be seen in pregnancy include nuclear atypia (**b**), mitoses, and atypical mitotic figures (not shown)

11.3 Uterine Lesions Associated with Pregnancy

11.3.1 Arias-Stella Reaction

The Arias-Stella reaction, named after the pathologist who first described it [2], is a pattern of exaggerated hypersecretory endometrium. It can be seen in association with intrauterine as well as ectopic pregnancies and does not indicate the location of the pregnancy. Histologically, the glands of the endometrium show cytologic atypia

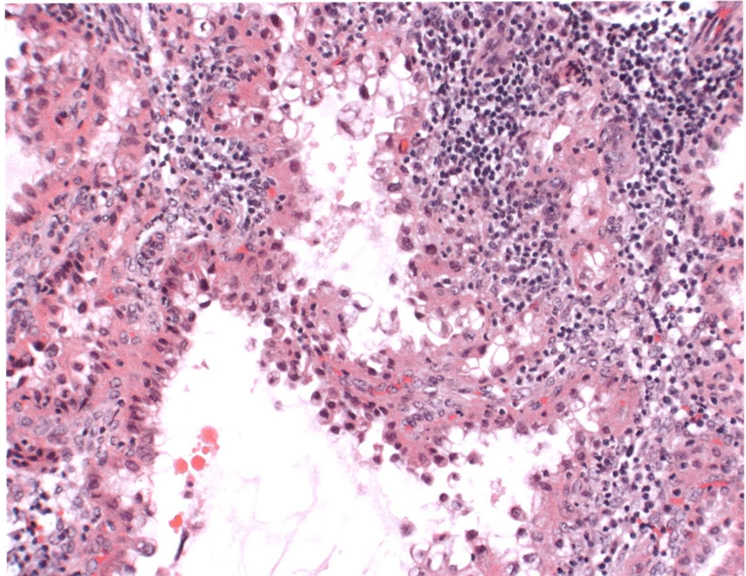

Fig. 11.2   Arias-Stella reaction in gestational endometrium from a partial mole. The glands show hobnail cells with nuclear atypia

with hobnail cells with prominent nuclei (Fig. 11.2). This can mimic one of the histologic patterns seen with clear cell adenocarcinoma, the tubulopapillary pattern, with which Arias-Stella change should not be confused. Clear cell adenocarcinoma of the endometrium generally occurs in a much older patient population and is not associated with pregnancy. Arias-Stella change can also be seen in the cervix, and in extrauterine sites, such as in endometriosis [2].

11.3.2 Spontaneous Abortion (Implantation Site)

With first trimester pregnancy loss, the pathologist reviewing the products of conception is tasked first and foremost with proving that an intrauterine pregnancy was present. When chorionic villi are present, this is a simple task. However, often with spontaneous abortion, the entire placenta has been passed prior to the patient's curettage. The pathologist then must seek evidence of an implantation site. While this does not completely rule out an ectopic pregnancy, it considerably lowers the risk, as heterotopic pregnancies are exceedingly rare, particularly in spontaneous gestations. Risk is greater in IVF pregnancies, but is still low. In curettings from a patient with a spontaneous abortion who has passed the placenta, the implantation site may be recognized by a fibrinoid layer on the decidua, Nitabuch's fibrin, the best place to identify the confirmatory implantation site trophoblasts (Fig. 11.3a, b).

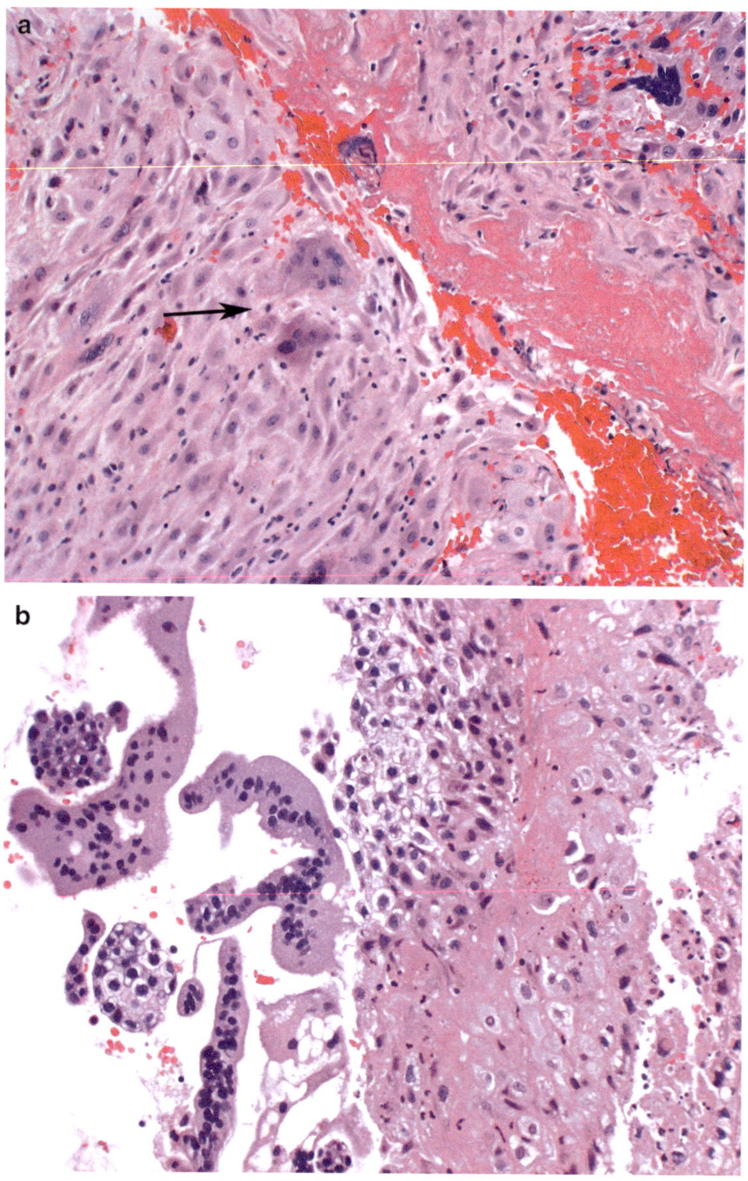

Fig. 11.3 Implantation site. Nitabuch's fibrin is seen adjacent to two implantation site intermediate trophoblasts (*arrow*). Occasionally syncytiotrophoblasts may also be seen (*inset upper right*) (**a**). Implantational intermediate and syncytiotrophoblasts can sometimes be seen in curettings without villi, adjacent to fibrin, confirming a recent intrauterine pregnancy (**b**)

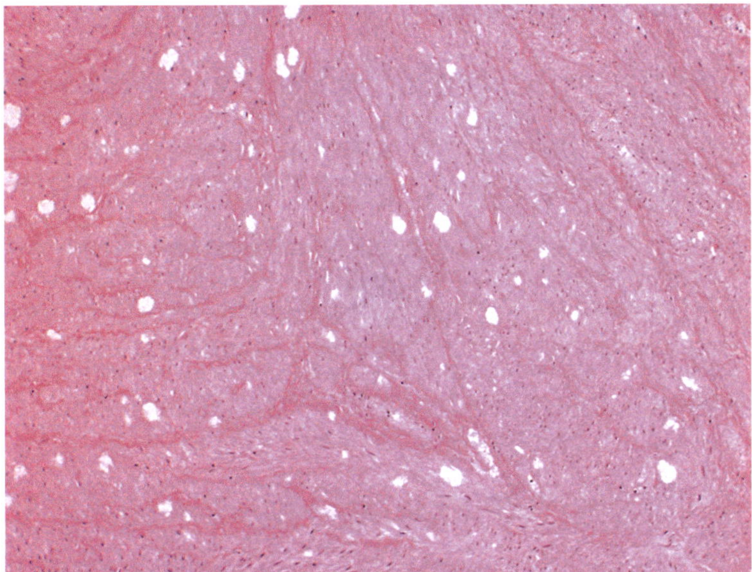

Fig. 11.4 Carneous degeneration. Grossly the myoma is *dark red*. Histologically, there is loss of nuclei and remaining nuclei are pyknotic

11.3.3 Pregnancy-Related Changes in Leiomyomata

Leiomyomas may grow rapidly in pregnancy, and then outgrow their blood supply. A change that may be seen grossly is carneous (red) degeneration. Histologically, necrosis can be appreciated by loss of basophilia in the nuclei (Fig. 11.4). This form of necrosis can be distinguished from the necrosis seen in leiomyosarcoma, which shows apoptotic debris, so-called "dirty necrosis."

11.4 Uterine Lesions Seen in Postpartum Hysterectomies

When a hysterectomy is performed for immediate postpartum hemorrhage, retained placenta or placenta creta are the first things the pathologist considers. However, other etiologies may lead to both early and late postpartum hemorrhage. In addition, other pregnancy-associated uterine lesions may occasionally be seen that do not lead to hemorrhage.

11.4.1 Placenta Acreta/Increta/Percreta

In association with the increased numbers of cesarean sections being performed, there is an increased incidence of placenta acreta/increta/percreta. The hallmark of this lesion, histopathologically, is the juxtaposition of placental villi to myometrium, without intervening decidua. If this is a surface change, it is placenta acreta. Increta goes into myometrium, and percreta goes through and through. This is not always a straightforward histopathological diagnosis. First, the placental/uterine interface is irregular to begin with and may have been further disrupted by attempts to remove an abnormally adherent placenta. Secondly, a layer of Nitabuch's fibrin and/or intermediate trophoblasts may be seen between villi and myometrium. This is diagnostic of creta as well, in the absence of decidua. For the ideal increta, one would see placental tissue within myometrium. However, both increta and percreta tend to expand and thin out the myometrium, rather than histologically "invade" it, and hence the section may show very thin (even only a few cells) myometrium external to the placenta. Inking of the uterine specimen may help, as the ink on the histology may serve to delineate the small amount of residual muscle (Fig. 11.5a–d).

11.4.2 Couvelaire Uterus

Seen in about 5 % of cases of placental abruption [3], a Couvelaire uterus ("uterine apoplexy") usually does not require a hysterectomy. Clinically, the uterus is dark purple red. This is due to the extensive intramyometrial hemorrhage (Fig. 11.6a). Another cause of hemorrhage, generally more focal, is secondary to laceration, as in a cervical laceration (Fig. 11.6b).

11.4.3 Subinvolution

The first thoughts with delayed postpartum hemorrhage are either retained placental tissue, or rarely, gestational trophoblastic disease; however, uterine subinvolution may also be associated with delayed postpartum hemorrhage [4]. Normal involution involves fibrointimal proliferation with obliteration of spiral arterioles at the implantation site. The trophoblast that had replaced spiral arteriolar endothelium during physiologic conversion disappears, and vessels are lined again by endothelium. Subinvolution is evidenced by persistence of extravillous trophoblast lining endomyometrial vessels of the implantation site, with dilated vessels showing thrombi of various ages [4] (Fig. 11.7a–d). Patency of uterine vessels with thrombi is normally present in the first 24 h after delivery, so the histopathologic diagnosis of subinvolution must take the clinical scenario into account [4].

11.4.4 Retained Placenta

Retained placental tissue may be a cause of postpartum hemorrhage, both early and late. With late postpartum hemorrhage, the retained products of conception are often necrotic (Fig. 11.8). In addition to chorionic villi, retained placental membranes may be seen. There may be associated endomyometritis.

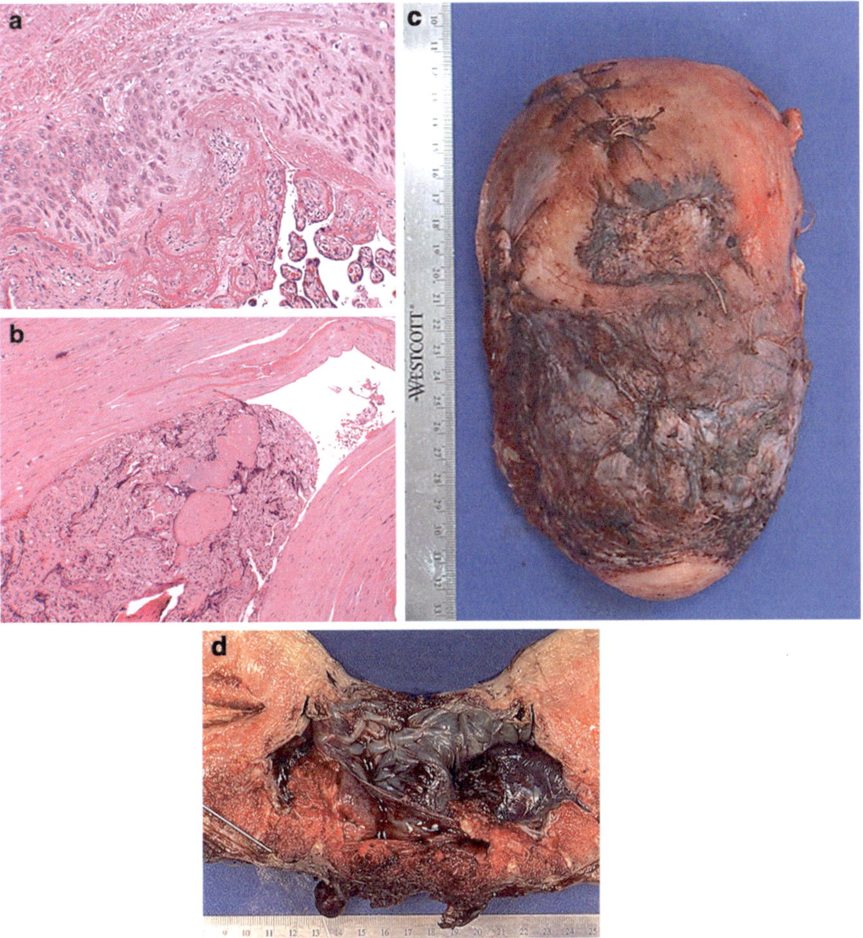

Fig. 11.5 Placenta creta. In acreta (**a**), placental tissue is shown with an intervening layer of Nitabuch's fibrin and intermediate trophoblast. The myometrium is below that (*upper left*). In increta (**b**), the placental tissue is within the myometrium. Placenta percreta (**c**, **d**), breaking through the myometrium. This is often better appreciated grossly

11.4.5 Puerperal Endomyometritis

Postpartum endomyometritis is a potential cause of postpartum fever. While this rarely leads to a hysterectomy, there have been cases of necrotizing uterine infection with group A streptococcus [5]. Histologically, acute inflammation and potentially abscess formation may be seen (Fig. 11.9). A similar histologic picture may be associated with myometritis due to uterine necrosis after uterine artery embolization [6].

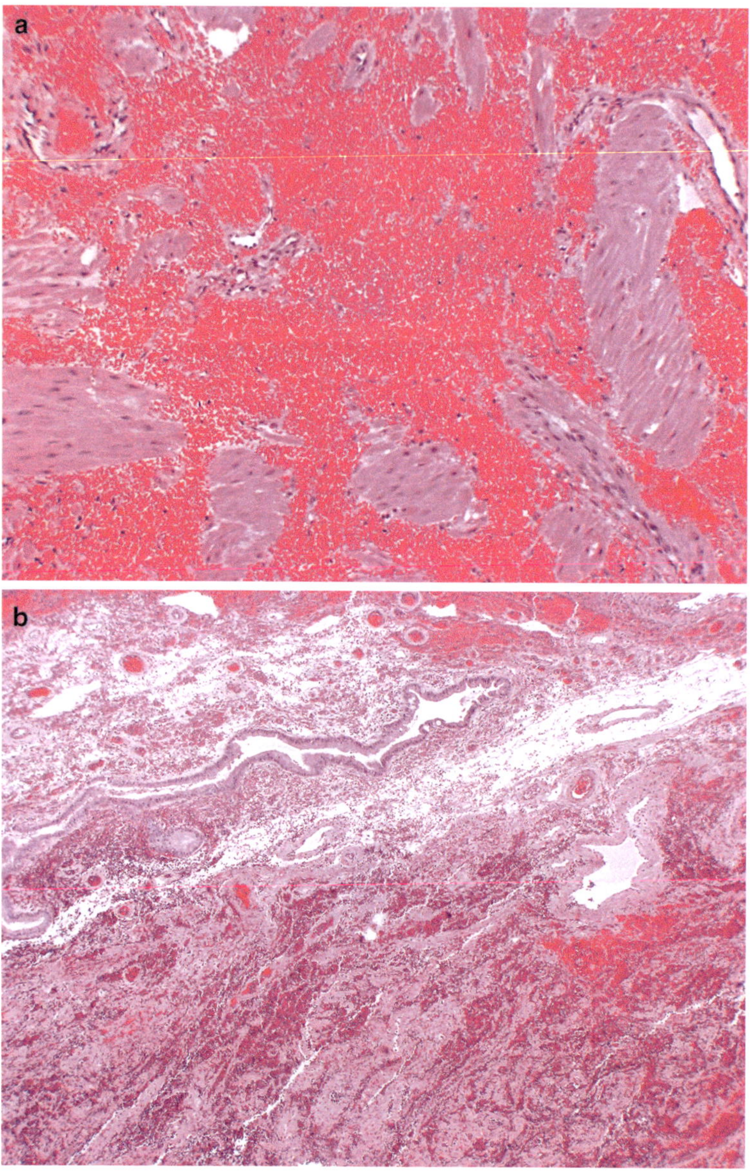

Fig. 11.6 Diffuse uterine hemorrhage (Couvelaire uterus) seen with abruption (**a**), or cervical hemorrhage seen is associated with a laceration (**b**)

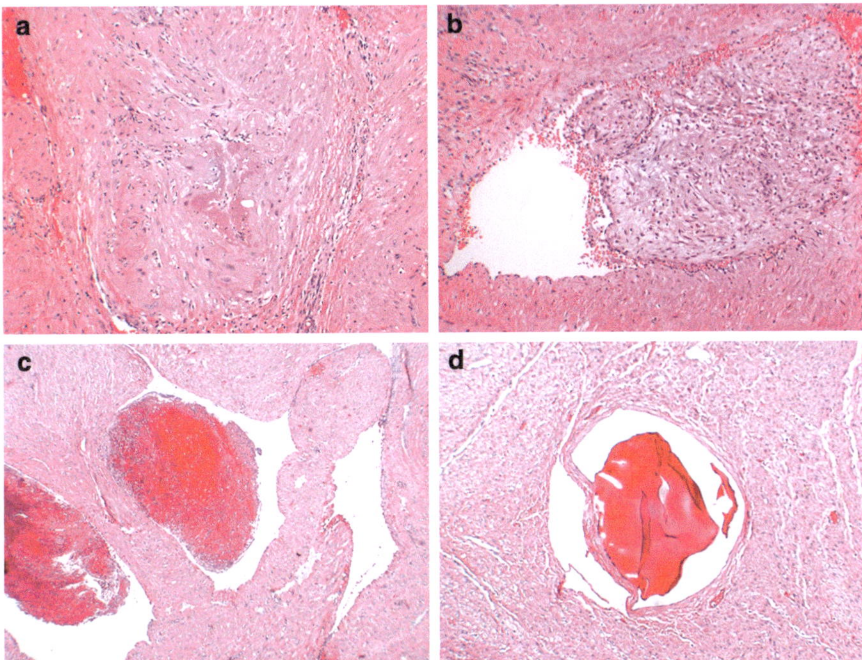

Fig. 11.7 Involution. Normal involution after a term pregnancy includes fibrointimal proliferation with obliteration of vessels in the myometrium (**a**, **b**). With subinvolution occurring weeks after the pregnancy, there are nonorganized thrombi in the myometrium (**c**). In addition, if embolization was performed to treat massive bleeding, embolic material may be seen in myometrial vessels (**d**)

11.5   Pseudoneoplastic Ovarian Lesions Associated with Ovulation Induction or Pregnancy

11.5.1 Luteoma of Pregnancy

The most important thing to be aware of with pregnancy luteomas is that they are hyperplastic, not neoplastic. As such, they are frequently but not always bilateral [7]. Considering this differential in the setting of pregnancy may prevent excision of a healthy ovary, however, the diagnosis is usually established histopathologically. Grossly, luteomas are usually brown multinodular solid lesions. Histologically, the lesion is composed of sheets of luteinized cells with abundant eosinophilic cytoplasm (Fig. 11.10). The gross and histologic appearances raise the main differential, steroid cell tumor. Steroid cell tumors occur in older patients who are not likely to be pregnant. However, a major histopathologic dilemma is distinguishing unilateral pregnancy luteoma from steroid cell tumor on a frozen section. Characteristic follicle-like spaces, if present, may assist in confirming pregnancy luteoma [7]. In addition, luteomas are brown, while steroid cell tumors are generally yellow. The corpus luteum of pregnancy may rarely be confused with

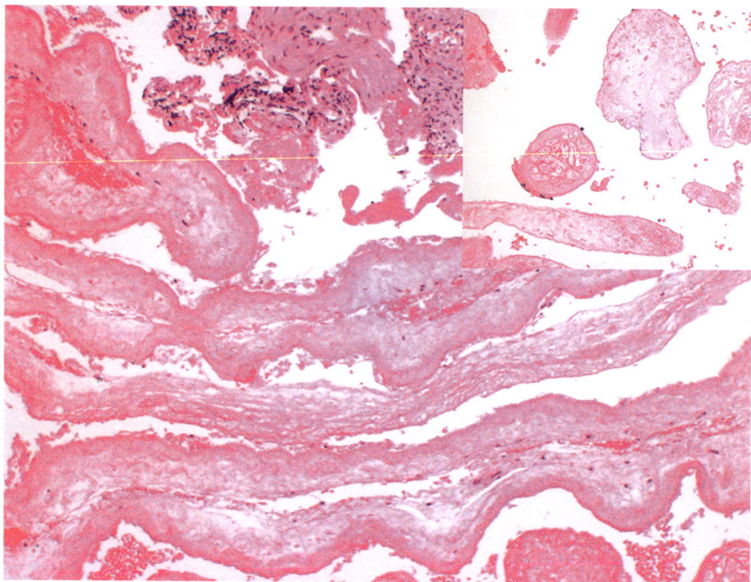

Fig. 11.8 Retained placenta showing necrotic membranes. A few ghost villi (*inset upper right*) were also seen

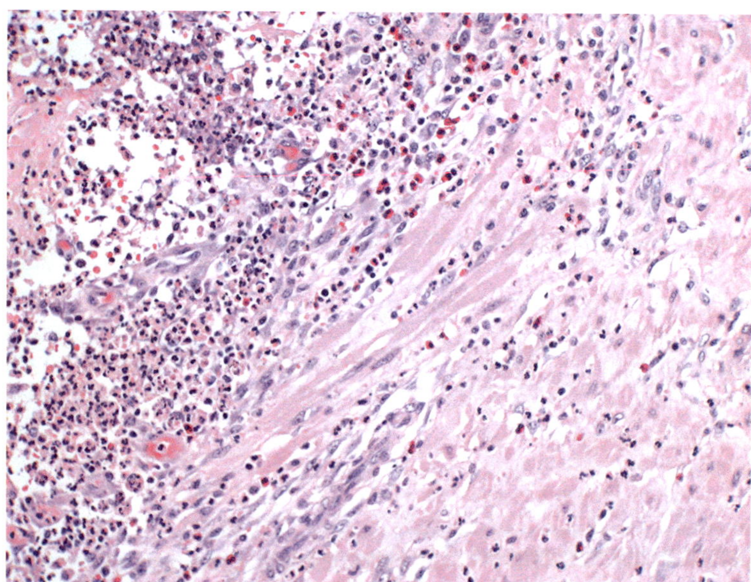

Fig. 11.9 Puerperal acute myometritis showing severe acute myometrial inflammation with focal necrosis

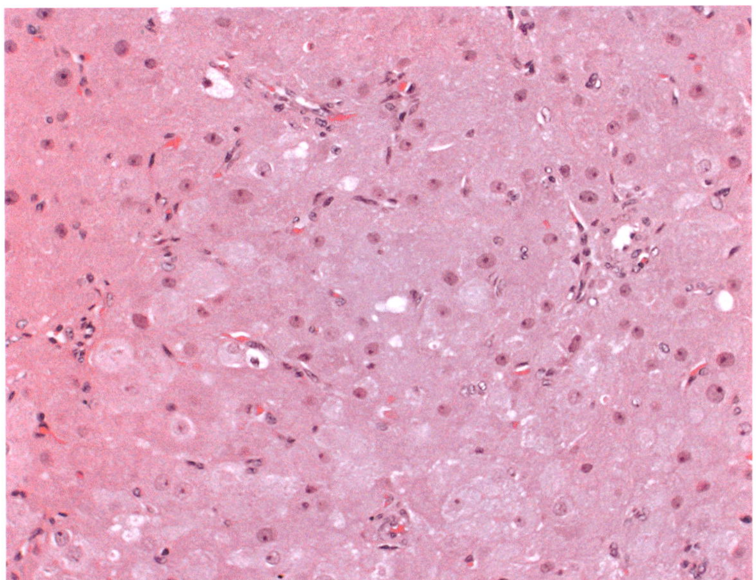

Fig. 11.10 Luteoma, composed of luteinized cells with abundant eosinophilic cytoplasm

a pregnancy luteoma; however, the corpus luteum is seen in early pregnancy and is yellow, while the luteoma is usually seen in late pregnancy and is brown [7]. Pregnancy luteomas regress after the pregnancy. Rarely, the lesions may masculinize the mother [7].

11.5.2 Hyperreactio Luteinalis

Hyperreactio luteinalis is secondary to ovarian hyperstimulation from b-HCG. This can occur in the setting of ovulation induction, or in association with increased b-HCG in cases of gestational trophoblastic disease, fetal hydrops, or multiple pregnancy [8]. The clinical scenario is important in establishing the diagnosis, as this condition does not usually lead to surgical intervention. The condition is bilateral and consists of multicystic enlarged ovaries containing numerous follicle cysts, which regress when the stimulus is removed. Occasional maternal masculinization has been reported [8].

11.5.3 Large Solitary Luteinized Follicle Cyst of Pregnancy and Puerperium

A rare condition is the large solitary luteinized cyst of pregnancy and the puerperium. As the name of the lesion states, it is a unilocular cyst, sometimes quite large, lined by luteinized follicle cells. The main differential diagnosis is a cystic granulosa cell tumor.

References

1. Nucci MR, Young RH, Fletcher CD. Cellular pseudosarcomatous fibroepithelial stromal polyps of the lower female genital tract: an underrecognized lesion often misdiagnosed as sarcoma. Am J Surg Pathol. 2000;24:231–40.
2. Arias-Stella J. The Arias-Stella reaction: facts and fancies four decades after. Adv Anat Pathol. 2002;9:12–23.
3. Rathi M, Rathi SK, Purohit M, Pathak A. Couvelaire uterus. BMJ Case Rep. 2014. pii:bcr2014204211. doi:10.1136/bcr-2014-204211.
4. Weydert JA, Benda JA. Subinvolution of the placental site as an anatomic cause of postpartum uterine bleeding. Arch Pathol Lab Med. 2006;130:153–42.
5. Castagnola DE, Hoffman MK, Carlson J, Flynn C. Necrotizing cervical and uterine infection in the postpartum period caused by group A streptococcus. Obstet Gynecol. 2008;111:533–5.
6. Tseng JJ, Ho JY, Wen MC, Hwang JL. Uterine necrosis associated with acute suppurative myometritis after angiographic selective embolization for refractory postpartum hemorrhage. Am J Obstet Gynecol. 2011;204:e4–6.
7. Burandt E, Young RH. Pregnancy luteoma: a study of 20 cases on the occasion of the 50th anniversary of its description by Dr. William H. Sternberg, with an emphasis on the common presence of follicle-like spaces and their diagnostic implications. Am J Surg Pathol. 2014;38:239–44.
8. Clement PB. Tumor-like lesions of the ovary associated with pregnancy. Int J Gynecol Pathol. 1993;12:108–15.

Pathology of the Placenta

12

12.1 Abnormalities and the Approach to Examination of the Placenta

The placenta can have numerous abnormalities, both gross and microscopic. The placenta may explain a poor pregnancy outcome, including growth restriction or stillbirth, and may provide information about future pregnancy risk. For many lesions, however, there is not a one to one correlation between the presence of a specific lesion and a negative fetal outcome. Epidemiologically, however, many of these lesions or groups of lesions are associated with poor outcomes (Table 12.1).

Examination of the placenta begins with a gross examination in the delivery room. The delivering provider may detect abnormalities that indicate that the placenta should be sent to the Pathology Laboratory. Some institutions send all placentas to Pathology; however, some reserve the evaluation for specific risk categories, which can be categorized as maternal, fetal, or placental issues.

On receipt of a placenta by the Pathology laboratory, a thorough gross examination is performed. Of note, by convention, placental weight is assessed after removal of the umbilical cord and membranes. A gross description is provided in the report, and then sections are selected, as with other pathology specimens. One way to think of the histopathologic evaluation of placentas is to remember to consider all the components; cord, membranes, villi, and decidua. There are many textbooks on placental pathology, which is an extensive topic. This short summary of some of the most concerning lesions will hopefully assist clinicians in interpreting their pathology reports.

© Springer International Publishing Switzerland 2015
D.S. Heller, *OB-GYN Pathology for the Clinician*,
DOI 10.1007/978-3-319-15422-0_12

Table 12.1 Key points about placental pathology

There are large numbers of lesions. Lesions don't always correspond directly with poor outcome, but may be epidemiologically associated with poor outcomes
Placental lesions can be separated into categories (infectious, ischemic, immune) to better evaluate the process associated with a poor outcome
Abruption may not always be detectible on pathology, and the gold standard for diagnosis is clinical
Candida funisitis warrants a phone call to the clinician due to possible associated fetal candidal sepsis

12.2 Gross Placental Abnormalities

12.2.1 Abnormalities of Placental Shape

The first part of placental evaluation is gross inspection of the placenta. Abnormal shapes may reflect a variety of genetic or mechanical issues. A circumvallate placenta (Fig. 12.1a) is thought to be secondary to chronic marginal abruption lifting up the peripheral membranes, with folding over of the membranes upon themselves. The fold in the membranes inserts internal to the edge of the placental disk. Circumvallation may be partial or circumferential. There is some association with preterm labor and abruption according to some authors [1]; however, the clinical significance is unclear [2]. Circummarginate placentas show a similar ridge of fibrin internal to the placental edge (Fig. 12.1b) on the fetal surface, but the placental membranes have not folded upon themselves. These lesions are not thought to be significant clinically in most cases.

Bilobed placentas consist of two lobes of fairly equal size (Fig. 12.2). Intervening vessels may be vulnerable to trauma. In succenturiate lobe, one lobe is smaller. The danger here is thinking the placenta is complete at delivery, with risk of postpartum hemorrhage from unsuspected retained placental tissue.

12.2.2 Abnormalities of the Membranes

Gross examination of the membranes may provide a clue to underlying pathology. Meconium staining, if recent and heavy, is a pea soup green color. Histologically, meconium may denude the amniotic epithelium entirely or may show as pigmented macrophages in the membranes (Fig. 12.3a). The timing of meconium spread from amnion to chorion to decidua is not reliable. The presence of meconium in and of itself does not have major clinical significance and is very common. However, meconium may cause vasospasm, which can cause fetal hypoxic stress (not discernable on histopathology), and if the placenta is exposed to prolonged meconium, myonecrosis of the vessels of the cord and chorionic plate may occur (Fig. 12.3b), significantly associated with fetal compromise.

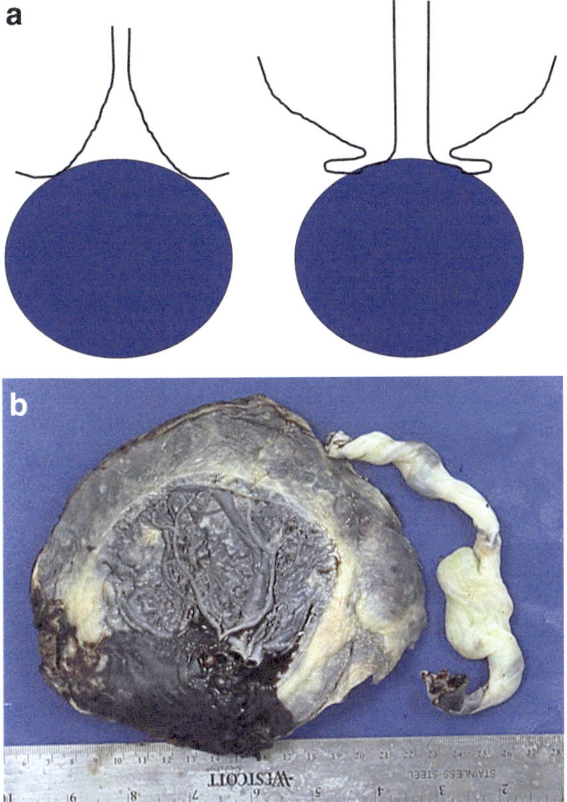

Fig. 12.1 Circumvallate placenta has folding over of the membranes, which then insert proximal to the placental edge (**a** *right*), while in circummarginate placenta, there is a ridge of fibrin; however, there is no folding of the membranes, which also insert proximal to the placental edge (**a** *left*, **b**)

Acute chorioamnionitis, if severe, may turn yellow, or membranes may opacify the membranes. Opaque membranes may also simply indicate a larger amount of adherent decidua to the membranes. For the histology of acute chorioamnionitis, see below section on infectious lesions.

Amnion nodosum may be seen as multiple small white nodules on the placental membranes and fetal surface. Amnion nodosum is comprised of clusters of fetal squamous cells and lanugo hairs that become adherent to the amnion, sometimes with amnion epithelium overgrowing, in cases of severe oligohydramnios (Fig. 12.4).

12.2.3 Abnormalities of the Cord

Many of the abnormalities of the umbilical cord are gross rather than microscopic diagnoses. Abnormal insertions, including velamentous insertion into the membranes, and battledore, which is marginal insertion into the disk, should be noted.

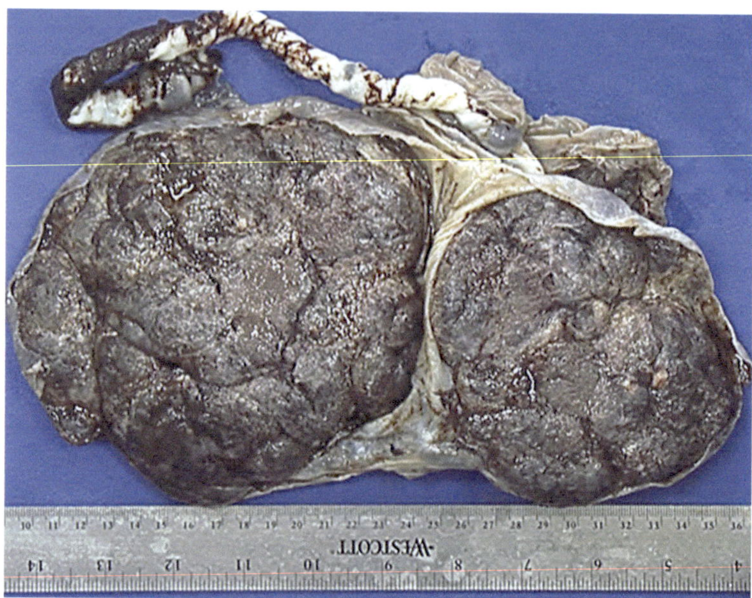

Fig. 12.2 Accessory lobes. If equal, the placenta is bilobed

Velamentous insertions are important because the exposed vessels are subject to trauma, which can compromise the fetus, as well as rupture, particularly if there is vasa previa. This can lead to fetal exsanguination. There may be increased twisting of the cord, with torsion along the length, or with stricture focally (Fig. 12.5). Hematomas of the cord are often iatrogenic, occurring during traction during the third stage of labor. However, if spontaneous, they may compress the fetal vessels and cause compromise (Fig. 12.6). Single umbilical artery can be recognized both grossly and microscopically. It is the most common placental anomaly. It is sometimes associated with abnormalities in the fetus, particularly genitourinary. True knots are common and are only significant if there is obstruction. This can be concluded from congestion of the cord on one side, or thrombi. False knots are varicosities due to the vessels being longer than the cord and are of no clinical significance.

One of the few placental lesions requiring a phone call from the pathologist to the clinician is candida funisitis. Grossly, the cord has multiple small yellow–white nodules on the amniotic surface, which represent histologic microabscesses. Stains can detect fungal organisms consistent with candida (Fig. 12.7). Although candida vaginosis is very common in pregnancy, candidal funisitis is uncommon and potentially signifies fetal candidal sepsis, hence the need for a phone call.

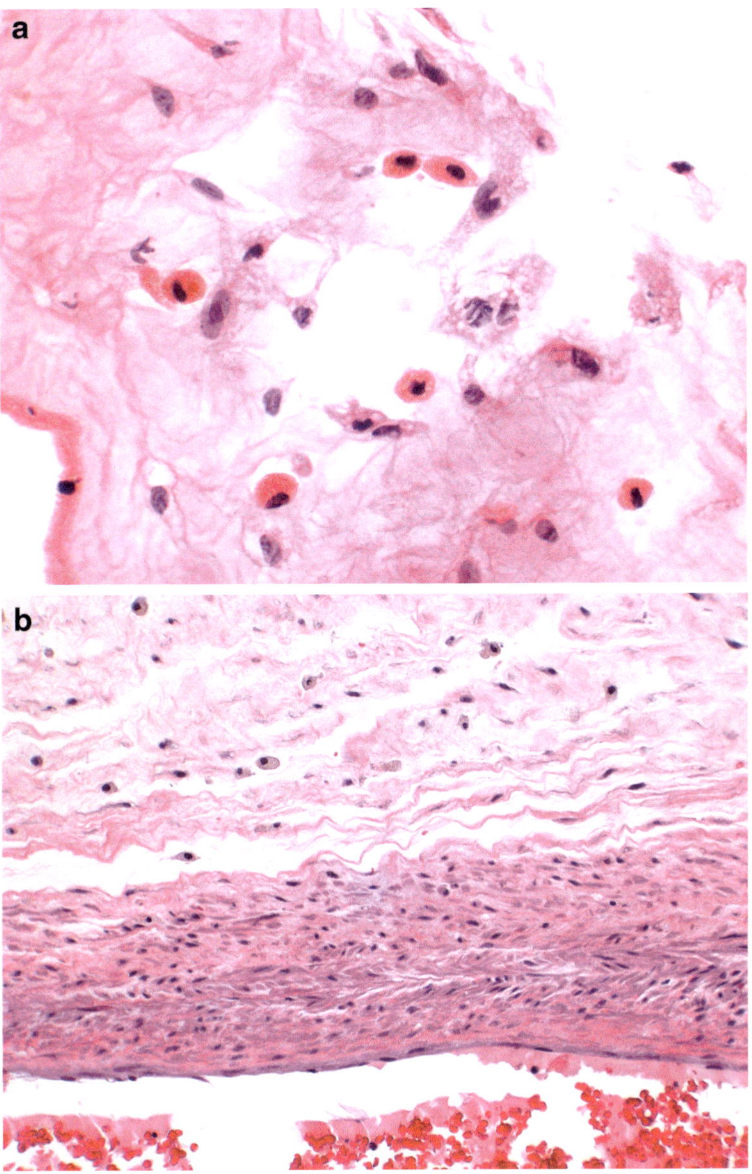

Fig. 12.3 Meconium. Meconium macrophages are seen in the membranes (**a**), as well as in the cord, where vascular myonecrosis is also seen adjacent in the vessel (**b**)

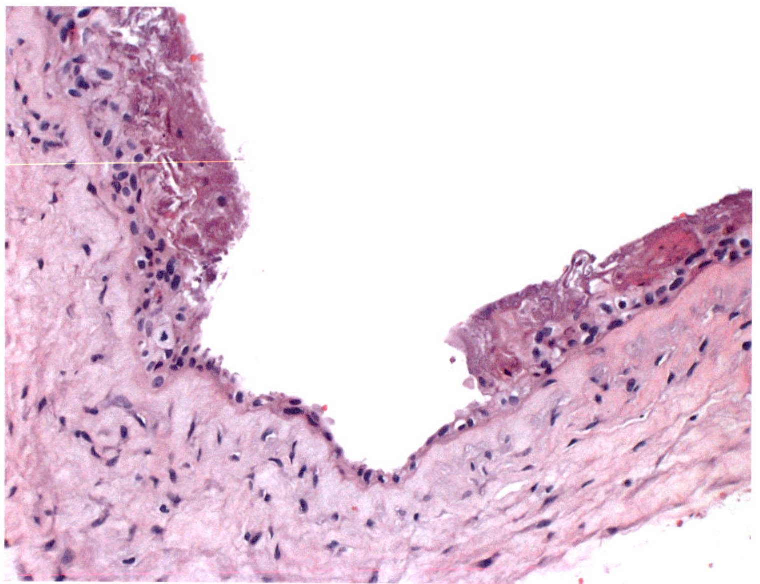

Fig. 12.4 Amnion nodosum. Numerous squames are adherent to the membranes

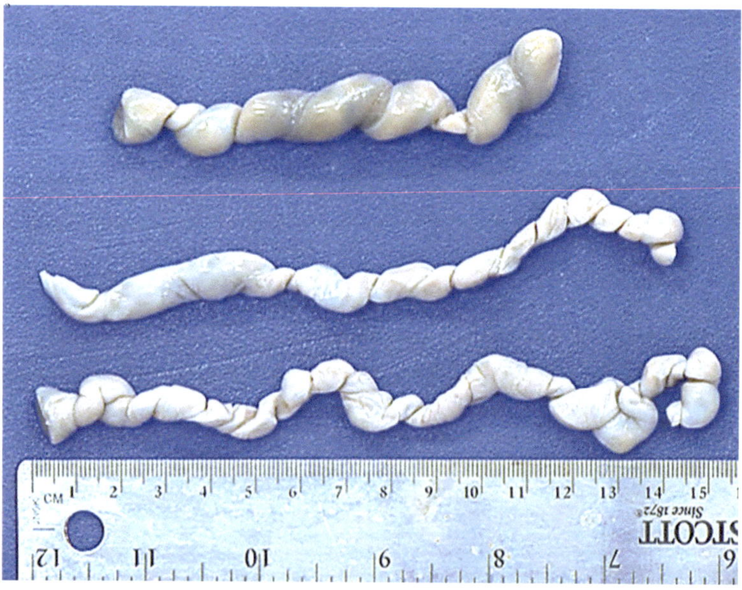

Fig. 12.5 Umbilical cords with increased twisting, and focal stricture at the top

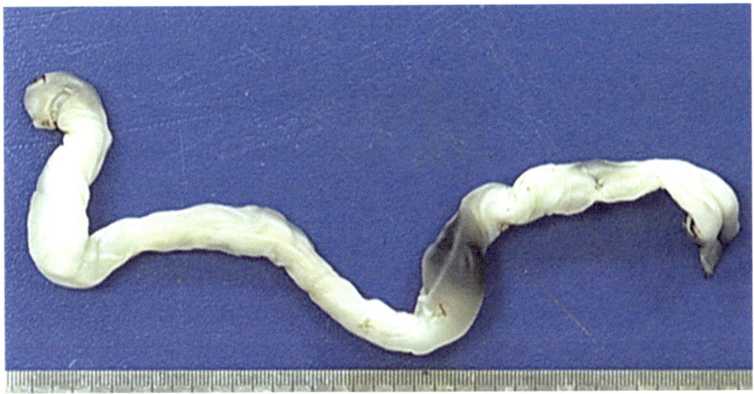

Fig. 12.6 Cord hemangioma is seen in the central portion of the cord

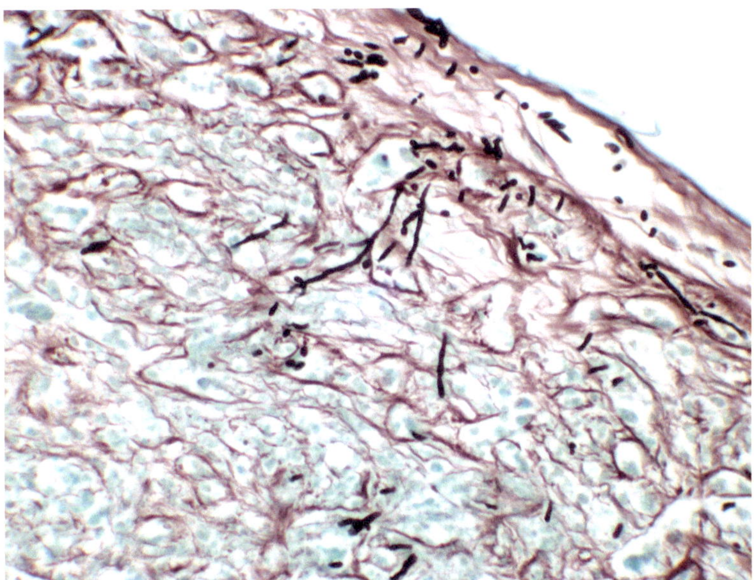

Fig. 12.7 Candida funisitis. GMS stain shows fungal organisms

12.2.4 Abnormalities of the Parenchyma

There are large numbers of parenchymal placental lesions. Lesions don't always correspond directly with poor outcome of an infant on a one to one basis, but may be epidemiologically associated with poor outcomes. Placental lesions can be separated into categories (infectious, ischemic, immune) to better evaluate the process associated with a poor outcome.

12.3　Lesions Associated with Ischemia

12.3.1　Abruption

The gold standard for the diagnosis of placental abruption is clinical. In order for the pathologist to confirm abruption, retroplacental hemorrhage must be retained behind the placenta long enough to indent the parenchyma (Fig. 12.8a, b). A densely adherent clot is suggestive, but not confirmatory. In the absence of indentation, the pathologist can support but not confirm abruption. If the hemorrhage escapes from behind the placenta, the blood may pass into the amniotic fluid if the membranes are intact ("port wine fluid"), or may pass vaginally, characteristically as dark blood, leaving no signs for the pathologist. There is a tendency for chronic processes associated with abruption such as chronic hypertension to be more likely to have parenchymal compression, as opposed to the more acute causes such as cocaine abuse, but in one study, this did not reach statistical significance [3]. If the abruption is of a more chronic nature, there may be some organization of the clot, with lines of Zahn present, and adjacent villi may be infarcted.

12.3.2　Decidual Vasculopathy/Atherosis

In order to accommodate the oxygenation and nutritional needs of the growing fetus, the spiral arterioles in the decidua undergo physiologic conversion, in which the endothelium is replaced by trophoblast in the first two trimesters. This physically converts the functioning of the vessels from contractile arterioles to passively open venous channels, providing greater flow to the pregnancy. If physiologic conversion doesn't occur, this is thought to set the stage for pre-eclampsia. Although not always present, the vascular lesion that may be seen with pre-eclampsia is decidual vasculopathy. The vessel wall may undergo hyalinization; there may be vasculitis, thrombosis, and/or infiltration of foamy macrophages, known as atherosis (Fig. 12.9a, b).

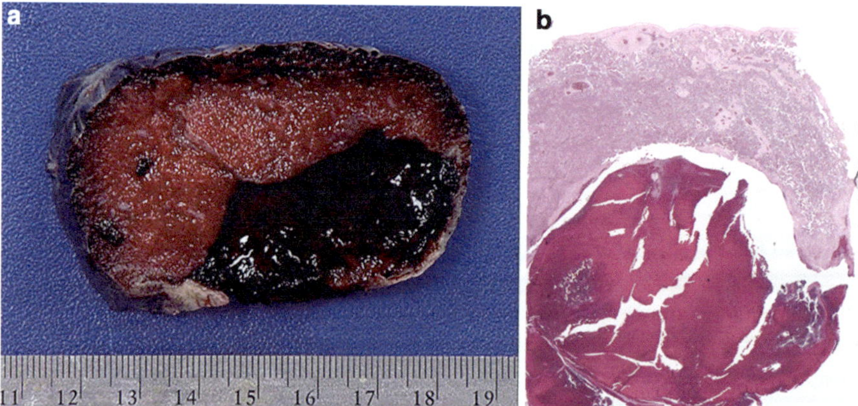

Fig. 12.8　Abruption, with large clot compressing parenchyma, which can be appreciated grossly (**a**), and microscopically (**b**)

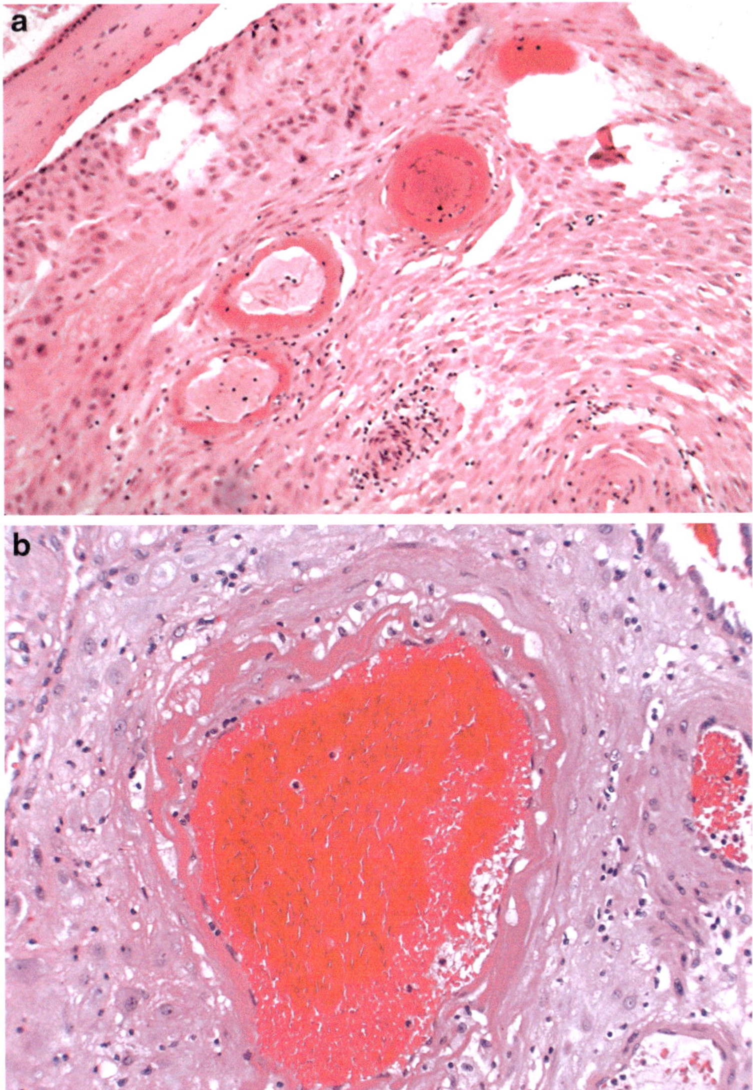

Fig. 12.9 Maternal decidual vasculopathy with hyaline degeneration of vessel walls (**a**) as well as atherosis (**b**)

12.3.3 Chorangiosis

The fetal unit may attempt to compensate for hypoxic stress in a number of ways. The presence of these compensatory changes only tells that compensation was made, not whether or not the hypoxia was sufficient to do damage to the fetus. Chorangiosis is one such compensatory mechanism, where there is an increased number of capillaries in the chorionic villi (Fig. 12.10a). Although the numerical criteria for number of

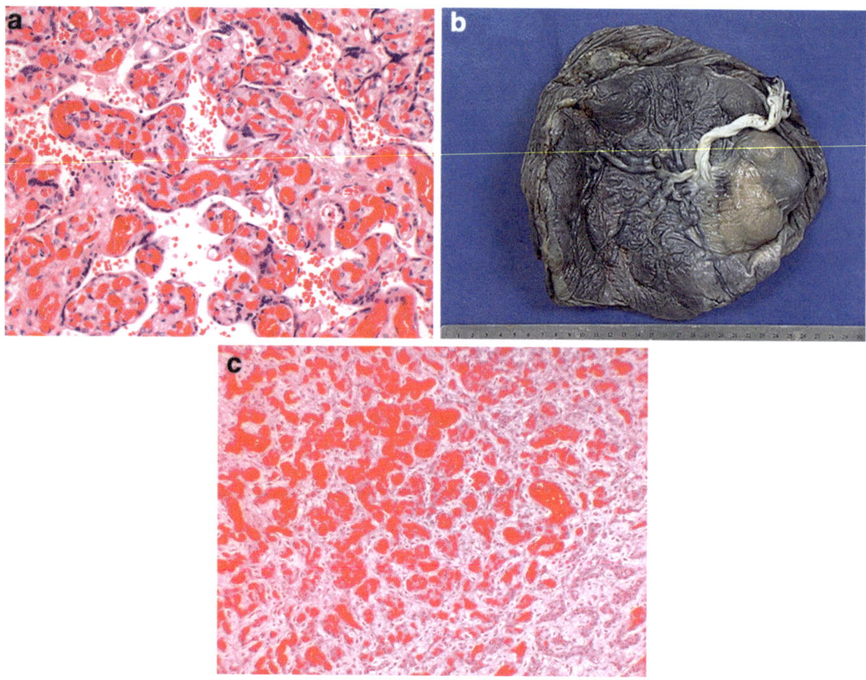

Fig. 12.10 Chorangiosis (**a**), showing increased numbers of capillaries in tertiary villi. This should not be confused with chorangioma (**b, c**), a discrete nodule (**b**) histologically consistent with a hemangioma (**c**)

vessels needed to diagnose chorangiosis have been established, most often the diagnosis is made by estimation. Chorangiosis may be confused with two other entities with similar sounding names, chorangiomatosis and chorangioma. Chorangiomatosis is also an increase in number of vessels, but in stem villi, rather than tertiary villi. The significance is uncertain. A chorangioma (Fig. 12.10b, c) is a capillary hemangioma. It may be seen grossly as a yellow nodule. Histologically, it resembles a capillary hemangioma elsewhere. It is usually not clinically significant unless very large, where it may compromise the amount of usable placenta, or may cause shunting.

12.3.4 Villous Malperfusion

Villous malperfusion (Fig. 12.11) manifests as increased branching of tertiary villi. Villi thus appear very small, with increased space in between. There may be hypovascularity as well.

12.3.5 Infarction

Infarction is not unusual in a term placenta, particularly if peripheral, as the placenta normally undergoes senescence at this age and beyond. Infarctions are abnormal if

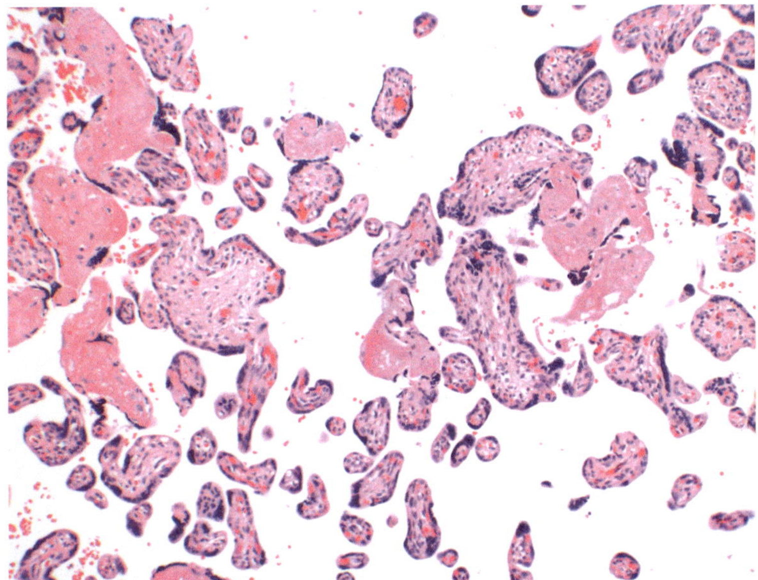

Fig. 12.11 Villous malperfusion. The villi are small due to increased branching, with increased space between

they take up a significant portion of the parenchyma (the placenta generally has a 20–30 % reserve) or occur in an immature placenta. Grossly, infarcts are usually wedge-shaped. They may be hard to appreciate grossly if recent, but older ones are usually tan-colored and more visible. Histologically, a recent infarct simply appears as crowding of the villi with loss of the intervillous space. The nuclei then become smudgy, and then finally by 48 h are nonviable (Fig. 12.12).

12.3.6 Myonecrosis

See discussion on meconium under membranes (Fig. 12.3b). Myonecrosis, caused by significant exposure of fetal vessels in the chorionic plate and cord to meconium, is associated with fetal hypoxic stress.

12.3.7 Increased Syncytial Knots

Another manifestation of hypoxic stress, often seen in association with preeclampsia, is increased syncytial knots (Fig. 12.13). Syncytial knots are formed by the aggregation of syncytiotrophoblast nuclei, which occurs as the fetal capillaries get closer to the outer portion of the villous parenchyma, in order to form the so-called "vasculosyncytial membranes," composed of the capillary endothelium and outer villous basement membrane and attenuated syncytiotrophoblast cytoplasm. This is the thinnest interface between the fetal and maternal intervillous

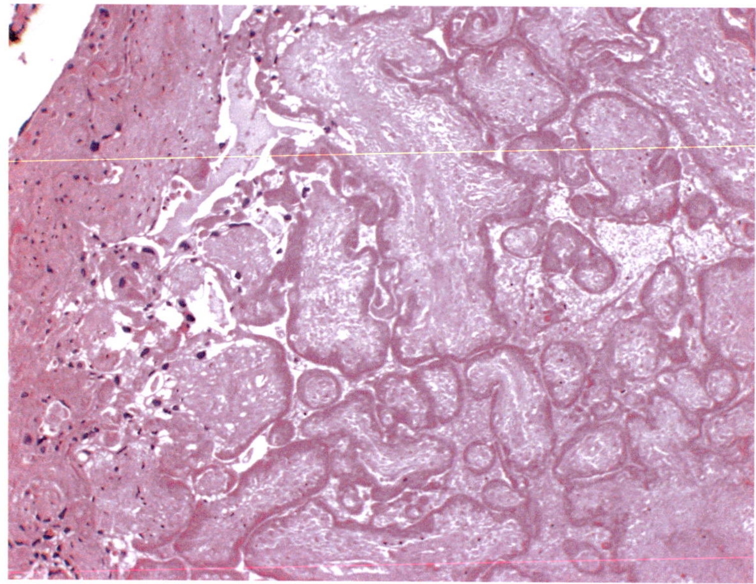

Fig. 12.12 Chronic infarct showing loss of viable nuclei, with only ghost villi seen

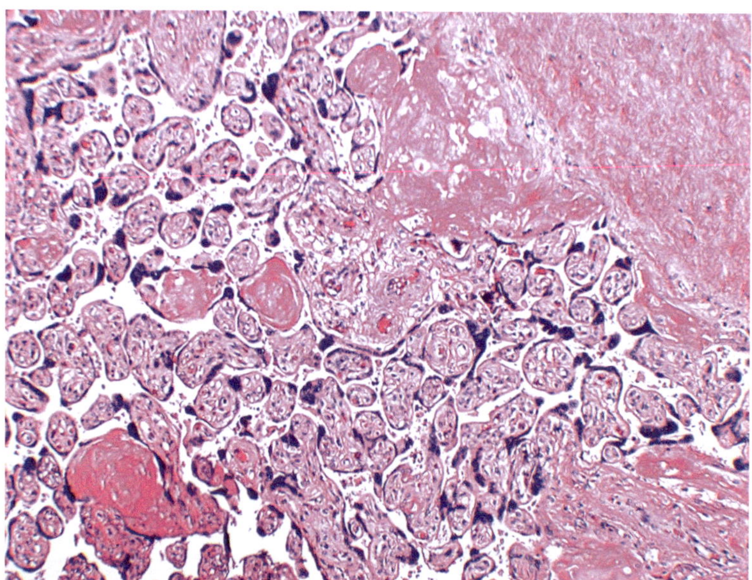

Fig. 12.13 Increased syncytial knots, thought to be due to increased numbers of vasculosyncytial membranes

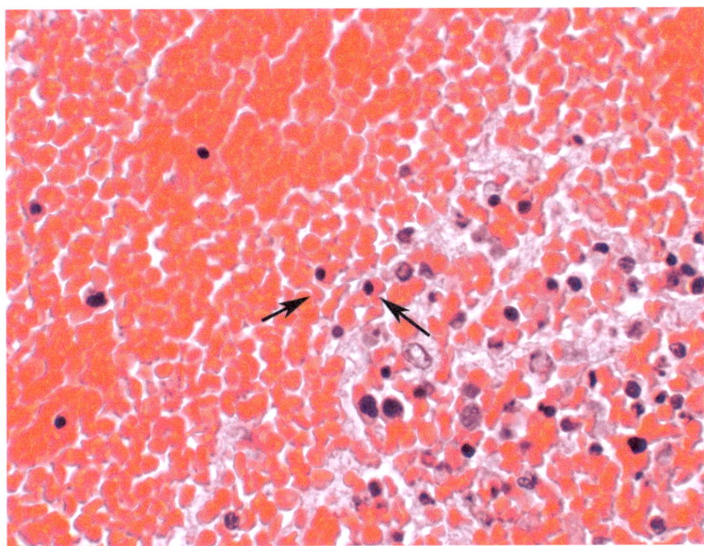

Fig. 12.14 Increased nucleated red cells (*arrows*), recognizable by the very round nuclei

circulations, analogous to the alveolar wall of the lung. In hypoxic states, there is a compensatory attempt to increase the vasculosyncytial membrane surface area, hence increased numbers of syncytiotrophoblast nuclei getting pushed into knots adjacent to these vasculosyncytial membranes.

12.3.8 Increased Nucleated Red Blood Cells in Fetal Vessels

It is normal to see nucleated red blood cells in fetal vessels in the first trimester, but after that, they decrease over time. In the third trimester, they are normally only occasional. A potential response to hypoxic stress is the release of increased numbers of nucleated red blood cells, normally found in the fetal liver, into the fetal circulation. These can be recognized and distinguished from white cell precursors by their very round nuclei (Fig. 12.14).

12.4 Infectious Lesions

12.4.1 Acute Chorioamnionitis and the Fetal Inflammatory Response

Acute chorioamnionitis is diagnosed by the finding of neutrophils in the free membranes and/or chorionic plate (Fig. 12.15a). The fetal inflammatory response (Fig. 12.15b, c) is diagnosed by the presence of neutrophils coming from inside large fetal vessels of the cord and chorionic plate, marginating outwards. In the chorionic plate, the inflammatory cells are markedly increased on the side of the vessel

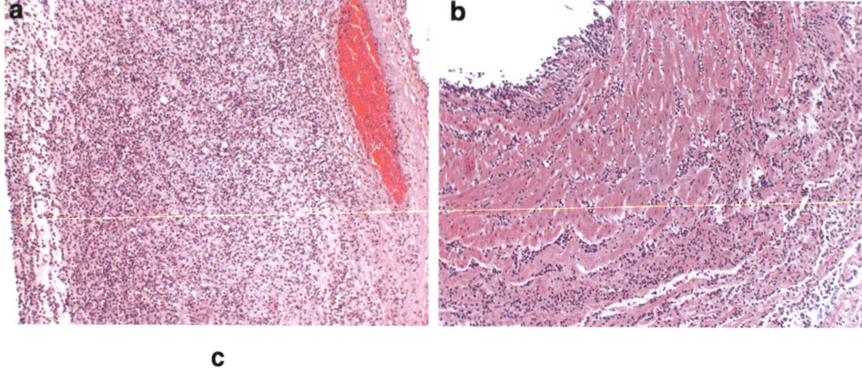

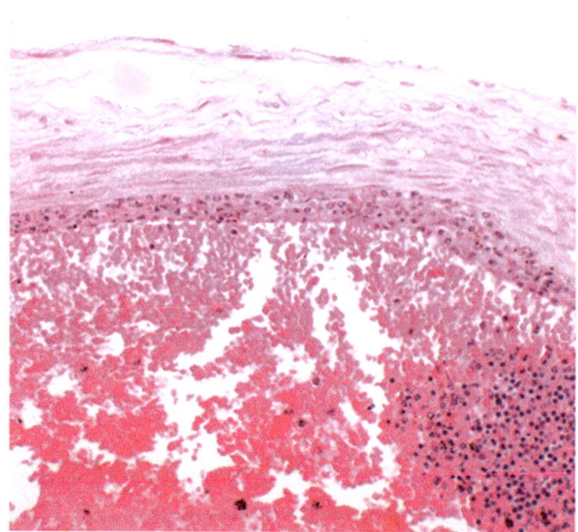

Fig. 12.15 Acute chorioamnionitis, with neutrophils in the membranes (**a**). When present, the fetal inflammatory response is manifested by neutrophils marginating from within the fetal vessels of the umbilical cord (**b**), and chorionic plate (**c**)

pointing towards the amniotic sac, the site of infection. The fetal inflammatory response is associated with increased cytokines. Evidence has suggested an association between the fetal inflammatory response and cerebral palsy, particularly in the preterm infant, but long-term studies are less conclusive.

12.4.2 Villitis

Hematogenous infections manifest as villitis, and this can be secondary to syphilis, bacterial, viral diseases, and protozoal diseases among other causes; however, most villitis is of unknown etiology and thought to be of immune origin (see below).

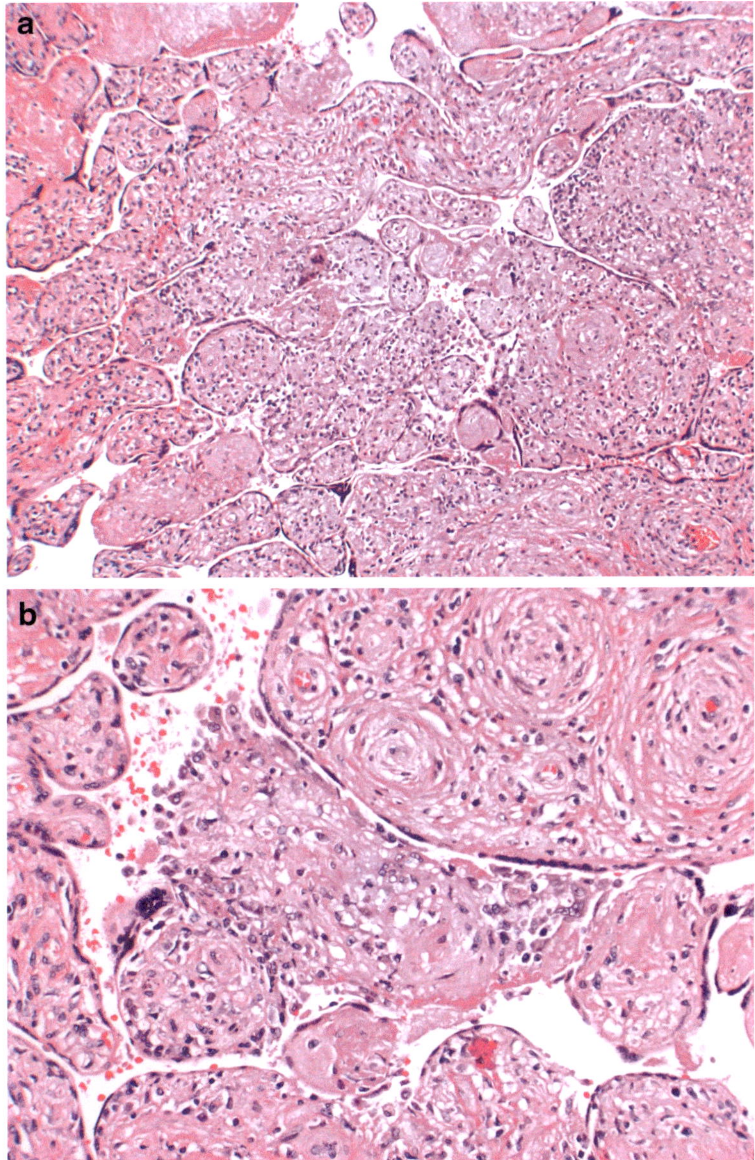

Fig. 12.16 Chronic villitis of unknown etiology. At low power, increased cellularity is seen (**a**). At higher power (**b**) this lymphohistiocytic infiltrate involves the villi

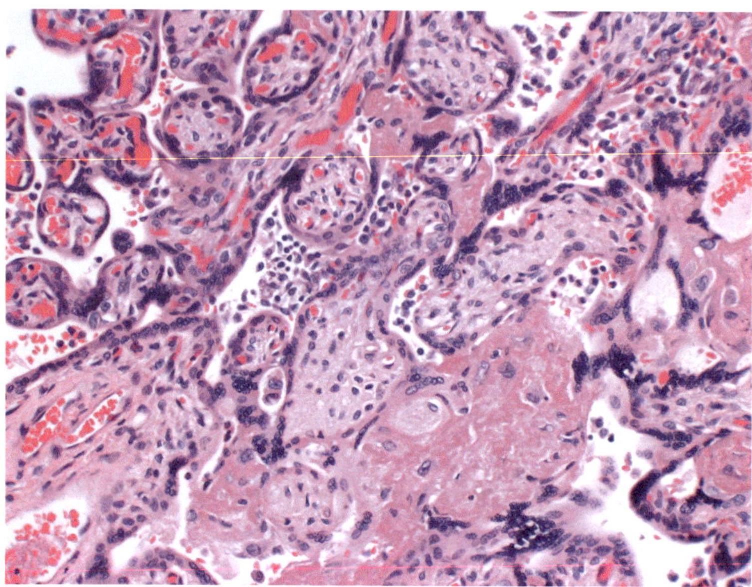

Fig. 12.17 Chronic lymphohistiocytic intervillositis. Here the inflammatory cells are between the villi

12.5 Lesions of Possible Immune Origin

Several lesions are thought to be of immune origin, possibly due to maternal rejection of the fetus. These lesions are associated with poor perinatal outcomes, including growth restriction and stillbirth. They have a high incidence of recurrence in future pregnancies, hence are important for the pathologist to report. Lesions in this group include villitis of unknown etiology (Fig. 12.16a, b), chronic histiocytic or lymphohistio-cytic intervillositis (Fig. 12.17), massively increased perivillous fibrin (Fig. 12.18a, b), and maternal floor infarction. Maternal floor infarction is a misnomer, as it is massively increased fibrin confined to the maternal surface, not a true infarct.

12.6 Miscellaneous Parenchymal Lesions

Intervillous thrombi are thought to be composed of a combination of fetal and maternal blood, hence representing fetal maternal hemorrhage (Fig. 12.19). They are common, and probably of no usual significance unless large or numerous. Potential complications in that case could include a symptomatic fetal-maternal hemorrhage, which would need a Kleihauer–Betke or other clinical modality to confirm. In addition, theoretically, a fetal-maternal hemorrhage could sensitize the mother to a fetal antigen.

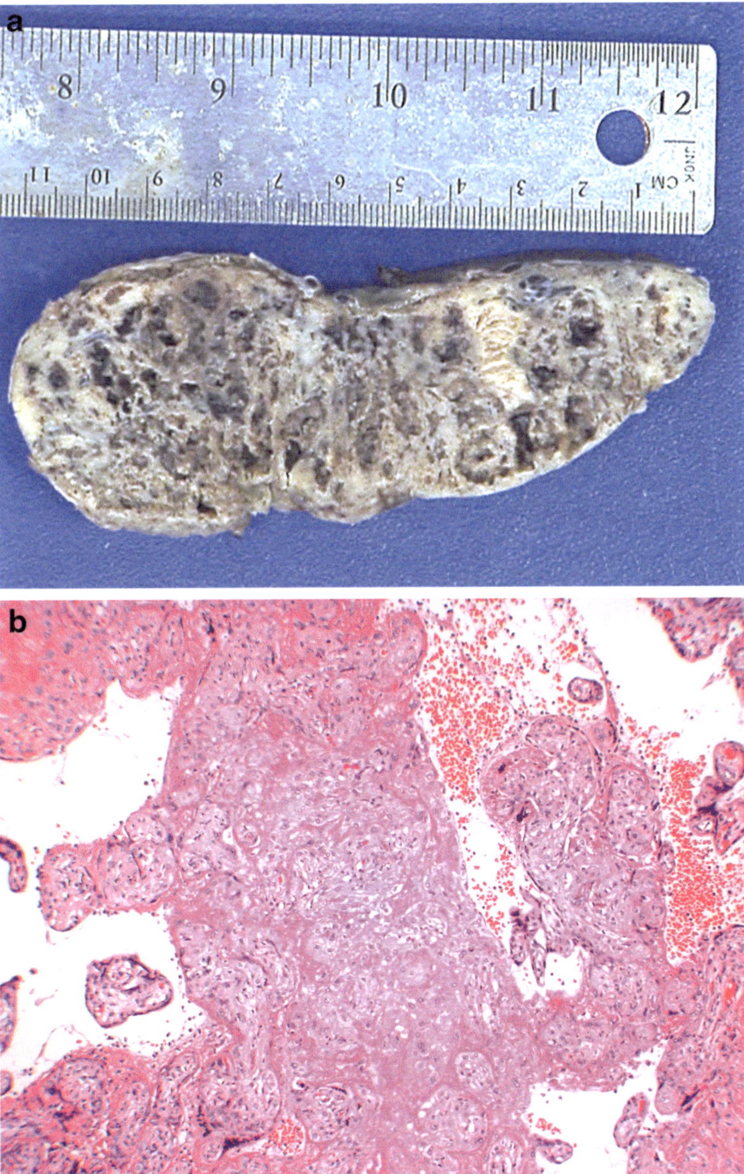

Fig. 12.18 Increased perivillous fibrin can be appreciated grossly (**a**) when massive and can be seen microscopically (**b**) as fibrin encasing the villi

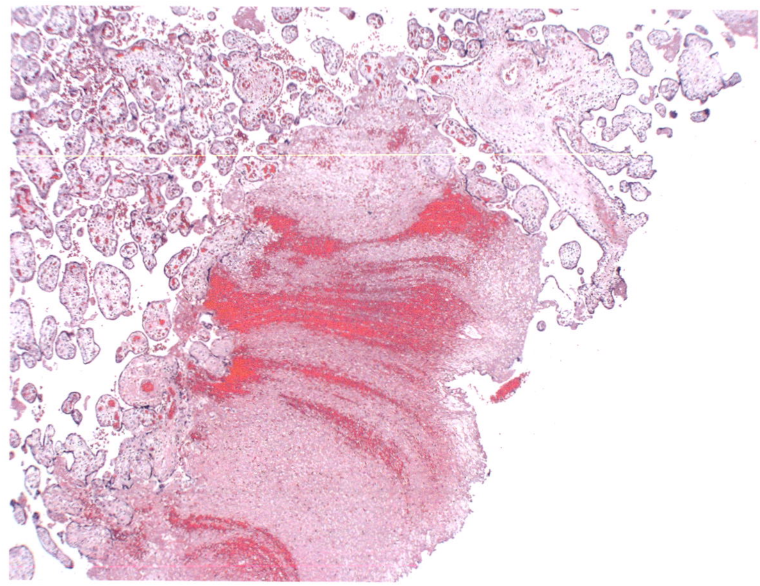

Fig. 12.19   Intervillous thrombus showing lines of Zahn

12.7   Twins

Dizygotic twins are "womb-mates," and as such, always dichorionic except in rare case reports. Monozygotic twins can be either monochorionic or dichorionic (Fig. 12.20a, b). Monochorionic twins are almost always monozygotic except in rare case reports. Depending on when the split occurs in monozygotic twins, the placentas get closer together the later the split. Hence, the earliest split twins have dichorionic, either separate or fused placentas. Later placentas are diamniotic monochorionic. The least common, occurring later, are monoamniotic monochorionic. As the cords are very close in these placentas, without the protection of a dividing membrane, entanglement and mortality is not rare. The best way to histopathologically evaluate chorionicity is to section a "t-section" of placental parenchyma with attached dividing membrane. A second membrane roll of the dividing membrane increases the chance of at least one section being well-oriented enough to interpret chorionicity.

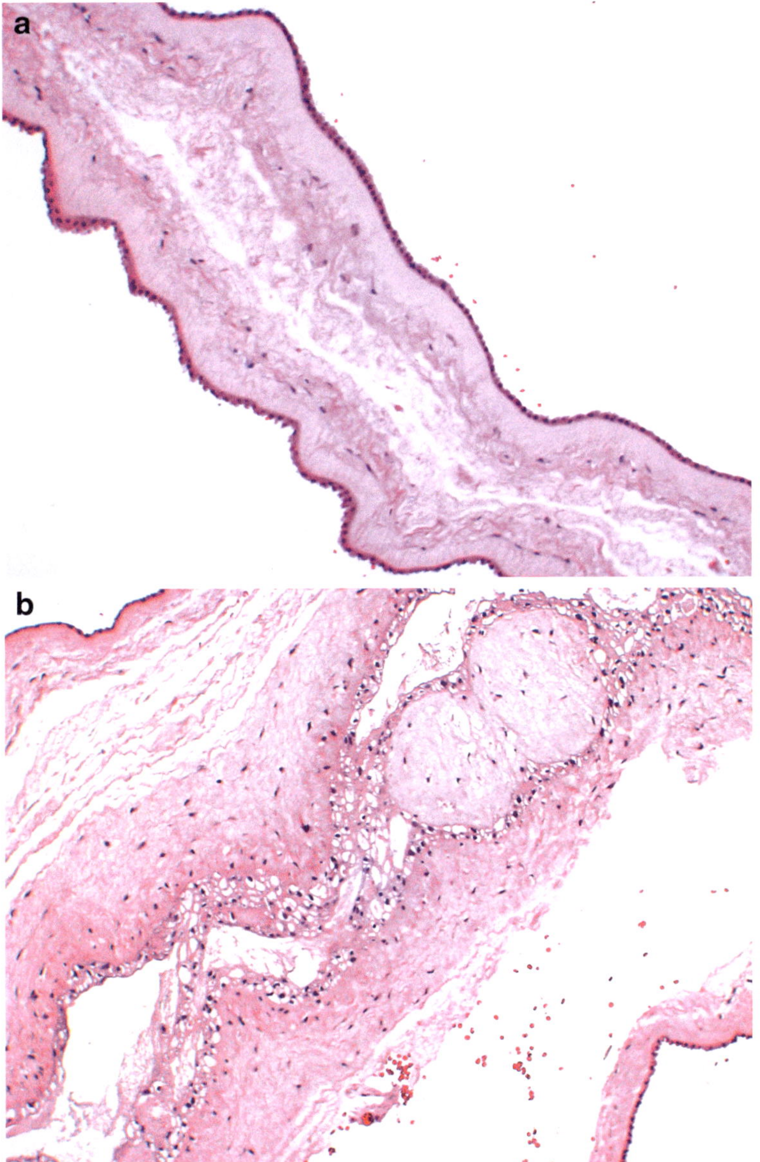

Fig. 12.20 The T-section of a monochorionic twin shows amnion on both sides with no intervening chorion (**a**), whereas the dichorionic placenta does show an intervening chorion (actually two fused chorions) between the two amnions (**b**)

References

1. Suzuki S. Clinical significance of pregnancies with circumvallate placenta. J Obstet Gynaecol Res. 2008;34:51–4.
2. Anyikam AL, Hull AD, Benke S, Trivedi N, Lacoursiere DY, Pretorius DH. Prenatal diagnosis of circumvallate placenta and pregnancy outcomes. Obstet Gynecol. 2014;123 Suppl 1:98S.
3. Heller DS, Keane-Tarchichi M, Varshney S. Is pathologic confirmation of placental abruption more reliable in cases due to chronic etiologies compared with acute etiologies? J Perinat Med. 2013;41:701–3.

13.1 Gestational Trophoblastic Neoplasia

Gestational trophoblastic neoplasia (GTN) is classified differently by the clinician and the pathologist. There may be treatment decisions made without tissue being obtained for histopathologic evaluation, particularly in GTN that follows a known hydatidiform mole. The clinical classification relates to tumor location and risk factors, not to histology. GTN may be uterine or extrauterine (invasive mole can rarely go to lungs, vulva, vagina), and tissue is not always available or needed to treat these patients. Clinical GTN is considered either benign (i.e., hydatidiform moles) or malignant. Malignant GTN is either nonmetastatic or metastatic. Metastatic disease is subdivided into good or poor prognosis based on specific risk factors. FIGO staging with a WHO scoring system [1] is utilized to make the prognostic determinations. The following discussion refers to the pathology of GTN where tissue is available for evaluation and some of the recent developments and challenges associated with diagnosis (Table 13.1).

13.2 Hydatidiform Mole

Hydatidiform moles may either be complete or partial. These present differently clinically, are genetically different, and have different risks for persistent GTN.

13.2.1 Complete Hydatidiform Mole

Complete moles are mostly 46XX, which can result from paternal duplication occurring after loss of maternal genetic material, or occasionally with dispermic fertilization of an empty egg. Geography and age have impact on risk, with the lesion being more common in Asian populations, as well as mothers under 15 years or over 45 years of age. Fathers over 45 years of age contribute to risk.

© Springer International Publishing Switzerland 2015

D.S. Heller, *OB-GYN Pathology for the Clinician*,

DOI 10.1007/978-3-319-15422-0_13

Table 13.1 Key points about gestational trophoblastic disease

Tissue may not be obtained in cases of GTN
There are areas of diagnostic difficulty for the pathologist:
Areas of pathological diagnostic difficulty
Early complete mole may not be recognized, or may be diagnosed as a partial mole
Partial mole is difficult to distinguish histologically from missed hydropic abortion
There is a risk of overdiagnosis of mole in tubal ectopic pregnancies due to exuberant trophoblast
There is a risk of overdiagnosis of exaggerated placental site as PSTT, particularly on curettage
There is a risk of overdiagnosis of atypical nonvillous trophoblast (often with a complete mole) as choriocarcinoma or PSTT
The best approach is to consider patient age, beta-hCG levels, history of recent or remote pregnancy, imaging findings, then perform in-depth histopathologic evaluation with appropriate immunohistochemistry

The older clinical presentation for a complete mole was in the second trimester, with bleeding, disproportionally elevated serum beta-hCG, uterine size greater than dates, and possible hyperemesis, toxemia, hyperthyroidism, or respiratory distress in some cases. Ultrasound showed absence of a fetus with a snowstorm pattern for the molar villi. Evacuation led to a specimen composed of "grapes," the hydropic villi. Patients may have ovarian theca lutein cysts at presentation (see Chap. 9).

However, patients present earlier in gestation than previously, and the first trimester specimens received by the pathology laboratory often lack the pronounced features of a second trimester complete mole (Fig. 13.1a–d). Second trimester moles show pronounced trophoblastic hyperplasia circumferentially around villi, and as extravillous clusters, with hydropic villi, enlarged, and some so edematous that cisterns have formed. With earlier terminations, uniform trophoblast hyperplasia and villous cavitation ("grapes") may not have developed yet. Five features have been identified as providing histologic evidence [2]: Redundant bulbous terminal villi, hypercellular myxoid villous stroma, labyrinthine network of villous stromal canaliculi, focal nonpolar cyto- and syncytiotrophoblastic hyperplasia of villi and undersurface of chorionic plate, and enlarged atypical hyperchromatic implantation site trophoblasts (Fig. 13.1e).

A significant number of complete moles go on to persistent GTN as evidenced by elevated serum beta-hCG, but most of these are probably persistent moles or invasive moles, with only a small percent going on to choriocarcinoma. Tissue in these cases may not be acquired, and the diagnosis and treatment may be based on clinical findings alone. Although the risk of persistent GTN is greater in complete moles than partial moles, recurrence risk of both complete and partial moles is less than 2 % in subsequent pregnancies [3].

13.2.2 Partial Hydatidiform Mole

Partial moles are triploid, usually XXY, which can result from dispermic fertilization of an egg. Clinically, partial moles present as missed abortions. Unlike complete

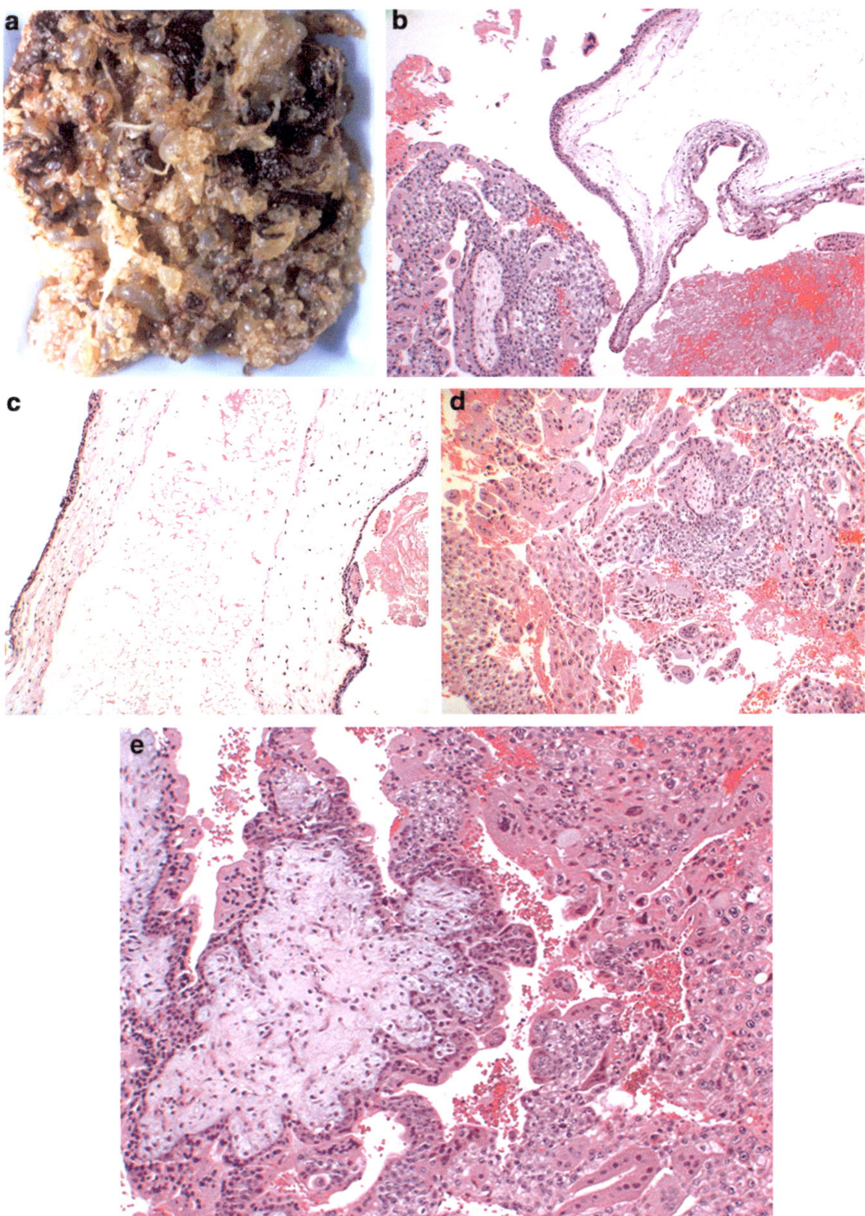

Fig. 13.1 Complete hydatidiform mole. Note the grape-like vesicular tissue (**a**). Histologically there is villous edema with cistern formation (*right*), and trophoblastic proliferation (*left*) (**b**). Higher power shows the cistern in the center of a markedly hydropic villus (**c**). Trophoblast proliferation is biphasic, with multinucleated syncytiotrophoblasts, and cytotrophoblasts with well-demarcated cell membranes (**d**). In early complete moles (**e**), hydropic change is less pronounced, but the villi show redundant bulbous outpouchings, hypercellular myxoid stroma with vascular anastomosing channels (*left*), and trophoblast proliferation (*right*)

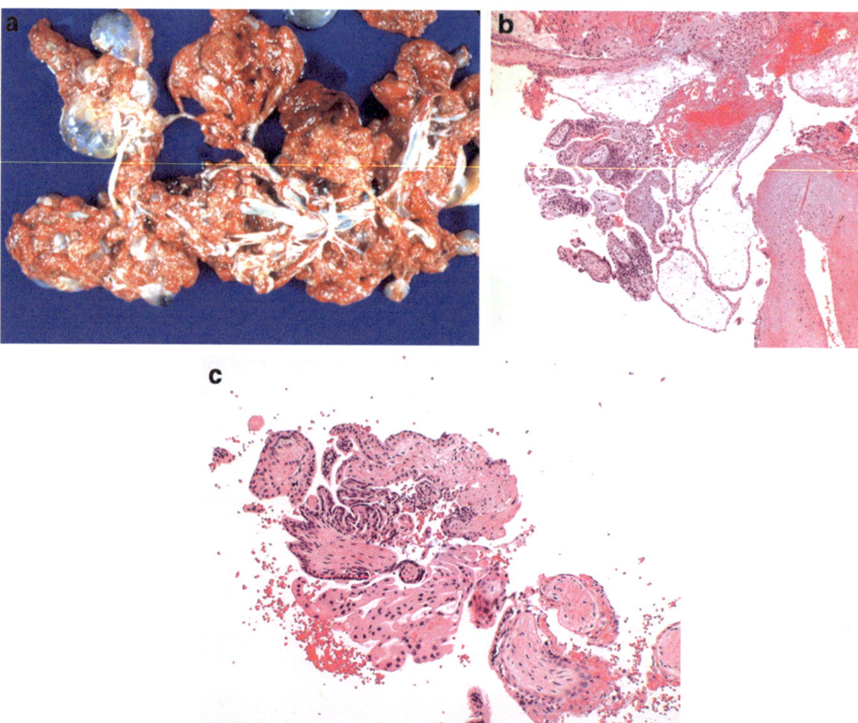

Fig. 13.2 Partial hydatidiform mole. Note that the tissue is less vesicular than in complete mole (**a**). The lesion is composed of a mix of enlarged molar villi and smaller normal appearing villi (**b**). Villi may be scalloped, with a lesser degree of trophoblast proliferation than complete mole (**c**)

mole, there is no age-associated risk. Grossly, molar changes are much less, and only occasional or no significantly hydropic villi may be seen. Histologically, there is usually evidence of a fetus. If the fetus develops, it is abnormal, but early termination may only show fetal tissue fragments or nucleated red blood cells in villous fetal vessels as evidence of a fetus. There is a mix of normal and molar villi. The molar villi are less edematous, irregular, and scalloped in shape, and there is less trophoblastic proliferation than complete mole (Fig. 13.2a–c). This makes the distinction from hydropic (missed) abortion a challenge at times, where there may be hydropic villi, but no trophoblast proliferation. Partial moles can persist in a small number of cases, but choriocarcinoma is rare. Recurrence of a partial mole in a subsequent pregnancy is similar to complete mole, with about a 2 % risk [3].

13.2.3 Distinguishing Complete Mole, Partial Mole, and Hydropic Abortion

Immunohistochemistry using antibody to p57 has proven very useful in distinguishing moles. p57 is expressed in maternally derived tissues, but not paternal tissues.

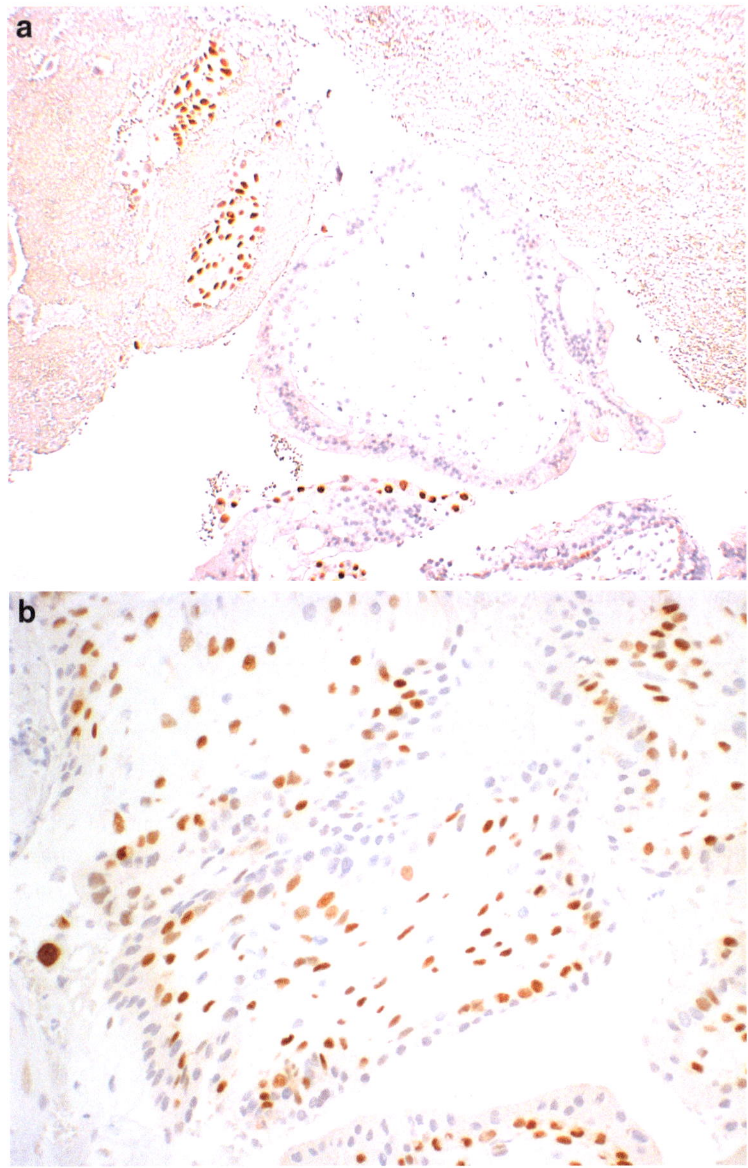

Fig. 13.3 p57 staining. p57 stains extravillous trophoblast but not villi in complete mole (**a**), and stains villous stromal cells and cytotrophoblast in partial mole (**b**)

As such, it has different staining patterns in complete and partial mole. As the villi are paternally derived in complete mole, they do not stain with p57, although staining may be seen in nests of extravillous trophoblast and in maternal decidua (Fig. 13.3a). In partial moles, as there is a maternal genetic component, villous staining in the cytotrophoblast and villous stromal cells may be seen (Fig. 13.3b). Missed hydropic abortions will stain similarly to partial moles, so that p57 is not helpful in this distinction.

Another group of modalities is flow cytometry, fluorescent in situ hybridization (FISH), or chromogenic in situ hybridization (CISH), used for ploidy. This would distinguish a diploid complete mole from a triploid partial mole. However, a missed abortion would also be diploid. In addition, a partial mole is due to diandric triploidy, where two of the three chromosome complements are paternal. Digynic triploidy, where two of the three chromosomal complements are maternal, would also read as triploid on ploidy studies, but digynic triploidy results not in a partial mole, but in an abnormal triploid fetus.

More recently, polymerase chain reaction (PCR) short tandem repeat genotyping has become a useful adjunct [4], although it is not universally available. It can distinguish androgenetic diploidy (complete mole), diandric triploidy (partial mole), and biparental diploidy (missed abortion). It can be used on formalin-fixed, paraffin-embedded tissue. It compares the placental tissue to the decidua, identifying what is "maternal" and "not maternal." It can also distinguish a new mole from a persistent one. There are pitfalls, including triploid androgenic complete moles and familial biparental complete moles, but these are rare cases.

13.3 Invasive Mole

Invasive mole is the most common form of persistent gestational trophoblastic disease, markedly more common than choriocarcinoma, and may occur both in the uterus (Fig. 13.4), where it must be distinguished from placenta increta, and in extrauterine locations, including lung. Histologically, the lesion is composed of molar villi in extrauterine locations, and as molar villi invading myometrium (Fig. 13.4) for intrauterine cases. When ruling out increta, the molar nature of the villi confirms invasive mole, versus increta, where the villi are not molar. Invasive mole is much more common as a clinical entity of "persistent GTN," rather than as tissue for the pathologist to evaluate.

13.4 Gestational Choriocarcinoma

Gestational choriocarcinoma is rare, representing only a fraction of persistent cases of GTN. Tissue may not be obtained in the evaluation and treatment of a patient, who may be followed by imaging and beta-hCG levels. While about half the antecedent pregnancies are hydatidiform moles, usually complete, any form of antecedent pregnancy can lead to a choriocarcinoma. Choriocarcinoma is an extremely hemorrhagic and angioinvasive tumor and may bleed profusely at biopsy. If tissue is obtained, what is seen is a very hemorrhagic tumor composed of a biphasic population of syncytiotrophoblasts, which are markedly beta-hCG-positive on immunostaining, and cytotrophoblasts (Fig. 13.5a, b). Although it is likely intermediate trophoblast are present as well.

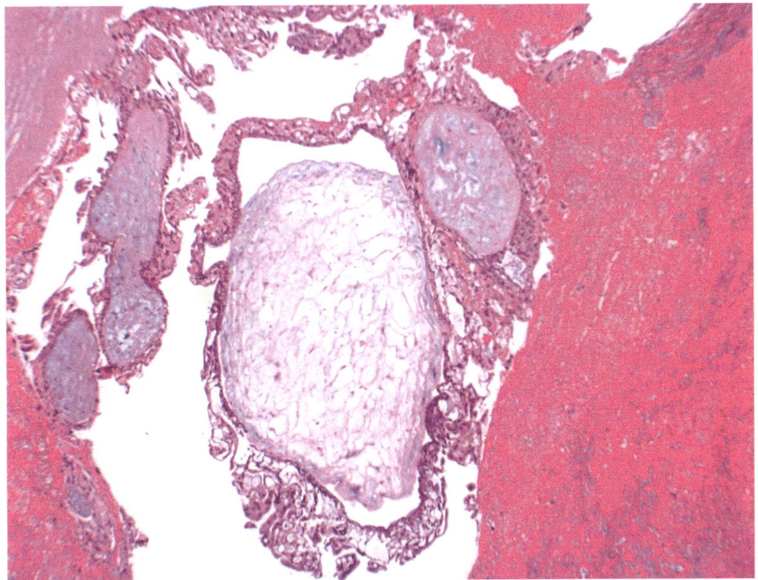

Fig. 13.4 Invasive mole. Molar villi may be seen invading myometrium

13.5 Tumors of Intermediate Trophoblast

It has come to be recognized that there are different subpopulations of intermediate trophoblast (IT), the villous type of IT, which anchors the chorionic villi to the basal plate via trophoblastic columns, implantation site IT which is seen infiltrating decidua and myometrium, and chorionic-type IT, seen in the free membranes in the chorion laeve. The different types of IT have different immunohistochemical staining profiles, which is helpful in identifying lesions arising from them. The last two, the implantation site IT and the chorionic type IT, give rise to both benign and potentially malignant lesions of IT [5]. Lesions of implantation site trophoblast include exaggerated placental site and placental site trophoblastic tumor (PSTT). Chorionic type IT gives rise to placental site nodules/plaques and epithelioid trophoblast tumor.

13.5.1 Exaggerated Placental Site

At the time of its description, this benign lesion of implantation site trophoblasts was thought to be due to "syncytial wandering cells," and given the term "Syncytial Endometritis," which is no longer applicable. Exaggerated placental site is a benign

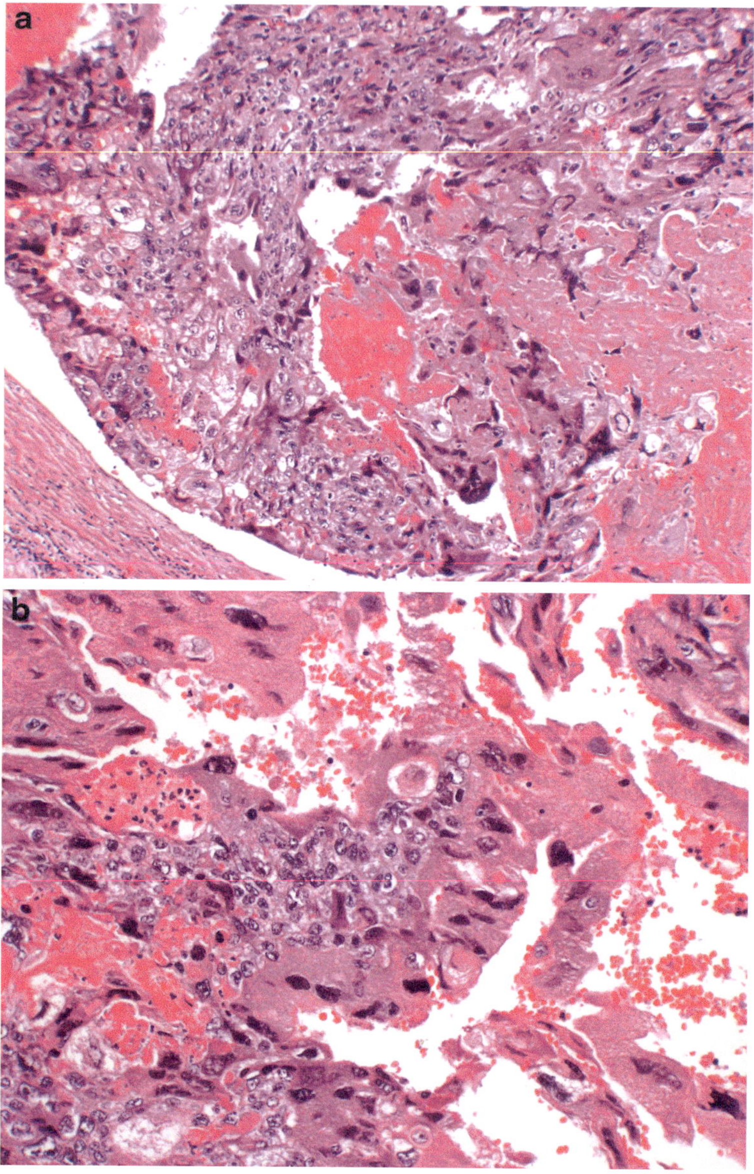

Fig. 13.5 Choriocarcinoma. The lesion is hemorrhagic with no villi present (**a**). Choriocarcinoma shows a biphasic population of syncytiotrophoblasts with multinucleation, and cytotrophoblasts (**b**)

lesion seen at or near the time of a pregnancy, normal, spontaneous abortion or molar, so villi are frequently seen. This temporal relationship is important to consider when differentiating this lesion from PSTT, a common dilemma, particularly on curettings.

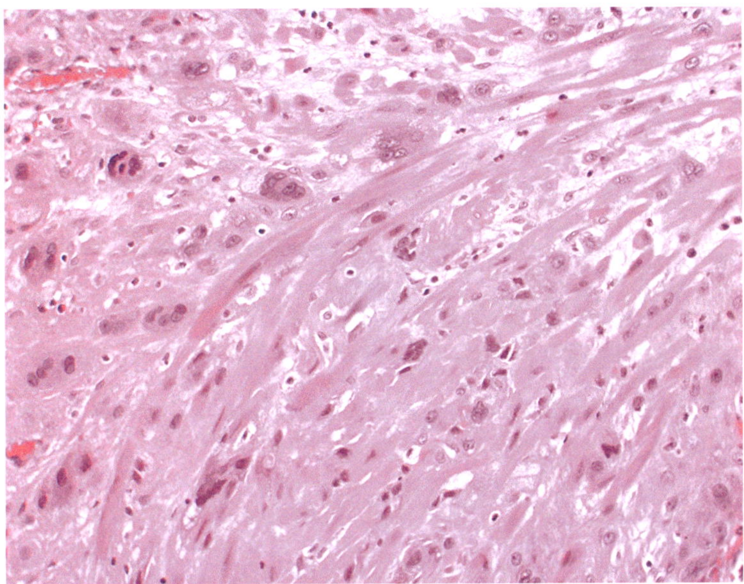

Fig. 13.6 Exaggerated placental site. Intermediate trophoblast cells are seen between fascicles of myometrium. This finding may raise concern for a PSTT, particularly on curettage

Exaggerated placental site is comprised of increased numbers of evenly distributed ITs infiltrating the decidua and myometrium without forming a mass, or exhibiting necrosis or architectural disarray (Fig. 13.6). Ki-67 proliferation index is usually <1 %, also helpful when evaluating lesions of IT. Lesions of implantation trophoblast are usually strongly positive for human placental lactogen, helpful in the differential [5].

13.5.2 Placental Site Trophoblastic Tumor

PSTT is also derived from implantation site trophoblast, and hence human placental lactogen tends to be strongly staining. P63 is negative, distinguishing PSTT from Epithelioid Trophoblastic Tumor (ETT), a lesion of chorionic IT (see next sections). While most PSTTs behave in a benign manner, a subset does exhibit aggressive behavior. They are usually treated by hysterectomy, although lesser excisions have been utilized. They tend to be chemoresistent, unlike the extremely chemosensitive choriocarcinoma. Distinguishing PSTT from an exaggerated placental site can be difficult histologically, particularly on curettings. PSTT usually presents in parous women around age 30, who present with abnormal bleeding or amenorrhea.

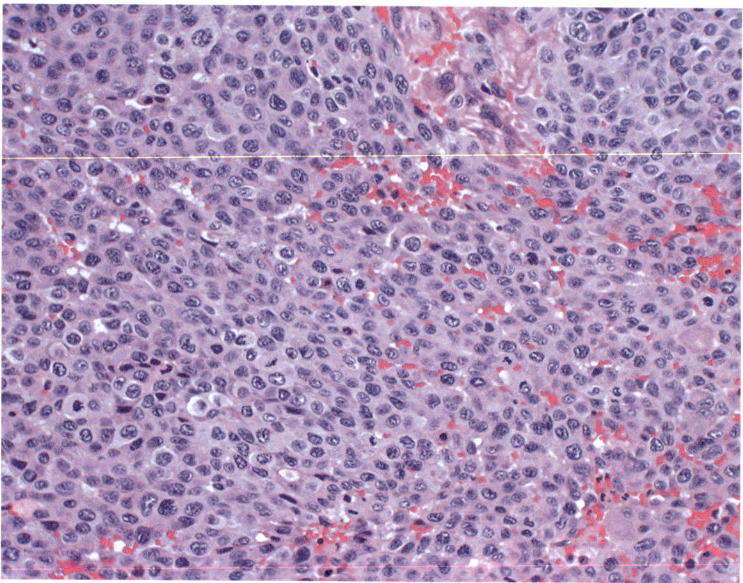

Fig. 13.7 PSTT. A monophasic proliferation of intermediate trophoblast cells is seen

The antecedent pregnancy is usually remote. Uterine size may or may not be increased. Beta-hCG may be mildly increased, but is not in the range of invasive mole or choriocarcinoma. The antecedent pregnancy is most often a normal gestation.

PSTT may show gross intramyometrial masses, or be infiltrative. Histologically, there is a monomorphic population of cells, with occasional bi- and multinucleate cells (Fig. 13.7). The tumor tends to split myometrial bundles, hence the histologic similarity to exaggerated placental site. The absence of villi in PSTT is helpful. There is variable atypia, focal necrosis, and an infiltrating margin. Occasional mitoses may be seen. Ki-67 proliferation index is >5–10 %, helping distinguish the lesion from exaggerated placental site, which is <1 % [5].

13.5.3 Placental Site Nodule and Plaque

Placental site nodules/plaques are derived from chorionic IT. They may represent the ghost of a blighted ovum or old implantation site. These benign lesions are seen during reproductive age, often discovered at curettage for bleeding, or they may be incidental. It is unclear if they are the actual cause of bleeding. Usually the lesions are not grossly visible, or rarely a nodule 1 cm or less, yellow/tan or hemorrhagic may be seen. Although they occur in parous women, they are generally remote from a known or undocumented pregnancy. On low power, the lesions are discrete and lobulated (Fig. 13.8a). Histologically on higher power, they are seen to be

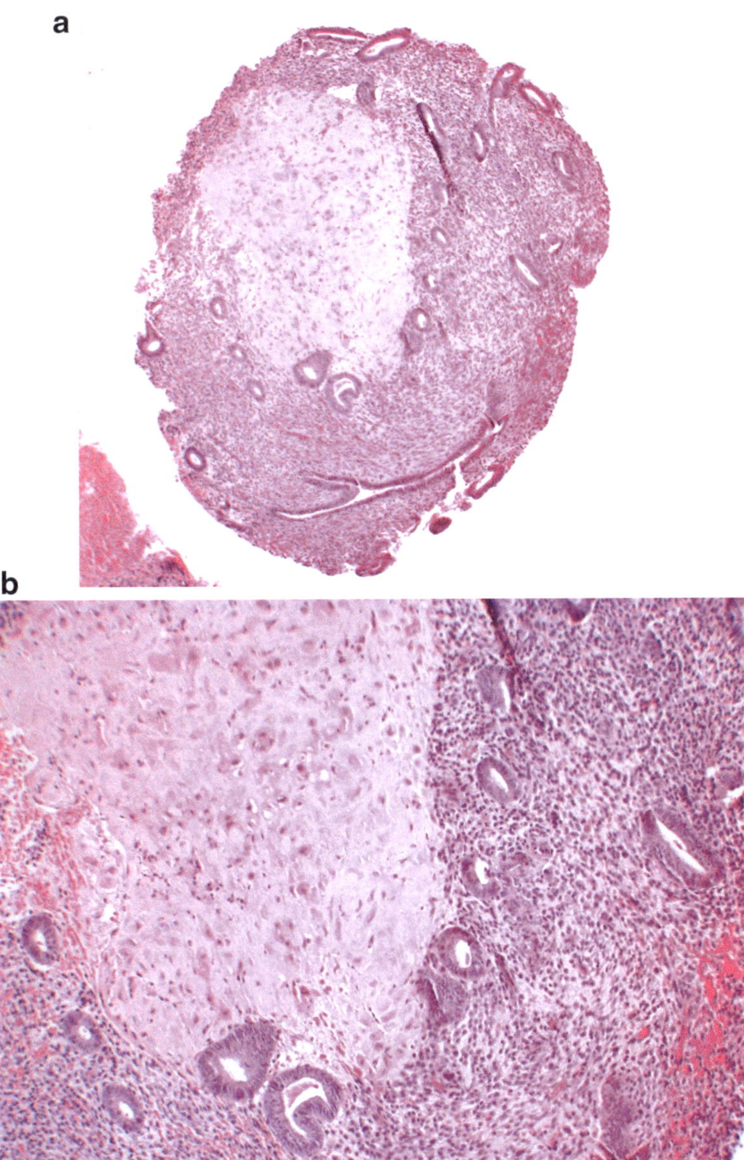

Fig. 13.8 Placental site nodule. At low power, the lesion is seen as a small circumscribed lesion (**a**). At higher power (**b**), placental site nodule shows rare IT cells in a paucicellular eosinophilic background

paucicellular, mostly comprised of eosinophilic material with rare intermediate trophoblast cells (Fig. 13.8b). They may stain focally for human placental lactogen, but not strongly, as seen in the implantation site trophoblastic lesions. The chorionic IT lesions stain for p63. Beta-hCG is usually negative immunohistochemically (as well as clinically). Ki-67 proliferation index is low but not 0.

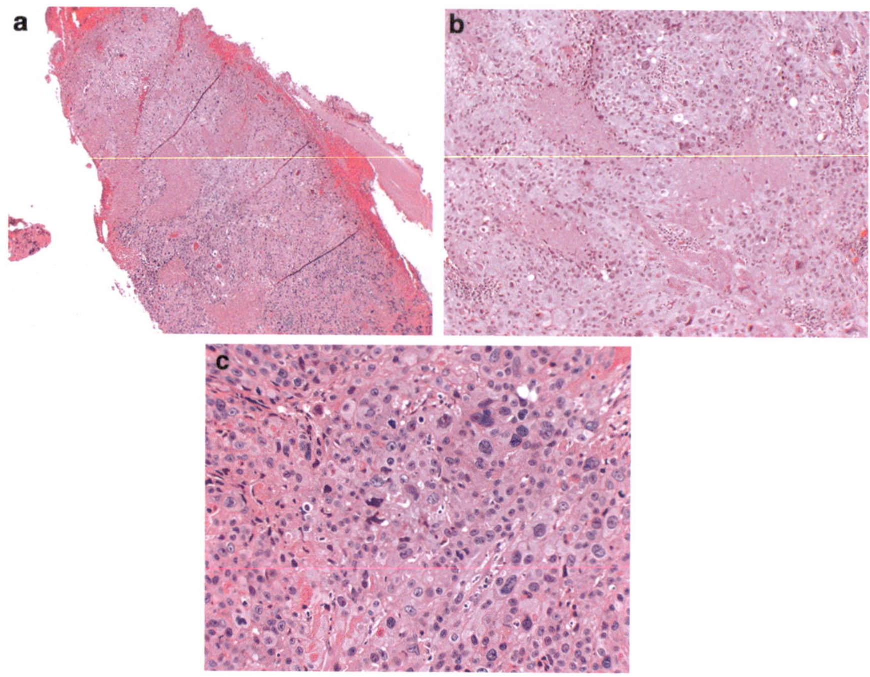

Fig. 13.9 Epithelioid trophoblastic tumor. At low power (**a**), geographic necrosis is seen. Higher power shows a monomorphous population of IT cells (**b**, **c**), with geographic necrosis (**b**)

13.5.4 Epithelioid Trophoblastic Tumor

A more recently described entity, ETT is a rare lesion of predominantly reproductive age women. It derives from the chorionic IT, and hence has the immunoprofile of that type of IT, with lesser staining for human placental lactogen, and strong positivity for p63. Behavior-wise, the lesions are similar to PSTT, with most lesions benign, but a potential for aggressive behavior. Beta-hCG levels may be elevated, but are not as high as seen in invasive mole/choriocarcinoma. There may be a long latency between the antecedent pregnancy and the presentation, which is often of abnormal bleeding. The lesions tend to be more nodular and discrete and less infiltrative than PSTT. ETTs have a tendency to reside in the cervix or lower uterine segment, and that location, along with the positive p63, means that the lesion needs to be distinguished from cervical squamous cell carcinoma, which would also stain for p63. Histologically, ETTs are composed of a monotonous population of IT with characteristic geographic necrosis (Fig. 13.9a–c) in nests, cords, and sheets. Central eosinophilic debris is seen. Unlike the infiltrative margins of PSTT, these margins are pushing in nature. Ki-67 index is usually over 10 % [5]. Like PSTT, primary treatment is usually surgical, and these lesions tend to be chemoresistent.

References

1. Lurain JR. Gestational trophoblastic disease II: classification and management of gestational trophoblastic neoplasia. Am J Obstet Gynecol. 2011;204:11–8.
2. Keep D, Zaragoza MV, Hassold T, Redline RW. Very early complete hydatidiform mole. Hum Pathol. 1996;27:708–13.
3. Sebire NJ, Fisher RA, Foskett M, Rees H, Seckl MJ, Newlands ES. Risk of recurrent hydatidiform mole and subsequent pregnancy outcome following complete or partial hydatidiform molar pregnancy. BJOG. 2003;110:22–6.
4. Ronnett BM, DeScipio C, Murphy KM. Hydatidiform moles: ancillary techniques to refine diagnosis. Int J Gynecol Pathol. 2011;30:101–16.
5. Shih IM, Kurman RJ. The pathology of intermediate trophoblastic tumors and tumor-like lesions. Int J Gynecol Pathol. 2001;20:31–47.

14.1 The Pap Smear

The pap smear is one of the best examples of the success of a screening test, with significant decreases in the incidence of cervical cancer since the availability of the test. It is not meant to be a diagnostic test, but a screening modality indicating that further evaluation may be warranted (Table 14.1).

14.2 The Bethesda System

Most laboratories utilize the Bethesda system for classification of pap smears (*nih.techriver.net/*). The report has several different components. Whether the slide is a conventional pap smear or liquid-based preparation is noted. Adequacy of the specimen is also noted. Interpretation includes negative for intraepithelial lesion or malignancy, epithelial cell abnormalities, and other malignancies. Also noted are any ancillary testing, automated review, and the option for educational notes or suggestions is included. Under negative for intraepithelial lesion/malignancy, organisms and other nonneoplastic findings can be reported.

14.3 Preparation of Cytology Slides

Most pap smears were previously prepared by obtaining the cells on the sampling device, smearing them directly onto the slide, and fixing the slide. This preparation can be difficult to interpret at times, due to thick areas and obscuring inflammation. Most laboratories now utilize liquid-based cytology, where the sampling device is placed in a preservative jar and the cells suspended in the liquid by swishing the sampling device around. The machines that prepare the slides filter out much of the

© Springer International Publishing Switzerland 2015
D.S. Heller, *OB-GYN Pathology for the Clinician*,
DOI 10.1007/978-3-319-15422-0_14

Table 14.1 Key points about gynecologic cytology

The pap smear has markedly decreased the incidence of cervical cancer
The pap smear is an excellent screening tool, but it is not a diagnostic tool. The purpose is to indicate that additional investigation is needed
The pap smear may have false positives and false negatives
Although an occasionally malignancy above the cervix (endometrium, ovary, fallopian tube) may shed and be detected on a pap smear, the pap smear is not a valid screening modality for these neoplasms

inflammatory debris and prepare thinner cell layers, making the slides prepared in this manner easier to read. In addition, the residual cytology preservative can be utilized for ancillary testing such as HPV testing.

14.4 Normal Pap Smear Findings

14.4.1 Normal Squamous Epithelium

Normal squamous epithelial cells as seen on a cytology preparation may be seen at different stages of maturation. Superficial cells contain small nuclei in abundant cytoplasm. Intermediate cells have slightly larger nuclei (Fig. 14.1). Parabasal cells are usually not seen during reproductive life, but show up on menopausal pap smears. The hormonal status of a woman used to be evaluated by pap smears, with estrogenic effect shifting the cell ratio towards superficial cells with intermediate cells and atrophic estrogen-deficient smears showing prominent parabasal cells with intermediate cells. This used to be used in clinical practice, expressed as the maturation index, expressed as percentages of parabasal:intermediate:superficial cells; however, has fallen by the wayside for the most part.

14.4.2 Normal Endocervical Cells

The presence of endocervical cells or metaplastic squamous cells indicates that the transformation zone was sampled. Endocervical cells can either have a picket-fence arrangement in strips, or sheets of cells may show a honeycomb pattern (Fig. 14.2).

14.4.3 Endometrial Cells

Abnormal endometrial cells can indicate neoplasia; however, it is not rare to see normal-appearing endometrial cells (Fig. 14.3a, b), particularly during or shortly after menses. As pathologists don't always have menstrual or menopausal status information, it is up to the clinician to determine if shedding endometrial cells are out of cycle or postmenopausal. The Bethesda system makes note of them in women over 40 to make sure to capture menopausal patients.

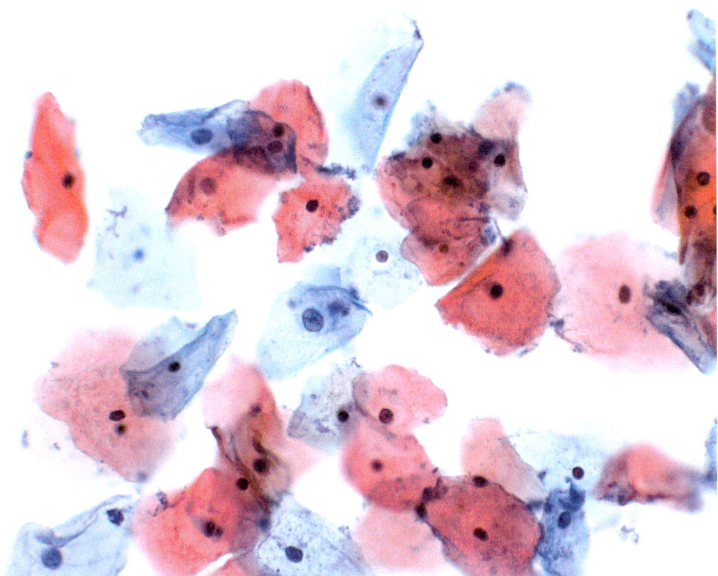

Fig. 14.1 Normal pap. Superficial cells with smaller nuclei, and intermediate cells (*center*) with larger nuclei are seen

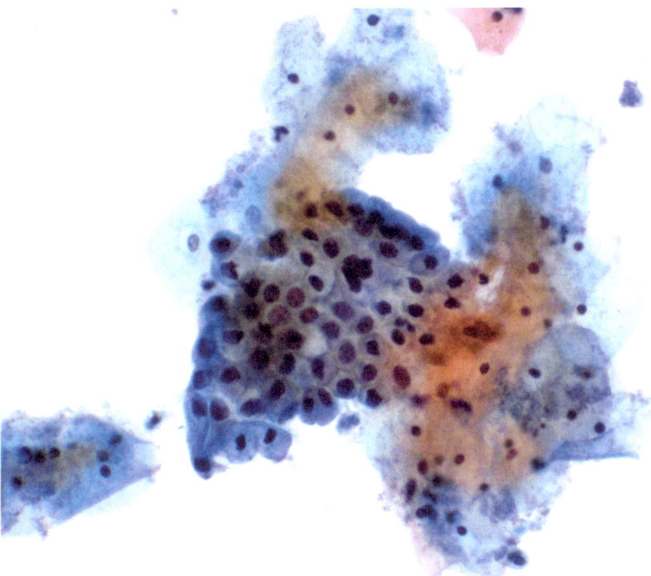

Fig. 14.2 Normal pap. Cluster of endocervical cells is seen showing a mix of the honeycomb configuration at the *left*, and the picket fence appearance at the *upper right* of the cell cluster

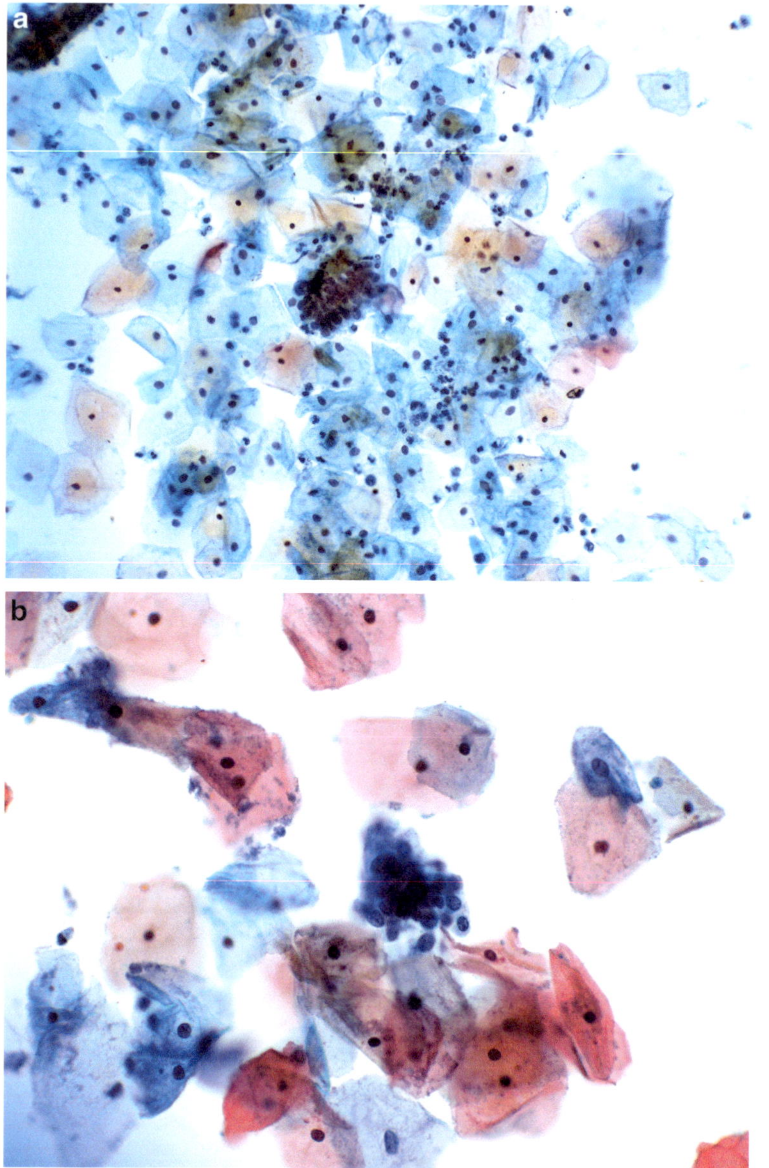

Fig. 14.3 Endometrial cells on pap. A cluster of endometrial cells is seen (**a**). The endometrial cells are much smaller than squamous and endocervical cells (**b**)

14.4.4 Atrophy

Atrophy associated with loss of estrogenic stimulus is a normal finding. It is characterized by a predominance of parabasal cells (Fig. 14.4). There may be abundant

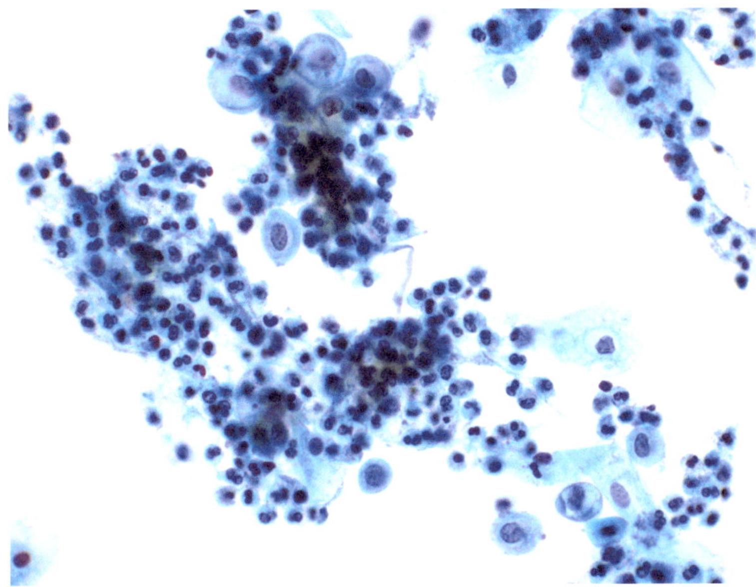

Fig. 14.4 Atrophy. The pap is composed of parabasal and occasional intermediate cells. Abundant neutrophils are seen, but do not correlate with symptomatology

inflammatory cells; however, the histologic diagnosis of "atrophic vaginitis" as opposed to "atrophic pattern" does not correlate with clinical symptomatology [1].

14.5 Infectious and Other Non-neoplastic Findings

14.5.1 Candida

Candida may be seen as either hyphae, or spores, depending on strain. Torulopsis appears as small spores in clusters. On liquid cytology preparations, the more common candida albicans appears as hyphae, with clumping of squamous cells described as a "shish kebab" appearance (Fig. 14.5a, b).

14.5.2 Bacterial Vaginosis

Bacterial vaginosis identified on a pap smear is described as consistent with a shift in vaginal flora. This finding does not necessarily correlate with patient symptomatology. The cytologic hallmark are "clue" cells, squamous cells covered by adherent bacteria (Fig. 14.6).

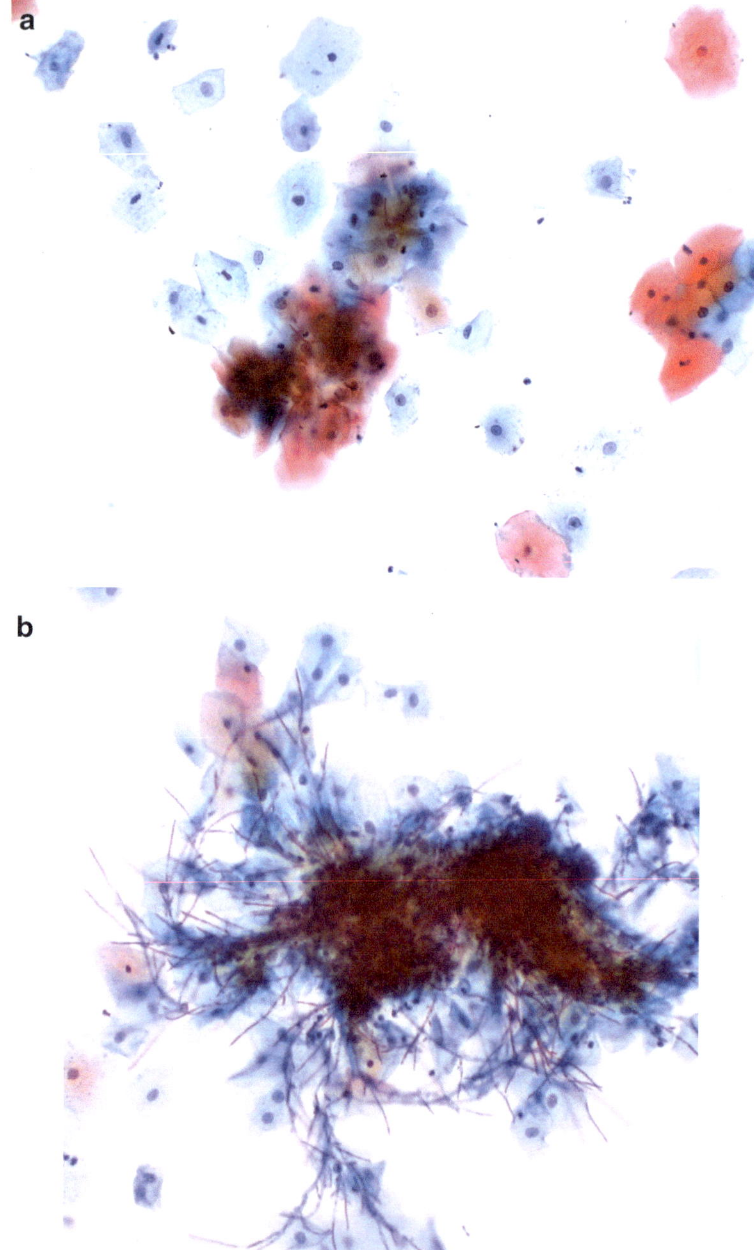

Fig. 14.5 Candida. A typical "shish kebab" cluster of squamous cells, agglutinated with candida are seen (**a**). Fungal hyphae of candida albicans are present (**b**)

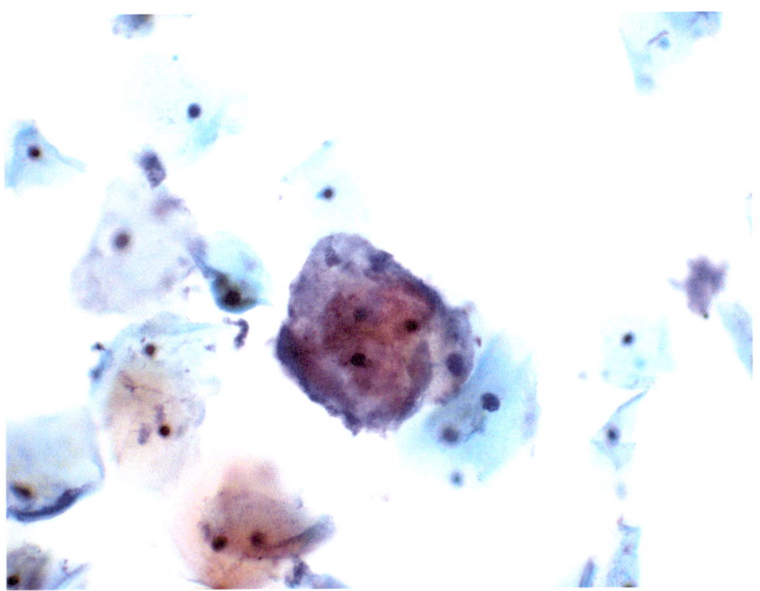

Fig. 14.6 Bacterial vaginosis. A "clue" cell, a squamous cell with adherent bacteria, is seen in the center

14.5.3 Trichomonas

Trichomonal organisms on traditional pap smears do not show the flagella seen on wet smears, although liquid-based cytology preps may show them. Liquid-based cytology is quite accurate in permitting the diagnosis of this organism [2]. The organisms are small and pear-shaped, with a small nucleus, with occasional cytoplasmic granules. The organisms may be associated with neutrophils and tend to cluster near squamous cells (Fig. 14.7).

14.5.4 Herpes

Occasionally herpes simplex is detected on paps and is seen as multinucleation with characteristic intranuclear inclusions (Fig. 14.8).

14.5.5 Actinomyces

Actinomyces, most often seen in association with an intrauterine device, is characterized by radiating clusters of filamentous organisms (Fig. 14.9), termed "sulphur granules," for the yellow color sometimes seen grossly.

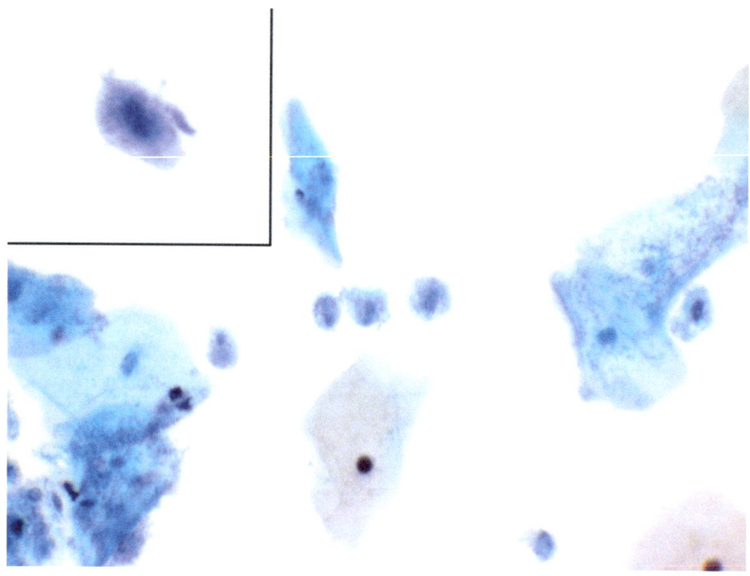

Fig. 14.7 Trichomonas. Several pear-shaped organisms are seen in the center of the field. The organisms have elongated nuclei (*inset*)

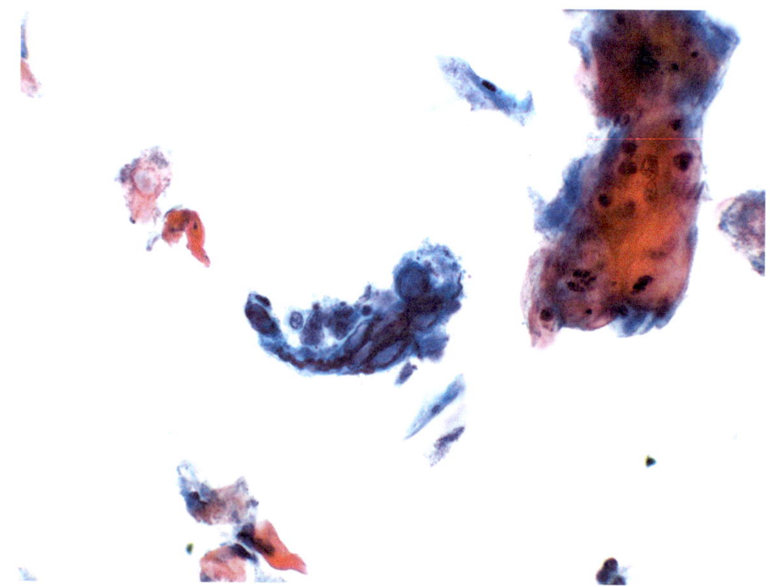

Fig. 14.8 Herpes. A multinucleated cell with ground glass nuclear inclusions characteristic of herpes

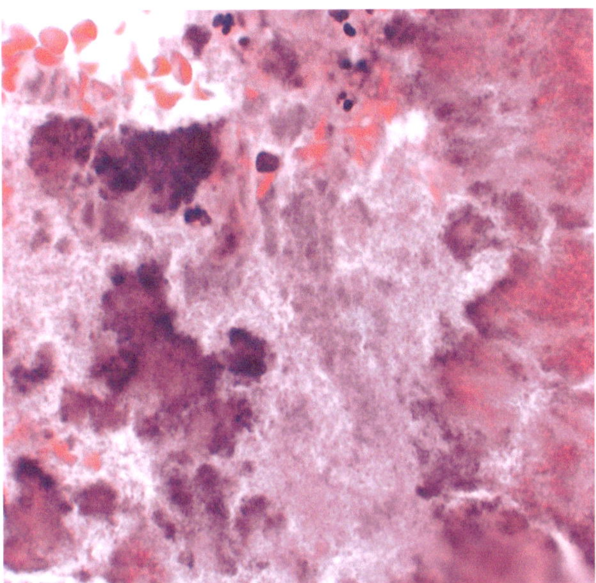

Fig. 14.9 Actinomyces. Filamentous organisms are seen in radiating configurations

14.5.6 Other Findings

Other findings optional to report in the Bethesda system include inflammation, repair, changes seen with an IUD, radiation changes, and glandular cells post-hysterectomy.

14.6   Atypical Squamous Cells of Uncertain Significance

Atypical squamous cells that do not sufficiently meet the criteria for a diagnosis of squamous intraepithelial lesion may be categorized as atypical squamous cells of uncertain significance (ASCUS) (Fig. 14.10). HPV reflex testing of the same liquid cytology residual fluid is often used to triage these cases. Many ASCUS paps represent low-grade squamous intraepithelial lesions (LSIL) that either don't rise to the diagnostic criteria or contain too few sufficiently atypical cells to confirm the diagnosis of LSIL.

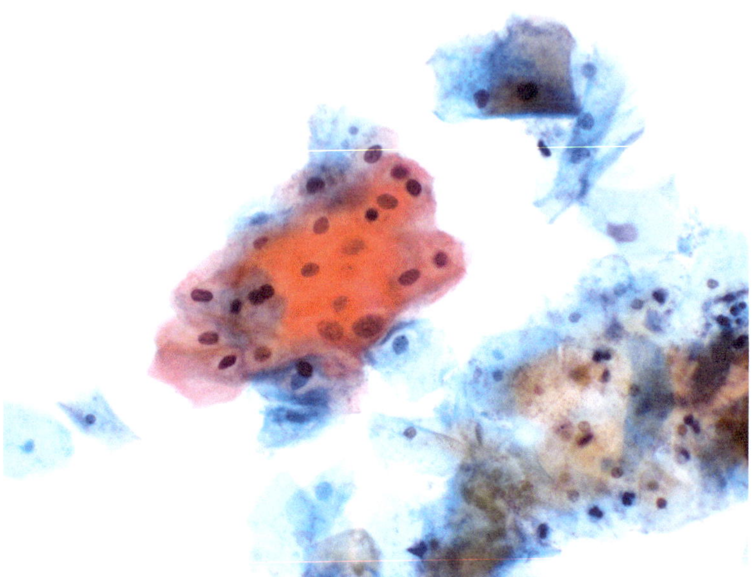

Fig. 14.10 ASCUS. A cluster of possible koilocytes is seen, but the nuclei are not sufficiently enlarged or atypical enough for a definite diagnosis of LSIL

14.7 Atypical Squamous Cells of Uncertain Significance, Cannot Exclude High-Grade Squamous Intraepithelial Lesion

This diagnosis, abbreviated ASC-H, is only applied occasionally, for ASCUS cases that are more worrisome. Often, it cannot be determined with certainty if the cells represent a high-grade squamous intraepithelial lesion (HSIL) or are atypical metaplastic cells, which can sometimes be difficult to distinguish.

14.8 Atypical Glandular Cells

Atypical glandular cells may be specified as endocervical, endometrial, or simply as atypical glandular cells, not otherwise specified (NOS) if it cannot be determined (Fig. 14.11).

14.9 Intraepithelial Neoplasia

Intraepithelial neoplasia, which refers to neoplasia that has not breached the basement membrane and therefore has no metastatic potential, may be squamous or glandular.

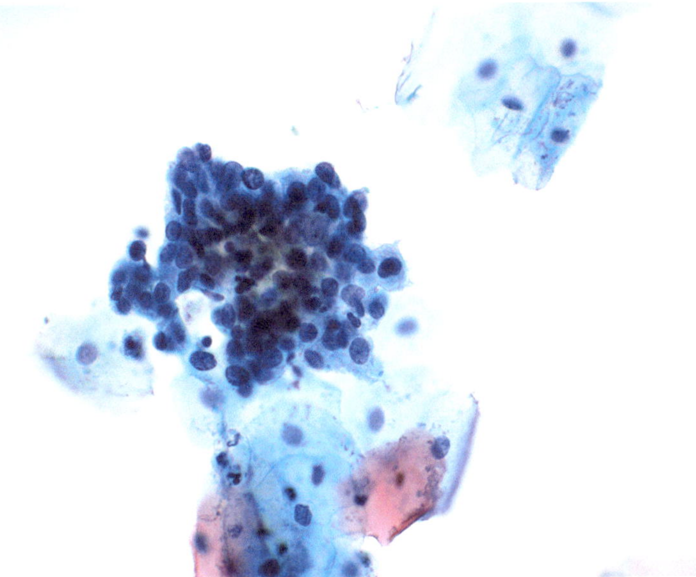

Fig. 14.11 Atypical glandular cells. A cluster of atypical glandular cells is seen

14.10 Low-Grade Squamous Intraepithelial Lesion

LSIL is characterized by koilocytes, squamous cells with enlarged nuclei with wrinkled nuclear membranes ("raisins"), as well as multinucleation, and perinuclear halos. Hyperkeratosis may be associated, but is not in and of itself diagnostic (Fig. 14.12a, b). Halos alone in the absence of nuclear atypia are insufficient for the diagnosis of LSIL, as they may be indicative of glycogen alone.

14.11 High-Grade Squamous Intraepithelial Lesion

HSIL can be a subtle finding on liquid-based cytology preparations, because the cells are quite small and resemble metaplastic cells. Hyperchromasia (increased nuclear staining) is helpful, but is not always present on liquid-based preparations, as it is on traditional paps. What are indicative are an increase in nuclear to cytoplasmic ratio, as well as nuclear membrane irregularities ("mouse bites" or "rat bites") (Fig. 14.13a, b).

14.12 Adenocarcinoma-In-Situ

Adenocarcinoma-in-situ (AIS) on a pap is characterized by atypical endocervical cells, often with a palisading of the cells around the edges of the cell groups (Fig. 14.14a, b). Distinction from frankly invasive endocervical adenocarcinoma on pap is extremely difficult at times, and it should be remembered that the pap is a screening test, not a diagnostic one.

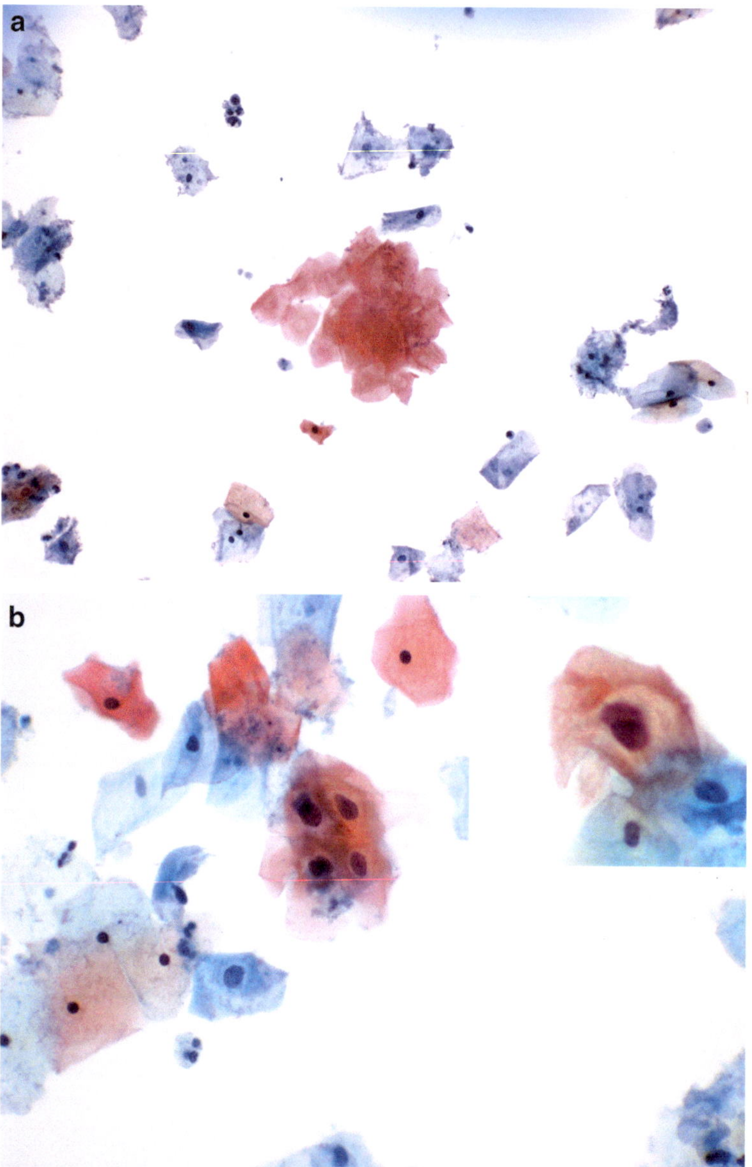

Fig. 14.12 LGSIL. Although not diagnostic, sometimes hyperkeratosis is seen accompanying LGSIL (**a**). Koilocytes are seen in this case of LGSIL (**b**), with binucleation, nuclear atypia, and a perinuclear halo (*inset*)

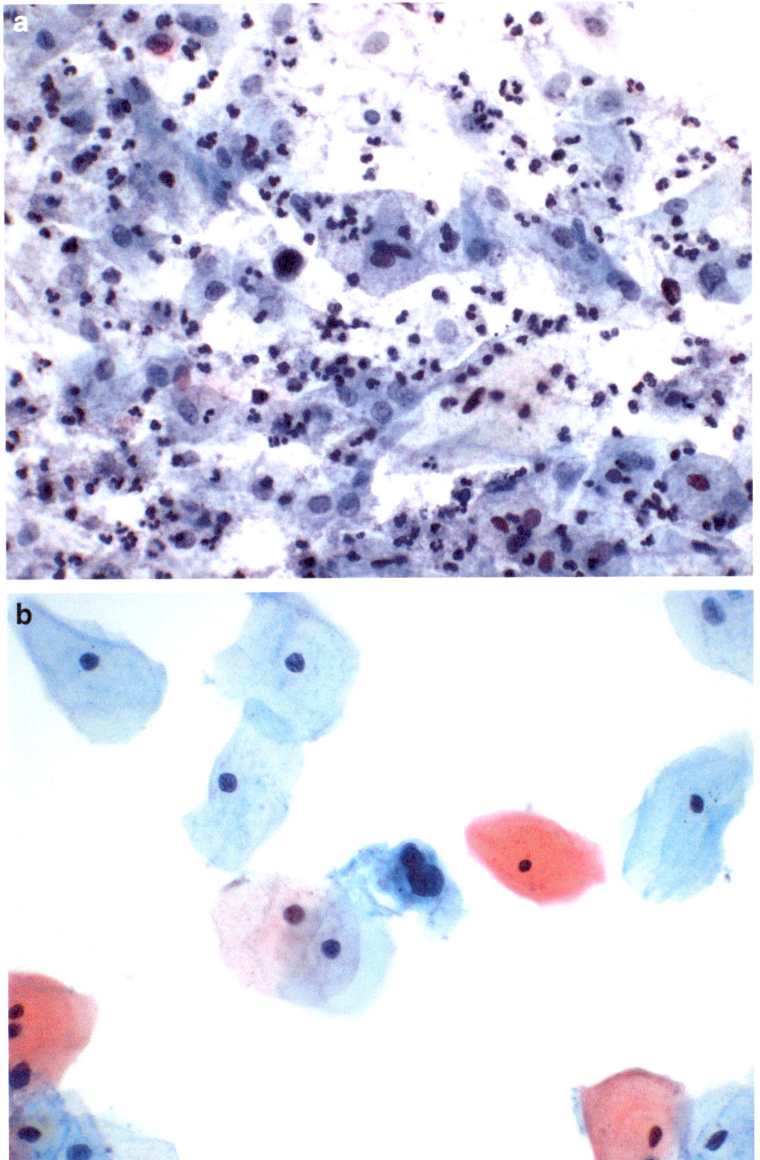

Fig. 14.13 HGSIL. On a conventional pap, the small HGSIL cell is partially obscured by inflammation and thick smear (**a**). On a liquid-based cytology preparation (**b**), HGSIL is easier to appreciate, with small cells with high nuclear to cytoplasmic ratio and nuclear atypia

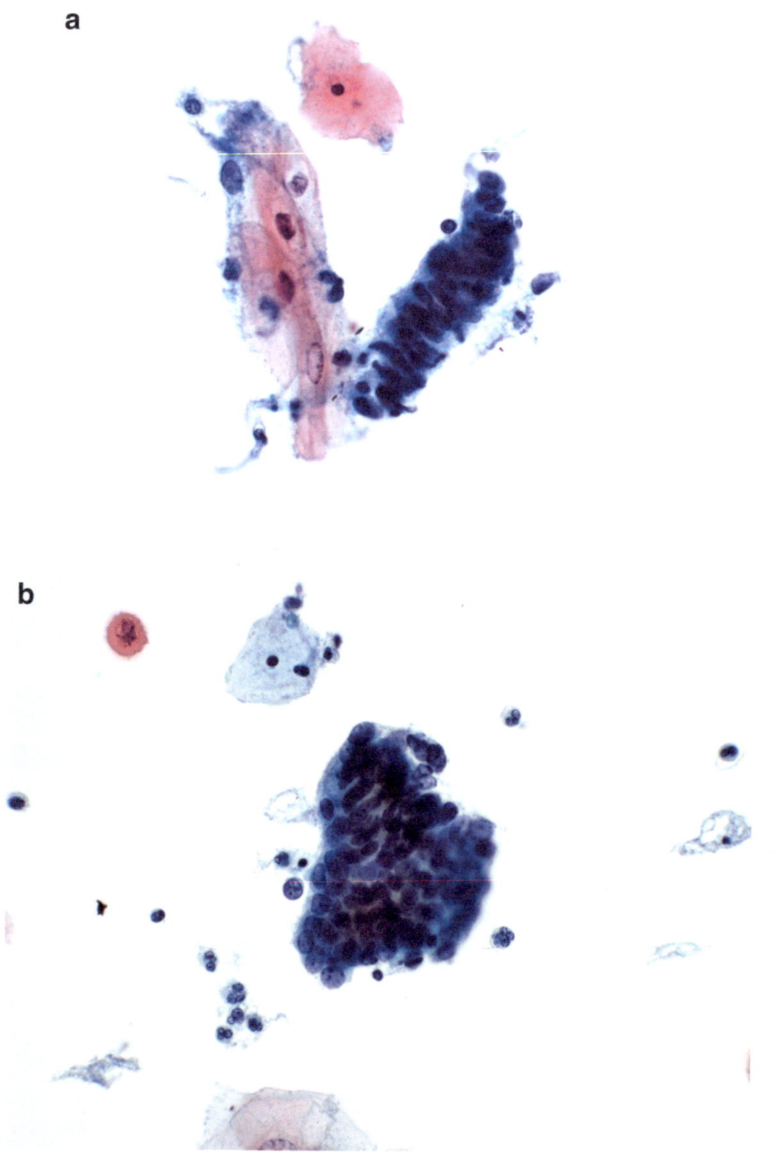

Fig. 14.14 Adenocarcinoma-in-situ. Atypical endocervical cells in strips (**a**) or clusters with palisading (**b**) may be seen

14.13 Invasive Carcinoma

Due to a lack of tissue on paps, there is no stroma to evaluate for invasion, and hence the diagnosis of invasion relies on other criteria (see below).

14.14 Squamous Cell Carcinoma

Frankly invasive squamous cell carcinoma shows more cytologic atypia than HSIL, with hyperchromatic nuclei, bizarre forms, and tadpole cells. The finding of tumor diathesis, necrotic debris associated with invasion, is helpful. In traditional pap smears, this is easier to detect, but may be washed away with liquid-based preparations. What may remain is a small amount of necrotic debris attached to cells as "clinging diathesis" (Fig. 14.15a–c).

14.15 Adenocarcinoma

Adenocarcinoma may be classified as endocervical, endometrial, extrauterine, or as NOS, depending on the diagnostic features present. The distinction of endocervical adenocarcinoma from AIS is difficult. Clues include the following features in invasive carcinoma: three dimensional clusters, prominent nucleoli, and clinging tumor diathesis (Fig. 14.16a, b).

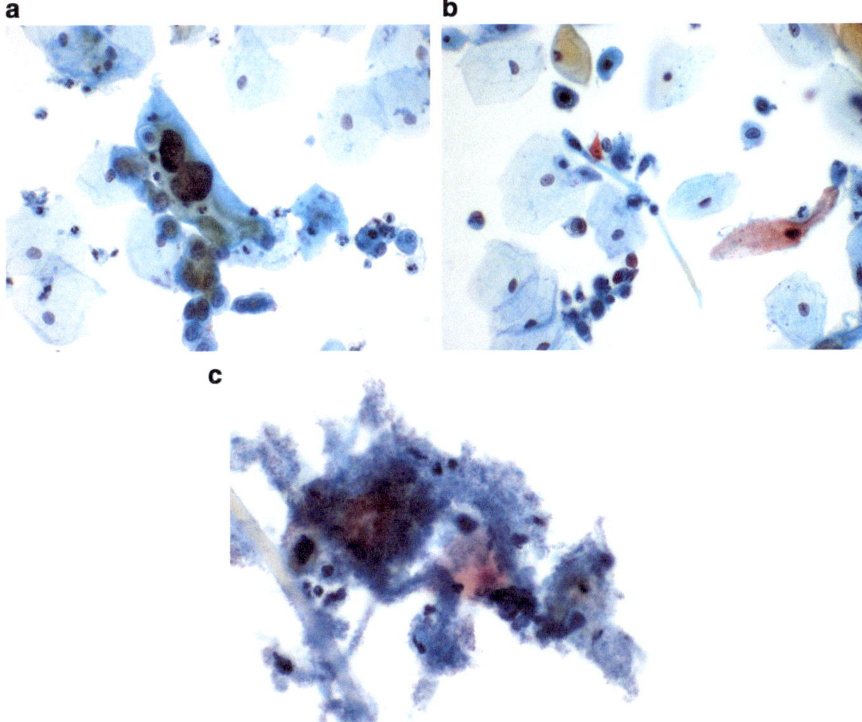

Fig. 14.15 Squamous cell carcinoma. There may be bizarre nuclei (**a**), tadpole cells (**b**), and the presence of clinging diathesis (**c**) is helpful

14.16 Peritoneal Washings

Peritoneal washings are submitted on many gynecologic surgical cases and used as part of the evaluation for extent of malignancies. An example is during a staging

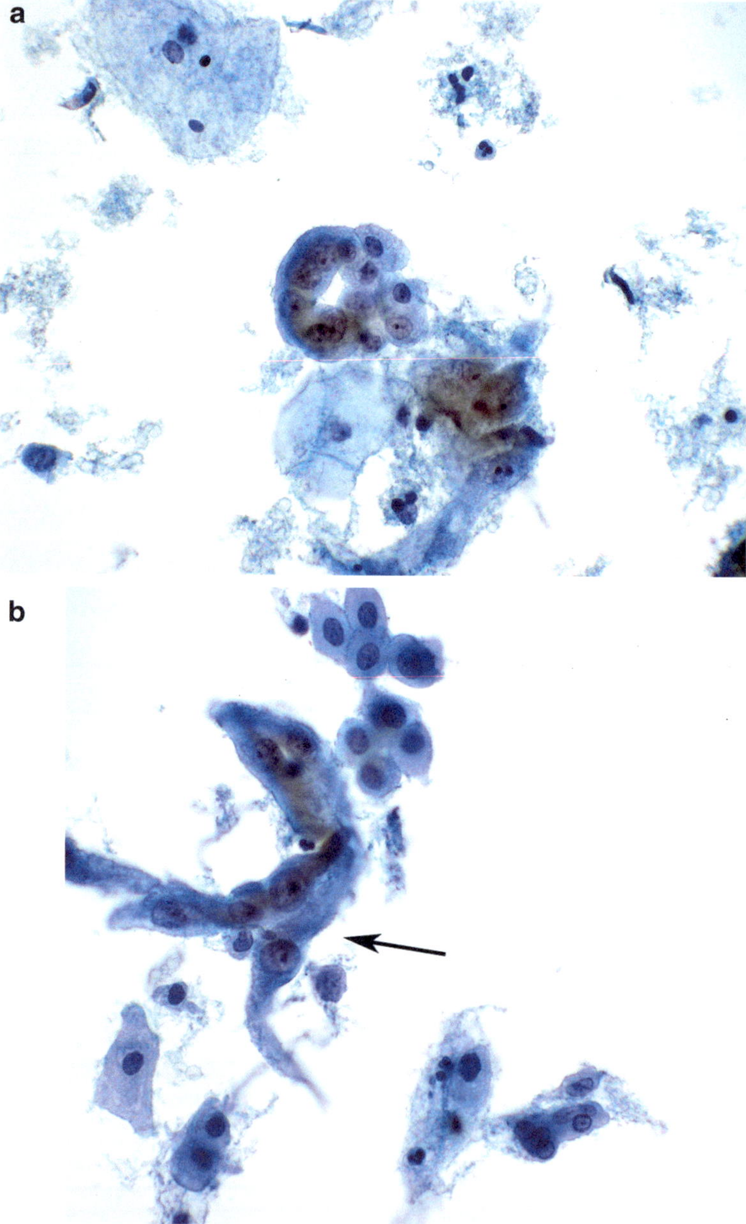

Fig. 14.16 Adenocarcinoma. A glandular cluster of cells (**a**) with prominent nucleoli, or a flat cell cluster (**b**) with atypical nuclei and prominent nucleoli (*arrow*) may be seen

procedure for an ovarian papillary serous cystadenocarcinoma (Fig. 14.17a, b), where washings can show the characteristic papillary atypical structures.

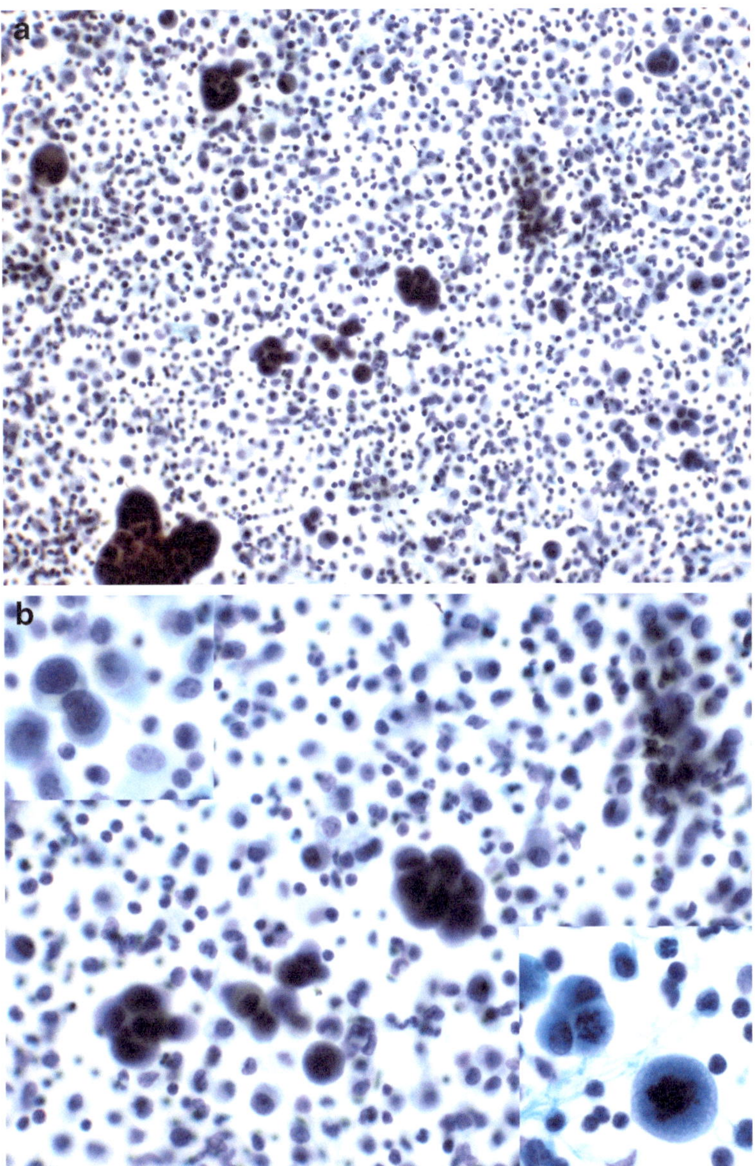

Fig. 14.17 Papillary Serous Carcinoma on a pelvic washing. Note the three-dimensional papillary cell clusters, which round up in the peritoneal fluid (**a**). On higher power, the cells may be seen to be larger and more atypical than the background lymphocytes and mesothelial cells (**b**, *insets*)

14.17 Fine Needle Aspiration

Another potential use for cytology in obstetrics and gynecology is fine needle aspiration. Aspirations performed on enlarged lymph nodes, for example, may confirm the presence of a metastasis, as may a fine needle aspirate of a distal site such as lung, suspected of harboring a metastatic gynecologic malignancy. Ovarian cysts may also be amenable to aspiration in some circumstances. The utility in breast masses is well established.

References

1. Heller DS, Weiss G, Bittman, S, Goldsmith L. Does a diagnosis of atrophic vaginitis on a pap smear signify the presence of inflammation? Menopause, in press.
2. Lara-Torre E, Pinkerton JS. Accuracy of detection of Trichomonas vaginalis organisms on a liquid-based Papanicolaou smear. Am J Obstet Gynecol. 2003;188(2):354–6.

Index

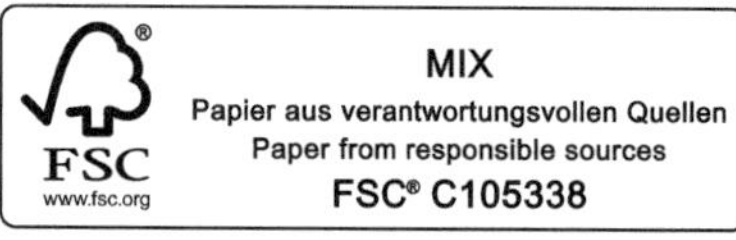

If you have any concerns about our products,
you can contact us on
ProductSafety@springernature.com

In case Publisher is established outside the EU,
the EU authorized representative is:
**Springer Nature Customer Service Center GmbH
Europaplatz 3, 69115 Heidelberg, Germany**

Printed by Libri Plureos GmbH
in Hamburg, Germany